EVIDENCE-GUIDED PRESCRIBING OF THE PILL

The International Workshop 'What is the appropriate level of
assessment of women using combined oral contraceptives in Europe'
was supported by Janssen-Cilag, NV Organon, Schering Health Care
and Wyeth Laboratories

EVIDENCE-GUIDED PRESCRIBING OF THE PILL

Edited by

P. C. Hannaford and A. M. C. Webb

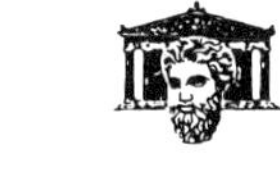

The Parthenon Publishing Group
International Publishers in Medicine, Science & Technology

NEW YORK   LONDON

Published in the USA by
The Parthenon Publishing Group Inc.
One Blue Hill Plaza
PO Box 1564, Pearl River,
New York 10965, USA

Published in the UK by
The Parthenon Publishing Group Limited
Casterton Hall, Carnforth,
Lancs. LA6 2LA, UK

ISBN: 1-85070-747-2

Typeset by Martin Lister Publishing Services, Carnforth, Lancs., UK

Printed and bound by Butler & Tanner Ltd., Frome and London, UK

Contents

Section 3 Genital tract disease and the pill

List of principal contributors

J. Austoker
Cancer Research Campaign
Primary Care Education Group
Department of Public Health
University of Oxford
65 Banbury Road
Oxford OX2 6PE
UK

D.J. Back
Department of Pharmacology and
  Therapeutics
University of Liverpool
PO Box 147
Liverpool L69 3BX
UK

T. Belfield
Family Planning Association
2–12 Pentonville Road
London N1 9FP
UK

V. Beral
Imperial Cancer Research Fund
Cancer Epidemiology Unit
Gibson Building
Radcliffe Infirmary
Oxford OX2 6HE
UK

K.W.M. Bloemenkamp
Department of Obstetrics,
  Gynecology and Reproductive
  Medicine
University Hospital Leiden
Building 1, H3-P
PO Box 9600
2300 RC Leiden
The Netherlands

D.R. Bromham
Academic Division of Obstetrics
  and Gynaecology
St. James's University Hospital
Beckett Street
Leeds LS9 7TF
UK

E. Buiatti
Epidemiology Unit
CSPO
Via di S. Salvi, 12
I-50135 Florence
Italy

L. Chasan-Taber
Channing Laboratory
Department of Medicine
Harvard Medical School and
  Brigham Women's Hospital
180 Longwood Avenue
Boston, MA 02115
USA

D. Crook
Wynn Division of Metabolic
  Medicine
21 Wellington Road
St. John's Wood
London NW8 9SQ
UK

H. Cuckle
Centre for Reproduction, Growth
  and Development
Research School of Medicine
University of Leeds
34 Hyde Terrace
Leeds LS2 9LN
UK

S. Franceschi
Servizio di Epidemiologia
Centro di Riferimento Oncologico
Via Pedemontana Occ.
33081 Aviano (PN)
Italy

M.D.G. Gillmer
Women's Centre
John Radcliffe Hospital
Headley Way
Oxford OX3 9DU
UK

A.K. Hackshaw
Wolfson Institute of Preventive
  Medicine
Department of Environmental and
  Preventive Medicine
St. Bartholomew's Hospital Medical
  College
Charterhouse Square
London EC1M 6BQ
UK

P.C. Hannaford
RCGP Manchester Research Unit
Parkway House
Palatine Road
Northenden
Manchester M22 4DB
UK

D.A. Hicks
Department of Genito-Urinary
  Medicine
Royal Hallamshire Hospital
Glossop Road
Sheffield S10 2JF
UK

K.L. Irwin
Division of HIV/AIDS Prevention
Mailstop E-45
Centers for Disease Control &
  Prevention
1600 Clifton Road
Atlanta, GA 30333
USA

J. Jespersen
Institute for Thrombosis Research
South Jutland University Center
Centralsygehuset i Esbjerg
Ostergade 80
DK 6700 Esbjerg
Denmark

R.J.E. Kirkman
University of Manchester
Palatine Centre
63/65 Palatine Road
Withington
Manchester M20 3LJ
UK

Ø. Lidegaard
Department of Obstetrics and
  Gynecology
Herlev Hospital
University of Copenhagen
DK-2730 Herlev
Denmark

P.-A. Mårdh
Institute of Clinical Bacteriology
University of Uppsala
S-75122 Uppsala
Sweden

J.S. McCormick
Department of Community Health
  and General Practice
Trinity College
University of Dublin
199 Pearse Street
Dublin 2
Ireland

B.J. Oddens
International Health Foundation
Avenue de Broqueville 116/9
B-1200 Brussels
Belgium

M. Oliveira da Silva
Calcada Palma de Baixo, 4-8B
1600 Lisbon
Portugal

N.R. Poulter
Department of Epidemiology and
  Public Health
University College London Medical
  School
1–19 Torrington Place
London WC1E 6BT
UK

M. Short
Women's Medical Clinic
34 Main Street
Blackrock
Co. Dublin
Ireland

S.O. Skouby
Department of Obstetrics and
  Gynecology
Frederiksberg Hospital
DK-2000 Copenhagen F
Denmark

L. Thomas
International Planned Parenthood
  Federation
European Network
Regent's College
Inner Circle
Regent's Park
London NW1 4NS
UK

M. Thorogood
London School of Hygiene and
  Tropical Medicine
Keppel Street
London WC1E 7HT
UK

G. Tolis
Endocrine Division
Hippokration General Hospital
114 Vas. Sofias
115 17 Athens
Greece

U.H. Winkler
Center of Obstetrics and
  Gynecology
University Hospital Essen
Hufelandstrasse 55
45122 Essen
Germany

P. Wølner-Hanssen
Department of Obstetrics and
  Gynecology
Kvinnokliniken
Universitetssjukhuset i Lund
221 85 Lund
Sweden

A.M.C. Webb
Abacus Centre for Contraception
  and Reproductive Health
16 Lord Street
Liverpool L2 1TA
UK

Preface

In March 1996, a group of individuals involved in contraceptive and reproductive health care met for an international workshop to determine the appropriate level of assessment required for the safe provision of combined oral contraceptives in Europe. For each subject area, the most current evidence about any relationship with combined oral contraceptive use, and the value of related screening procedures, was presented by participants with a particular expertise in that area. This information was then discussed by the entire group, following which a consensus about the most appropriate level of assessment emerged. This book documents the evidence which formed the basis for the group's conclusions and recommendations. The consensus statement will be published separately in a peer-reviewed medical journal.

Much of our understanding of the effects of combined oral contraceptives comes from the work of Dr Clifford Kay, former director of the Royal College of General Practitioners' Manchester Research Unit. We are pleased to be able to dedicate this book to Clifford in recognition of his 30 years of combined oral contraceptive-related research.

Manchester, May 1996   *Philip Hannaford*
Anne Webb

Introduction

P.C. Hannaford

As we approach the next millenium, there is a growing awareness that sustainable global development is unlikely to be possible without restraints on the number of humans inhabiting the Earth[1,2]. Otherwise, *Homo sapiens* is in danger of outstripping the world's vast natural resources of land, energy and water. For the foreseeable future, combined oral contraceptives (COCs) will be a major component of many modern, effective family planning programs.

Over 60 million women are currently thought to be using COCs throughout the world[3]. In some countries, such as the United Kingdom, most women are thought to use this method of contraception at some time during their reproductive lives[4]. Indeed, researchers wishing to examine the effects of COCs are now faced with the dilemma of deciding who constitutes a suitable comparison group. Women who have never used COCs may be a rather peculiar, self-selected group and, therefore, not a suitable choice. Widespread usage, however, does not necessarily mean universal popularity. Certainly, the effects of COCs continue to be of immense interest to women, their medical advisors, the media and, increasingly, the legal profession. Some women continue to be reluctant users, seeing themselves as having to make the best of a bad lot.

There are probably a number of reasons why the pill still attracts interest and opinion, even after more then 35 years of availability. First, contraception is inextricably associated with sexuality, still a taboo subject in some parts of society. Exaggerated concerns about the safety of the pill are sometimes used in a moralistic way to try and force a greater restriction on its availability. Second, because COCs are mostly used by healthy young women to prevent a natural event, their safety profile must be exemplary. Consumers have the understandable desire to expose themselves to the smallest of risks. Third, there is some disquiet that even now there are important gaps in our knowledge of the pill's effects[5]. For instance, we still await definitive answers to questions about the relationship with breast and cervical cancer. Neither do we yet fully understand the mechanisms by which the pill exerts its effects, particularly on the vascular system. Fourth, the public's perception of the pill's safety is dominated by reports of its adverse effects whether real or perceived. Important benefits associated with COC use, such as protection against endometrial and ovarian cancer[6], tend to be ignored. This is partly because pill users who are prevented from developing these conditions are unaware that they were at risk in the first place. Thus, stories from women whose lives were saved or improved by the pill tend not to appear in the media. Last, the medical profession is guilty of conveying mixed messages. On the one hand, we claim that COCs are safe, while on the other we sometimes subject potential users to a battery of clinical tests. Consumers quite understandably ask, 'If the pill is so safe, why do I need to have all these investigations?'

During the past four decades, much has been learnt about how COCs affect women. Some effects, suspected when the pill first became available, have proved to be unfounded. For instance, we no longer believe the pill causes overt diabetes mellitus[7]. Other concerns have been substantiated. For example, the pill has been linked with vascular events such as thrombotic strokes and heart attacks with remarkable consistency[6]. Even these risks, however, do not affect all pill users uniformly; smokers appear to have a greater risk than non-smokers[8–10]. Major shifts in the hormonal content of COCs[11], and the prescribing habits of physicians[11], have also probably resulted in material changes in the risks associated with using the pill. In addition, there have been major advances in our understanding of the value and limitations of screening procedures for disease in young women.

Against this background of growing scientific knowledge, there continue to be wide variations in clinical practice when prescribing COCs. Some physicians adopt a minimalist approach, even to the point of questioning whether the blood pressure of potential pill users should be checked at all. Others take a more interventionist line, advocating the checking of the blood pressure, urine, blood, breasts and pelvis of women wishing to use this method of birth control. Each clinician believes, often vehemently, that he or she is doing the correct thing. But what is the right thing? What is the evidence to support the stance of either clinician?

Ideally, there should be a balance between avoiding unnecessary interventions, particularly if they put barriers in the way of women who wish to use COCs, while simultaneously providing safe contraception. In order to determine what this balance might be, Anne Webb and I have assembled a group of experts working in epidemiology, gynecology, family planning, metabolic and hemostatic research, nursing and sociology. The task of the group is to evaluate whether today's pills are associated with a number of important clinical events, and, if so, whether this risk can be reduced by the prudent evaluation of women prior to their receipt of a prescription for the pill. On some issues, the evidence will be woefully sparse. In addition, other considerations such as social, economic, psychological and cultural factors will contribute to decisions about contraceptive choices. It is hoped, however, that a careful appraisal of all the available information will guide our clinical practice, and perhaps narrow some of the variations that currently exist.

REFERENCES

1. Smith, R. (1993). Overpopulation and overconsumption. Combating the two main drivers of global destruction. *Br. Med. J.*, **306**, 1285–6
2. United Nations Population Fund (1994). In Marshall, A. (ed.) *The State of World Population 1994. Choices and Responsibilities.* (New York: UNFPA)
3. Population Information Program (1988). *Lower-dose Pills. Series A, No. 7. Oral Contraceptives.* (Baltimore: Population Information Program)

4. Royal College of General Practitioners' Manchester Research Unit (1986). New oral contraception study: pilot trial report. *J. R. Coll. Gen. Pract.*, **36**, 545–6

5. Hannaford, P.C. (1995). Combined oral contraceptives: do we know all of their effects? *Contraception*, **51**, 325–7

6. Vessey, M.P. (1990). The Jephcott Lecture, 1989. An overview of the benefits and risks of combined oral contraceptives. In Mann, R.D. (ed.) *Oral Contraceptives and Breast Cancer*, pp. 121–35. (Carnforth, UK: Parthenon Publishing)

7. Hannaford, P.C. and Kay, C.R. (1989). Oral contraceptives and diabetes mellitus. *Br. Med. J.*, **299**, 1315–16

8. Royal College of General Practitioners' Oral Contraception Study (1981). Further analyses of mortality in oral contraceptive users. *Lancet*, **1**, 541–6

9. Croft, P. and Hannaford, P.C. (1989). Risk factors for acute myocardial infarction in women: evidence from the Royal College of General Practitioners' Oral Contraception Study. *Br. Med. J.*, **298**, 165–8

10. Hannaford, P.C., Croft, P.R. and Kay, C.R. (1994). Oral contraception and stroke. Evidence from the Royal College of General Practitioners' Oral Contraception Study. *Stroke*, **25**, 935–42

11. Thorogood, M. and Vessey, M.P. (1990). Trends in use of oral contraceptives in Britain. *Br. J. Fam. Plann.*, **16**, 41–53

Section 1

Why do we need this workshop?

1

The need for effective contraception: a global and European perspective

L. Thomas

INTERNATIONAL

Although there are encouraging signs that both access and acceptability of modern contraception including the pill are on the increase, the fact remains that there as many as 400 million couples in the developing world who do not have access to modern family planning services. Most would like to delay or space their pregnancies, or stop having children altogether[1]. According to the World Health Organization, more than 500 000 women die every year of pregnancy-related causes, and a further 5–10 million are left severely disabled as a result of pregnancy. Inadequate birth spacing is the cause of death for 5.6 million children every year.

These figures do not necessarily illustrate the very real individual choices and dangers that women without access to adequate services have to make on a daily basis. Despite advances and international consensus generated from the International Conference on Population and Development in Cairo in 1994 and the Beijing Women's Conference in September 1995, it is still an uphill struggle to put words into action and ensure that all women have access to effective, acceptable and affordable family planning and reproductive health services. There are still as many as 52 million abortions performed every year, of which 21 million are performed in countries where the procedure is not legal[2]. Many of the 70 000 deaths each year as a result of illegal abortion could be averted with greater access to effective contraception[3].

Access to contraception is not a priority for governments. The United Nations has estimated that US$ 2.5 billion is required to meet existing family planning needs, rising to US$ 9 billion by the end of the decade. Before the Iraqi conflict, the nations of the world were spending US$ 2.5 billion every day on peacetime armaments. The all too apparent marginalization of women's health, limited services outside capital and major cities, and inadequate funds for development of new methods of contraception have also had a detrimental effect upon women's access to services they want. There is also the increasingly vocal and desperate anti-choice movement, whose task it is to scare and intimidate women into risking their health and safety.

Anyone in any doubt about the need for effective contraception need only look at the oppression of family planning and reproductive rights during the Ceausescu regime to see how women suffer without access to contraception and reproductive health services. During Ceausescu's rule, the risk of death by illegal abortion was 29% in Ethiopia, 20% in Bangladesh, and 86% in Romania[4]. Romanian women were reduced to paying for the services of back-street abortionists, risking their lives and health because the dictatorship had no interest in women's needs and rights. An estimated 20 000 Romanian women died from illegal abortion between 1966 and 1989. Maternal deaths from abortion fell by 317% in the first 3 years following Ceausescu's death after the introduction of access to safe abortion and family planning services in Romania[5].

EASTERN EUROPE AND THE FORMER SOVIET UNION

Progress in Eastern Europe and the former Soviet Union is being measured in terms of economic development, not in access to health services, particularly women's health services – 'democracy with a male face' according to the Yugoslavian novelist Slavanka

Drakulic. The need for family planning is acute in Eastern and Central Europe and the former Soviet Union including the Central Asian Republics. Abortion accounts for 13% of maternal deaths in Eastern Europe and 23% in the former Soviet Union. In the former Soviet Union, only 25% of women use any methods of contraception, many of which are outdated or unreliable. The fragile economic situation in a number of these countries has resulted in increasing cuts in health expenditure. Of the little funding that is available, most is devoured by the cost of running curative services, leaving little or no funds for preventative health care such as contraception and human immunodeficiency virus prevention. Much of the medical profession in this region is either inadequately trained and badly informed, or limited in their work by lack of resources. In many Eastern European countries, services are provided only by obstetricians and gynecologists rather than by general practitioners and nurses. Services that are taken for granted in the UK are still either a luxury or a dream throughout many parts of the region.

Lack of funds to distribute what contraceptives may be in stock and to replace them is adversely affecting both maternal and infant mortality rates. Lack of modern contraception is causing continued reliance on abortion services, often performed without anesthetic. Eastern Europe may be developing western style forms of economy, politics and advertising, but the region does not as yet have the resources or the political will to create comprehensive family planning services. Where comprehensive services are available, women's health is directly and quickly improved, and at very low cost.

Between 1985 and 1994, in the Altaisko region of Russia, the contraceptive prevalence rate among women in the fertile age rose from 6.8% using intrauterine devices to 47.5%, and less than 1% using the pill to 14.4%. During the same 9-year period, the abortion rate fell from 116.0 per 1000 women to 47.8 per 1000 women[6].

Between 1991 and 1994 in the Czech Republic, the number of women using the pill increased by 71%. In the same 4 years, the abortion rate per 1000 women between the ages of 15 and 44 decreased from 45.8 to 23.3[7].

WESTERN EUROPE

In Western Europe, where relatively good services are available, there have b een concerted attempts to limit access to those services. In the past 12 months, in The Netherlands and Britain (two ostensibly advanced countries within the context of reproductive and sexual health), attempts have been made to bring the pill off the prescription list, thus depriving poorer women of access to one of the most effective methods of contraception. Thankfully, both these moves were unsuccessful primarily because of vocal and organized lobbying from the women's movement and from the pharmaceutical industry. Over the last few years in the Republic of Ireland, there have been positive changes in attitude towards sexual health and the government is looking to provide comprehensive funding for family planning services and sex education. However, in the same country, the extremes of the anti-choice movement almost succeeded in forcing a 14-year-old girl – the X case – to bring to term to an unwanted and certainly unplanned pregnancy. In France, a return to nationalism has dragged with it an outdated and oppressive attitude to women's rights which include a woman's right to choose abortion. In some European countries, pronatalism is being sold as patriotism. Eastern Europe presents particular new challenges, but we must make sure that already established rights and freedom throughout the rest of Europe are not eroded by smaller health budgets and the work of extreme right-wing and anti-women parties.

DEFINITION OF EFFECTIVE

There is no doubt that there is need for contraception, but we must be careful in our definitions of effective. There are effective contraceptive methods available, one of the most effective being the pill, but effectiveness is not just about technology and efficacy of actual methods. For a method of contraception to be effective, it must be affordable and acceptable; acceptable for the user, not the distributor or the medical profession. In years to come, we may develop the 'perfect' contraceptive – 100% efficacy, no side-effects, inexpensive –

but again it is the user who must outline her (or maybe in the future, his) actual needs. If the pill is not available to young women because they cannot afford it or fear that their confidentiality will be breached, then it is an ineffective method. If a woman does not have a guaranteed continuous supply of her chosen method, then it is ineffective.

What must not be forgotten in the development and provision of contraceptives is a much greater emphasis and empathy for those people who are actually choosing to use contraception. Any future medical and sociological research into access to contraception must be centered on those women who are exercising their human right to family planning and reproductive health. Each individual must make her own choice regarding her reproductive health, and it is up to all of us here to respect that choice and act upon it accordingly. At the same time, research into improvement of the existing methods and development of new methods must continue

Effective contraception allows women to live their lives as they wish. It frees them from the anxiety of unplanned pregnancy. It allows them to decide when and if they wish to have children. It makes a pregnancy a cause for celebration not fear.

REFERENCES

1. Sadik, N. (1992). Family planning: impact on the individual and the family. *Family Planning: Meeting Challenges, Promoting Choices.* Proceedings of the IPPF Family Planning Congress, New Delhi, October 1992, pp. 7–14. (Carnforth, UK: Parthenon Publishing)
2. Ashford, L.S. (1995). New perspectives on population: lessons from Cairo. *Pop. Bull.*, **50**, March
3. World Health Organization (1995). *WHO Position Paper.* (Geneva: WHO)
4. World Health Organization (1987). Safe Motherhood Fact Sheet, February. (Geneva: WHO)
5. *Entre Nous: The European Family Planning Magazine*, **16**, September, 1990
6. Family Planning and Reproductive Health in Altaisko Krai: Problems and Policies, Russian Family Planning Association, 1995
7. Uzel, R. (1995). Czech Family Planning Association, July

2

The pill: an historical overview

M.D.G. Gillmer

HISTORY OF 'THE PINCUS PILL'

Prehistory

The earliest demonstration that fertility could be influenced by hormonal manipulation is attributed to Ludwig Haberlandt, of Innsbruck, who in 1921 performed ovarian transplants between pregnant animals and non-pregnant animals of the same species. By this means, he was apparently able to render five out of eight rabbits and three out of eight guinea-pigs infertile. Otfried Otto Fellner, working in Vienna, at about the same time, reported infertility following injection of a lipid extract of the ovary which he called 'Feminin'. When he used this material on 30 rabbits, only three remained fertile. Fellner is thought to be the first scientist to suggest that estrogen could be used for fertility control[1]. Much later in 1937, Makepeace and co-workers reported inhibition of ovulation in rabbits following progesterone injection[2], while Sturgis and Albright in 1940 reported the inhibition of ovulation in women with dysmenorrhea treated with estradiol injections[3].

Shortly before this, in 1938, Hans Inhoffen, a German chemist, working for Schering in Berlin had produced a potent synthetic estrogen, ethinylestradiol, and the progestogen, ethisterone, by the addition of an acetylene group at the 17-carbon position of the naturally occurring hormones, estradiol and testosterone, respectively[4]. This modification changed the activity of testosterone from

15

an androgen into an orally active progestogen. Research was, however, seriously hampered because of the scarcity of these hormones which could only be obtained from animal sources. Four tons of sows' ovaries were required to extract 25 mg of pure estradiol[5]!

Synthesis of progestogens

In 1939, an enigmatic chemist Russell Marker, who was Professor at the State College in Pennsylvania, managed to synthesize small quantities of progesterone from extracts of the root of the sarsaparilla plant. Although this proved to be a poor source of the hormone, in 1942 he succeeded in adapting the process to synthesize progesterone in kilogram quantities from the root of the wild Mexican yam, *cabeza de negro*[6]. The following year Marker joined two European refugees, Dr Emeric Somlo and Dr Frederico Lehmann who owned a small pharmaceutical company, Laboratorias Hormona, in Mexico City and with them, in 1944, founded Syntex (a name derived from the words *syn*thesis and Me*x*ico!). Their intention was to produce progesterone on a commercial basis but the partnership was short lived, as Marker left Mexico after a quarrel with his colleagues and took with him all details of the production process! In 1945, George Rosenkranz, also of Hungarian origin, joined Syntex from Cuba and restored the manufacture of progesterone[7].

In 1949, Carl Djerassi joined Syntex, at the invitation of George Rosenkranz, to work on the synthesis of cortisone. He became preoccupied, however, with the idea of synthesizing an orally active progestogen. Two years later, on 15 October 1951, using the same plant source that Marker had used for the synthesis of progesterone, Luis Miramontes, working under Djerassi's supervision, removed the 19-methyl group from Inhoffen's ethisterone, producing 19-nor-17α-ethinyltestosterone or norethisterone[8]. Syntex, however, lacked any biological test facilities and this material was therefore sent to a number of laboratories for further investigation. These included Roy Hertz at the National Cancer Institute, Alexander Lipschutz in Chile, Edward Tyler in Los Angeles, Robert Greenblatt in Augusta, Georgia, and Gregory Pincus at the Worcester Foundation for Experimental Biology in Massachusetts[1].

Early studies with progestogens

The previous year, Pincus had been introduced by the birth control pioneer Margaret Sanger to the wealthy heiress Mrs Katherine McCormick to whom his book *Control of Fertility* is dedicated[9]. Both women had impressed upon Pincus their view that new methods of contraception were desperately required to help with third world overpopulation and it is reputed that the possibility of oral treatment was considered. At about this time, he received samples of norethisterone from Syntex in Mexico City and is reputed to have told his wife Lizuska of his ideas for a contraceptive pill[11]. Certainly, his assistant M.C. Chang became actively involved in the animal testing of a variety of progestogens in 1951, and within a year or two these studies had extended to women with infertility under the care of John Rock, a Catholic gynecologist, from Brookline, Massachusetts.

Just over a year after Djerassi and colleagues filed their patent for norethisterone in 1952, Frank Colton of G.D. Searle and Co. filed a patent for the progestogen norethynodrel[12]. Although this compound was apparently manufactured by an entirely different chemical process, it differs structurally from norethisterone only in the position of the double bond in the A ring of the basic steroid molecule and is apparently converted to norethisterone by dilute acid such as that in the stomach[8]. Norethynodrel, the patent for which was filed in 1953, was also available to Pincus for biological study as he was a consultant to G.D. Searle and Co.

The first clinical study of these progestogens was initiated in December 1954 and preliminary results were presented by Pincus at the Fifth International Planned Parenthood Conference held in Tokyo in October 1955[13]. Having given evidence that both compounds administered by the oral route appeared to inhibit ovulation, he concluded, 'We cannot on the basis of our observations thus far designate the ideal antifertility agent, nor the ideal mode of administration. But a foundation has been laid for the useful exploitation of the problem on an objective basis.' Further information from these ongoing studies was presented to the Laurentian Hormone Conference in September 1956[14] and published as a preliminary report in the journal *Science*[15], later the same year, by Rock and Pincus together with a young American gynecologist Celso Ramon Garcia who was working with Rock. In these studies, norethisterone and norethynodrel were 'administered in doses ranging from 5 to 50 mg per day usually from the 5th through the 25th days of three menstrual cycles', to 50 women with unexplained infertility. This regimen was shown to inhibit ovulation. No mention of side-effects of the treatment is made in either paper, but, in the discussion which follows the definitive paper, Rock is reported as saying, 'I am not prepared to state the kind or frequency of side-effects in women, …I do know, however, that they were minimal.' Later Garcia adds that '…the only significant things noted were a few breast changes as manifested by engorgement, tenderness, or fullness…' He also reports, '…an overall average weight gain of about 5 pounds per patient…' and that, '…a few patients noted irritability and nervousness.' but, 'As far as androgenic properties are concerned, none of our patients on this regime complained of any factors which we might consider an androgenic response.'

CLINICAL TRIALS

The Puerto Rican trials

A field trial using the Searle product norethynodrel commenced in Puerto Rico shortly after the publication of these reports[16]; '265 Puerto Rican wives from the low income population living in a housing development project in a slum clearance area' were recruited. Norethynodrel was apparently chosen in preference to other progestogens because in '…animal experiments it appeared to be somewhat more potent…'. Although the preparation was found to be extremely effective as a contraceptive, 27% of the women enrolled in the study discontinued because of 'troublesome symptoms'. These were listed by the authors as breast tenderness, nausea, dizziness, vomiting and pelvic pain, side-effects that would appear with hindsight to be due at least in part to the estrogen supplement that was apparently used for the first time in this trial. It is, however, of interest that no mention whatsoever was made of estrogen supplementation in any earlier report on the animal or human use of norethynodrel or indeed of any of the other progestogens studied by this group. They state in this paper that, 'The most effective estrogen supplement appeared to be the 3-methyl ether of ethinylestradiol' (mestranol), and that 'In 1467 of the cycles studied in this investigation, the subjects received tablets each containing 10 mg of norethynodrel and 0.22 mg ethinylestradiol 3-methyl ether, or, in a very few instances, 0.23 mg. In the remaining 390 cycles reported, the estrogen supplement was somewhat lower, i.e. 0.08 mg in 157 cycles, 0.15 mg in 61 cycles, and 0.18 mg in 172 cycles.' Although no mention is made in this paper or in any other of the publications of these workers that the 'estrogen supplement' was in fact an estrogen contaminant, there seems little doubt that this was the case and that this group originally intended to use a pure progestogen for 'oral medication' and that the combination of progestogen with estrogen was due purely to chance. In short, the 'combined oral contraceptive' pill was a product of serendipity! Evidence for this appears in letters written by Pincus in 1956 (Pincus papers, Library of Congress, Washington – personal communication, Dr Lara Marks). The estrogen impurity is also mentioned by Paul Vaughan[11] in his book *The Pill on Trial* and by Clifford Kay[5] in his *James Mackenzie Lecture* in 1979, but neither author provides any reference source for this information. Indirect evidence, however, derives from the bizarre range of doses and cycles of observation of the 'estrogen supplement' in the Puerto Rican trials. These can be most easily explained as the results of retrospective analyses of the estrogen content of the batches of tablets that *had been used*, in the study *after* Searle had recognized the problem of estrogen contamination. In addition Cook and colleagues[17] in their paper 'Oral contraception by norethynodrel: a 3 year field study' published in 1961 state, 'Information available in 1957 suggested that 9.85 mg of norethynodrel combined with 0.15 mg of the synthetic estrin, ethynylestradiol-3-methyl ether, was the optimal daily dosage.' This would imply that of the 10 mg norethynodrel, thought initially by Pincus and colleagues to be in each tablet, the average estrogen contaminant was 0.15 mg mestranol and this would correspond to the *average* of the 'supplements' listed in the report of the Puerto Rican field trial! It is also the dose of mestranol finally included in Searle's 'Enovid'. A drug which, despite near complete ignorance of its metabolic effects, was licensed in 1957 by the Food and Drug Administration (FDA) in the USA for '... the treatment of a variety of disorders associated with the menstrual cycle'. The era of oral contraception did not, however, begin until 3 years later in May 1960 when Enovid was approved by the FDA for the cyclic control of ovulation and immediately afterwards marketed by Searle as the 'Pincus Pill'! Two years later, norethisterone in combination with mestranol was also marketed as the oral contraceptive Ortho Novum by the Ortho division of Johnson and Johnson under license from Syntex[12].

The British experience

The first reference in Britain to the successful studies performed by Pincus and colleagues in Puerto Rico appeared in the *British Medical Journal* of 12 April 1958 as an extract from an article by Dr A.S. Parkes, 'Towards Oral Contraception'[18]. It concluded, '...It seems, however, that treatment is necessary over some 20 days in each cycle, probably in order to ensure that ovulation is prevented and not merely postponed, and for this and other reasons this work cannot yet be said to have put oral contraception on a practical basis.' This was followed in January 1960 by a brief statement at the end of the second part of a review article on 'Progestogens and their clinical uses' by Dr Gerald Swyer, in which he observed[19], 'The strikingly successful results of the use of Enovid as an oral contraceptive in the Puerto Rico experiment conducted by Pincus and his colleagues are now well known. It is perhaps doubtful if in its ultimately perfected form the contraceptive pill will be a progestogen, but certainly the reported results are so encouraging that renewed interest in the problem has been aroused and further advances are now inevitable. Comment beyond this need not be made here.' Within weeks an appeal for volunteers to try the 'Pincus Pill' was made in Birmingham, leading Dr Eleanor Mears, Medical Secretary to the Family Planning Association and Council for the Investigation of Fertility Control to write to the *British Medical Journal* to provide information about the proposed trial[20]. With great enthusiasm she wrote that, 'Experts are agreed that the investigations so far carried out indicate: (a) administration of these pills for three or four years is harmless; (b) there is no decrease in subsequent fertility; fertility is restored to normal, or even improved, as soon as the administration is stopped; (c) they are not carcinogenic.' Considering that the pill had, at this time, been used for a maximum of 4 years in only a few hundred women these statements can, with hindsight, only be viewed as somewhat optimistic if not unrealistic! She also stated that, 'Although these steroids are harmless, a number of patients drop out because of unpleasant side-effects, notably nausea, headaches and upset in the menstrual rhythm.' Two months later in the 'Medical News' section of the *British Medical Journal* it was reported that, 'About 40 women, half in Devon and half in London, are at present the subjects of a trial of oral contraceptives, and it is hoped to extend the trial now to 100 volunteers in Birmingham'[21].

British trials

The first British trial commenced in Birmingham in March 1960 and the results were published in November 1961[22]. The preparation under study was initially presumed to be norethynodrel 2.5 mg and mestranol 0.05 mg. Of the 48 women recruited 14 became pregnant, seven in the first cycle and three in the second. Subsequent analysis of the pills used, revealed that they actually contained 2.3 mg norethynodrel and only 0.036 mg of mestranol. The pregnancies were therefore assumed to be due to the inadequate dose of progestogen and estrogen in the tablets supplied by Searle. Despite this setback the trial continued but the dose of progestogen was increased to 5.0 mg norethynodrel and 0.075 mg mestranol. This combination was eventually marketed as Conovid in early 1961. We now know that the original, but incorrect, trial formulation *is* an effective oral contraceptive combination. It therefore seems, with hindsight, to be more likely that the failure of the lower dose preparation was in fact due to the protocol that the women in the study were advised to follow, rather than to the reduced hormonal content of the pills. The women recruited for study in Birmingham were, like the Puerto Rican women, instructed to take one pill daily from the 5th day of the cycle for 20 days and then to stop, await a withdrawal bleed (usually 1–4 days later) and start the new bottle on the 5th day of the next menstrual cycle. However, whereas the Puerto Rican women were advised to control breakthrough bleeding by taking two pills for the remainder of the cycle, the Birmingham women were told to stop taking the pills if bleeding equivalent to a period

Table 1 Efficiency and acceptability of early combined oral contraceptives – based on patients under trial in the UK up to July 1962. (Source FPA *Handbook on Oral Contraception*, 1962, courtesy of Dr Lara Marks)

| | | | Pregnancies | | Withdrawals | |
| | | | | | | |
Products	*Number of women*	*Number of cycles*	*Tablet failure*	*Patient failure*	*Reasons connected with tablets*	*Reasons not connected with tablets*
Conovid	208	1900	Nil	2	34	12
Conovid-E	183	1228	Nil	2	33	12
Anovlar	166	1023	Nil	Nil	15	5

occurred, and then to resume the tablets on the 5th day of bleeding. In addition, the Birmingham women were not advised to use other precautions during the first 14 days of pill taking. This combination of factors would almost certainly have created a situation where the pill was omitted for in excess of 7 days in many women during the early cycles of treatment enabling 'escape' ovulation, and pregnancy, to occur.

A second trial with the 2.5 mg dose of norethynodrel commenced in Slough in August 1960[23], this time in combination with a still higher (0.1 mg) dose of mestranol. Like the 5 mg dose this proved to be extremely effective in preventing pregnancy (Table 1) and was marketed the following year as Conovid-E. The third major British trial commenced in London in May 1961. The progestogen was norethisterone acetate 4 mg and the estrogen 0.05 mg of ethinylestradiol. This very effective preparation was marketed in 1962 by Schering as Anovlar[24].

The menstrual and other side-effects of these preparations are shown in Tables 2 and 3.

All adverse symptoms were noted to be more common in the first cycle, and most, especially nausea, had resolved by the second cycle of treatment. It is also notable that the incidence of nausea appears to be related to the estrogen content of the preparations while the tendency to weight increase is a reflection of the progestogen content. Breast tenderness was, however, similar with all three preparations. The incidence of spotting and breakthrough bleeding

Table 2 Side-effects of early combined oral contraceptives – based on patients under trial in the UK up to July 1962. (Source FPA *Handbook on Oral Contraception*, 1962, courtesy of Dr Lara Marks)

Products	Number of cycles	Nausea (%)	Breast discomfort (%)	Head-ache (%)	Weight increase 3 lb (%)	Weight increase 7 lb (%)
Conovid						
1st cycle	208	36	24	13		
all cycles	1900		16	11	20	14
Conovid-E						
1st cycle	183	46	21	14		
all cycles	1228		4	3	12	5
Anovlar						
1st cycle	166	22	26	18		
all cycles	1023		7	6	45	13

Table 3 Effect on the menstrual cycle of early combined oral contraceptives – based on patients under trial in the UK up to July 1962. (Source FPA *Handbook on Oral Contraception*, 1962, courtesy of Dr Lara Marks)

Products	Number of cycles	% Cycles of spotting	% Cycles of BTB*	% Cycles without bleed	In-crease in flow (%)	De-crease in flow (%)
Conovid						
1st cycle	208	29	28	4		
all cycles	1900	18	20	4	8	22
Conovid-E						
1st cycle	183	24	31	2		
all cycles	1228	10	30	1	9	18
Anovlar						
1st cycle	166	18	8	Nil		
all cycles	1023	5	3.8	1	8	74

*BTB, breakthrough bleeding

was highest with the more estrogenic preparations while the greatest improvement in menstrual blood loss occurred with the most progestogenic combination. Although the side-effects in the Birmingham trial were described as '... generally slight and tolerable ...', the later studies identified increased premenstrual symptoms in a small number (11%) of women, and a cluster of other rarer problems such as dizziness, headaches and acne[22]. The incidence of side-effects was, however, much lower than that observed in the original 'high-dose' Puerto Rican studies.

EARLY CLINICAL EXPERIENCE

In early 1961 the combined oral contraceptive pill was generally considered to be harmless and the only contraindications listed in the FPA *Handbook on Oral Contraception,* of the time were: gross overweight, liver dysfunction, jaundice or gallstones, menopausal irregularity and lactation.

The first case report of a serious side-effect was described in a letter to the *Lancet* on 18 November 1961. The patient was a 40-year-old nursing sister with endometriosis who had been treated with Enovid. This caused such severe vomiting that she had to stop treatment after a few days and shortly afterwards had a bilateral pulmonary embolus. This experience was followed by a cluster of similar reports, which were noted to occur particularly in women who had a past history of venous thromboembolism in pregnancy. Despite growing evidence to the contrary, the proponents of 'the pill' and the manufacturer Searle concluded that the '... available statistics are not adequate to determine whether or not there is a causal relationship between Enovid administration and the occurrence of thrombophlebitis ...'. It was, however, recommended by the FPA that women inclined to venous thrombotic conditions or with a past history of thromboembolic complications in pregnancy should not be given the combined oral contraceptive pill, 'Until it has been determined by clinical study and statistical survey whether the incidence of these complications is related to the use of oral contraceptives ...'. It was not until the late 1960s that this evidence became available and an estrogen dose-dependent relationship was demonstrated[25]. Long before this, however, in the mid-1960s, laboratory studies began to appear in the literature demonstrating that these preparations not only had a pro-coagulant effect similar to that observed in pregnancy[26] but also that they might have adverse effects on both lipid and carbohydrate metabolism that could predispose women taking them to an increased risk of diabetes and atherosclerosis[27-30].

On 10 February 1968, it was announced in the *Lancet*[31] that, 'The Royal College of General Practitioners has received a grant of up to £38 000 from the MRC to conduct a 5-year controlled prospective study into the effects of oral contraceptives on health. The college has appointed Dr Clifford Kay as recorder of the study which will be co-ordinated from Manchester.' The search for sound epidemiological evidence had commenced!

REFERENCES

1. Robertson, W.H. (1990). *An Illustrated History of Contraception*, pp, 122–3. (Carnforth, UK: Parthenon Publishing)
2. Makepeace, A.W., Weinstein, G.L. and Freedman, M.H. (1937). The effect of progestin and progesterone on ovulation in the rabbit. *Am. J. Physiol.*, **119**, 512–6
3. Sturgis, S.H. and Albright, F. (1940). The mechanism of estrin therapy in the relief of dysmenorrhoea. *Endocrinology*, **26**, 68–72
4. Inhoffen, H.H., Logemann, W., Hohlweg, W. and Serini, A. (1938). Untersuchungen in der sexualhormon-Reihe. *Chem. Berlin*, **71**, 1024–32
5. Kay, C.R. (1980). The happiness pill? *J. Roy. Coll. Gen. Pract.*, **30**, 8–19
6. Lehmann, F.P.A. (1992). Early history of steroid chemistry in Mexico: the story of three remarkable men. *Steroids*, **57**, 403–8
7. Rosenkranz, G. (1992). From Ruzicka's terpenes in Zurich to Mexican steroids via Cuba. *Steroids*, **57**, 409–18
8. Djerassi, C. (1992). Steroid research at Syntex: "the pill" and cortisone. *Steroids*, **57**, 631–41
9. Pincus, G. (1965). *Control of Fertility*. (New York: Academic Press)
10. Chang, M.C. (1968). Mammalian sperm, eggs, and control of fertility. *Perspec. Biol. Med.*, **11**, 412–19
11. Vaughan, P. (1970). *The Pill on Trial*, pp. 5–6. (Middlesex: Penguin books Ltd)
12. Colton, F.B. (1992). Steroids and 'the pill': early steroid research at Searle. *Steroids*, **57**, 624–30

13. Pincus, G. (1956). Some effects of progesterone and related compounds upon reproduction and early development in mammals. *Acta Endocrinol. Suppl.*, **28**, 18–36

14. Rock, J., Garcia, C.R. and Pincus, G. (1956). Synthetic progestins in the normal human menstrual cycle. *Rec. Prog. Horm. Res.*, **13**, 323–46

15. Rock, J., Garcia, C.R. and Pincus, G. (1956). Effects of certain 19-nor steroids on the normal human menstrual cycle. *Science*, **124**, 891–3

16. Pincus, G., Rock, J., Garcia, C.R., Rice Wray, E., Paniagua, M., Rodriguez, I. and Pedras, P.R. (1958). Fertility control with oral medication. *Am. J. Obstet. Gynecol.*, **75**, 1333–46

17. Cook, H.H., Gamble, C.J. and Satterthwaite, A.P. (1961). Oral contraception by norethynodrel: a 3 year field study. *Am. J. Obstet. Gynecol.*, **82**, 437–45

18. Parkes, A.S. (1958). Towards oral contraception. *Br. Med. J.*, **1**, 859

19. Swyer, G.I.M. (1960). Progestogens and their clinical uses: Part II. *Br. Med. J.*, **1**, 121–2

20. Mears, E. (1960). Trial of oral contraceptives. *Br. Med. J.*, **1**, 491–2

21. Medical News (1960). *Br. Med. J.*, **1**, 1145

22. Eckstein, P., Waterhouse, J.A.H., Bond, G.B., Mills, W.G., Sandilands, D.M. and Shotton, D.M. (1961). The Birmingham oral contraceptive trial. *Br. Med. J.*, **2**, 1172–8

23. Pullen, D. (1962). 'Conovid-E' as an oral contraceptive. *Br. Med. J.*, **2**, 1016–19

24. Mears, E. and Grant, E. (1962). 'Anovlar' as an oral contraceptive. *Br. Med. J.*, **2**, 75–9

25. Inman, W.H.W., Vessey, M.P., Westerholm, B. and Engelund, A. (1970). Thrombo-embolic disease and the steroidal content of oral contraceptives. A report to the Committee on Safety of Drugs. *Br. Med. J.*, **2**, 203–9

26. Egeberg, O. and Owren, P.A. (1963). Oral contraception and blood coagulability. *Br. Med. J.*, **1**, 220–1

27. Aurell, M., Cramer, K. and Rybo, G. (1966). Serum lipids and lipoproteins during long-term administration of an oral contraceptive. *Lancet*, **1**, 291–3

28. Wynn, V. and Doar, J.W.H. (1966). Some effects of oral contraceptives on carbohydrate metabolism. *Lancet*, **2**, 715–9

29. Wynn, V., Doar, J.W.H. and Mills, G.L. (1966). Some effects of oral contraceptives on serum lipid and lipoprotein levels. *Lancet*, **2**, 720–3

30. Gillmer, M.D.G. (1989). Metabolic effects of combined oral contraceptives. In Filshie, M. and Guillebaud, J. (eds.) *Contraception: Science and Practice*, pp. 11–38. (London: Butterworth and Co.)

31. Oral contraceptive study (1968). *Lancet*, **1**, 312

3

Current accessibility and perceptions about the pill in Western Europe

B. J. Oddens

INTRODUCTION

Given their efficacy in preventing pregnancy and comparative ease of use, oral contraceptives (OCs) have been accepted rapidly since the 1960s. Currently, an estimated 22 million women use OCs in the more developed countries[1]. Among young women, they constitute the principal method of family planning. The benefits of OCs outweigh their possible health risks by far, and, in particular, because of prevention of ovarian and endometrial cancer, OC use reduces mortality in the long term[2]. Dutch general practitioners consider it no longer necessary to give (medical) follow-up to OC users. Several proposals have been voiced to make OCs available without medical prescription in pharmacies and/or drugstores[3,4]. Women generally associate OCs with side-effects and health risks, and believe they should not use them for 'too long' since this might be detrimental to their health. These negative perceptions might be taken as an argument against a reduction of the role of health-care professionals as advisers to OC users. On the other hand, medical prescription may limit accessibility.

27

CONTRACEPTIVE PRACTICE

In Table 1, data on contraceptive practice among sexually active, fertile women who were not pregnant or trying to get pregnant at the time of the survey ('exposed' women) are presented for a number of West European countries. Such data allow us to estimate that approximately 9 million women in Western Europe use traditional and generally less effective contraceptive methods (rhythm, withdrawal and no method). The large majority of unintended pregnancies result from contraceptive failure or non-use. Half of the unintended pregnancies are terminated, resulting in 700 000 abortions being officially recorded each year in Western Europe (and the statistics are far from complete)[14]. Moreover, some 60% of women with occasional sexual partners report not using condoms for protection against sexually transmitted diseases (including HIV/AIDS)[10–13].

According to Evert Ketting[15], the quality of family planning and contraceptive use depends primarily on three factors:

(1)   Ample availability of contraceptives;

(2)   Easy accessibility and good quality of services; and

(3)   Sufficient knowledge of contraception and motivation for use.

The availability of contraceptives is no longer a major problem in Western Europe. However, accessibility, knowledge and motivation warrant further scrutiny. Since young women constitute a special risk group for unintended pregnancy and abortion, I will first discuss this specific population in more detail.

ADOLESCENTS AND WOMEN IN THEIR EARLY TWENTIES

Prevention of pregnancy

Compared with older women, women aged 15–24 years old have a relatively limited contraceptive choice. Since intrauterine devices and sterilization are inappropriate in most cases, OCs are the most effective contraceptive method available to them, followed by injectable steroids and condoms[2].

Table 1 Percentage of 'exposed' women* aged 15–45 in selected West European countries currently using contraception by method

	Spain 1984[5]	Austria 1987[6]	Denmark 1988[7]	France 1988[†8]	Nether-lands 1989[‡9]	Great Britain 1992[10]	Germany 1992[11]	Italy 1993[12]	Sweden 1994[13]
Oral contraceptives	19	42	36	44.9	44.0	39.3	53.3	30.3	38.4
Injectable steroids	nr	nr	nr	nr	0.6	0.4	0.2	0.0	2.1
Intrauterine device	13	7	14	25.1	9.8	7.3	12.2	8.1	20.7
Barrier methods**	23	16	25	4.5	13.4	20.8	12.6	30.5	22.6
Sterilization	3	5	14	7.7	24.7	26.1	10.2	1.1	5.1
Periodic abstinence	7	7	1	6.6	1.7	1.5	7.4	6.4	6.2
Coitus interruptus	9	5	3	6.4	0.6	1.1	1.2	18.3	2.8
No method	26	18	8	2.2	4.1	3.6	2.7	4.9	1.9

nr = not reported. *'Exposed': sexually active, not pregnant or wishing to get pregnant and non-infertile; [†]women aged 18–44; [‡]women aged 20–40; **barrier methods: condoms, diaphragms and spermicides

Table 2 Age-specific abortion rates per 1000 women and percentage distribution of abortions in selected West European countries (1986–88). Data from reference 16

	Age (years)						
	<20	20–24	25–29	30–34	35–39	>39	Total
Denmark	15.7 14.1%	29.9 29.1%	24.8 22.5%	18.8 16.2%	13.5 11.8%	6.8 6.4%	18.3 100%
England and Wales	20.9 24.9%	23.8 31.5%	16.4 20.0%	11.3 12.1%	7.2 8.1%	3.0 3.3%	14.2 100%
Finland	15.4 18.9%	19.0 26.6%	12.2 17.3%	9.5 14.3%	8.2 13.3%	7.0 9.6%	11.7 100%
France*	10.3%	23.9%	23.8%	20.7%	15.3%	6.0%	100%
German Federal Republic*	7.5%	24.0%	25.5%	20.1%	15.5%	7.4%	100%
Netherlands	4.2 13.7%	7.4 25.4%	6.7 22.0%	6.2 19.1%	4.4 14.0%	2.2 5.7%	5.3 100%
Norway	22.1 23.3%	29.0 30.1%	18.3 18.2%	14.2 14.0%	10.2 9.8%	4.9 4.6%	16.8 100%
Scotland	14.0 28.1%	14.9 31.9%	9.5 18.6%	6.7 11.6%	4.2 7.2%	1.6 2.7%	9.0 100%
Sweden	21.5 17.1%	31.2 26.9%	24.6 19.3%	19.0 15.4%	15.6 13.8%	8.2 7.5%	19.8 100%

*Rate not reported

Teenagers and women up to 25 years are generally recognized as being at risk of unintended pregnancy: the number of abortions carried out in young women each year is disproportionately high (Table 2), as is the number of sexually active women who do not use any contraception. During their first sexual experiences, 20–30% of adolescents do not use any contraception[17]. Thereafter, 10–25% continue to have sex without using any method. Eventually, however, most sexually active adolescents use OCs by the time they reach their twenties.

Difficulty of access to effective contraception is often held responsible for non-use of contraception among adolescents. Indeed, their perceptions in this respect point to the same conclusion. In Britain, nearly three-quarters of adolescents asked were worried that their consultation for family planning would not be confidential[18]. Many of them also reported that they were deterred from consulting by 'unfriendly' attitudes of general practitioners (GPs). The question remains, however, whether these perceptions reflect actual accessibility problems. Lack of awareness of existing contraceptive services does not seem to be an issue[19]. Most (unintended) pregnant adolescents were found to have consulted a GP or family planning clinic in the past and most of them (92%) had used a contraceptive method previously[19]. Probably most sexually active adolescents find their way to contraception counselling[20], although improvements to the services offered could be made (Table 3).

Studies on specific interventions also shed light on these issues. In the US increased provision of family planning clinics did not improve adolescent contraceptive practice: the number of sexually active adolescents not using any method remained unchanged, as did the number getting pregnant[21]. In contrast, improvements in the quality of services (special training of providers with a focus on adolescent counselling) reduced abortion rates in Sweden[22], although the effects of quality improvement could not be disentangled entirely from those of improvement of sex education or subsidies on OCs. The finding that contraceptive use is more effective in districts where family planning clinics play a larger part in delivering the service than GPs[23] is consistent with the view that special, more anonymous family planning services offering a wide range of contraceptives can contribute to more effective contraceptive use among

Table 3 Percentages of pregnant adolescents who reported negative experiences with their visit to a general practitioner (n = 100) or family planning clinic (n = 50) for contraceptive counselling. Data from reference 19

	General practitioner	*Family planning clinic*
Unfriendly	6	4
Embarrassing	13	22
Not helpful	12	14
Not private	21	5
Not easy to access	8	4

adolescents. These various observations indicate that current family planning services do not constitute a barrier to contraceptive use for most adolescents. However, assurance of confidentiality, adaptation of the services to adolescents' needs and outreaching efforts to bring adolescents to the services could perhaps improve contraceptive use among those who remain reluctant to attend. Information to parents, that sex education does not necessarily lead to early sexual experiences[24], and that their children know how to have sex but need to learn how to deal with sexuality and contraception, is another issue that warrants attention.

Adolescents' contraceptive problems should not focus only on accessibility. Knowledge, communication and interaction competence play important roles as well. Adolescents exhibiting more effective contraceptive behavior are more sexually experienced, have deeper and more stable partner relationships, are better able to communicate and interact with their partners and peers in relation to sexuality and contraception, evaluate contraception in a practical rather than a normative way, and have more control over the course of contacts with a partner than other adolescents[25]. Furthermore, a realistic estimation of the chances of conception from unprotected intercourse determines their contraceptive use[26]. Young people pass through a phase of 'trial and error' (in terms of contraceptive use) when they become sexually active. Given the fact that each year a new cohort enters the field, efforts must be continued to help young people to keep this phase as short as possible. Access to contraception must be easy (while also ensuring that only those without contraindications use the method concerned), and knowledge and interaction competence improved. Sex education programs focusing on these issues can result in more effective contraceptive use and fewer unintended pregnancies[27,28]. They also result in more explicit attitudes towards sexuality and sometimes postponement of first intercourse[29]. Finally, postponement of a pelvic examination until after a first family planning visit may make young women less reluctant to consult[30].

Prevention of sexually transmitted diseases: 'double-method' use

No longer can we address OC use without considering sexually transmitted diseases, including HIV/AIDS. Young people are at particular risk of these diseases due to their so-called sequentially monogamous relationships. More than one in three new cases of sexually transmitted diseases in the Netherlands occurs in young people (aged 15–24)[31]. Young people generally perceive that they have a single sexual partner (rather than a sequence of partners), and believe they are less likely to be at risk of infection than 'others with multiple partners'. Awareness of AIDS has grown substantially over the past decade[10,11,13], but people generally underestimate their own risks and have insufficiently changed their behavior[31]. In Great Britain and Germany, but perhaps in other countries also, condom use among women aged 15–24 doubled between 1984 and 1992[10,11]. However, about 60% of those at risk still did not use condoms. Several authors have related higher rates of condom use induced by AIDS campaigns to the increases in the occurrence of unintended pregnancies[32,33]. This underlines the relevance of promoting the 'double-method' use (OCs for contraception and condoms for AIDS/STD prevention) rather than advising the young people to use condoms only. Among women aged 15–24, double-method use rates currently amount to 10–15% in the Netherlands, 15% in Sweden, 12% in Great Britain and 3% in Germany[10,11,13,34].

EXPERIENCES WITH AND PERCEPTIONS OF THE PILL

Many family planning providers consider OCs to be effective, easy to use, reasonably safe for health and not disturbing to sex life[35,36]. Women share these perceptions[10–13] with one exception: they generally associate OCs with side-effects and some serious health risks (Table 4). This latter discrepancy between the perceptions of providers and women is highly relevant, since providers who no longer view the health risks of OCs as significant may tend not to counsel their patients explicitly on these issues. Many women receive their OC prescription without any additional explanation or information[9], the prescriber assuming that they know what OCs are for, what their advantages and disadvantages are, how they work and how they should be used. I have commented previously on the role of adverse media publicity (pill scares) on the perceptions of women[17]. The good news about OCs (for example, prevention of specific cancers, no relation with coronary heart disease in non-smokers) has not reached the lay public to the same extent as the scare stories of the past (cancer and cardiovascular disease) or present (thromboembolism during use of particular OCs). However, apart from the selective attention of the mass media to spectacular bad news stories, the role of physicians who underestimate the psychological needs of their clients to be reassured in this respect must not be overlooked.

Of all women who use OCs during a 1-year period, 10–15% will be starters, 12–15% will stop and about 10% will switch their OC brand[37]. Most women who stop OC use do so in order to get pregnant, but some stop because of side-effects, poor cycle control or fears of health risks. Not all women who have stopped subsequently use another contraceptive method (viz. 25% of all women who stopped OCs during the 1-year period). Furthermore, 30–37% of users of barrier methods in Great Britain, Germany and Sweden report problems with a previous method (predominantly OCs) as their motive for choosing barrier methods[10,11,13]. The corresponding percentages for periodic abstinence users in Germany and Sweden were 32–36%. These data show that use of less effective methods of contraception may quite often be related to OC issues.

Women who switch OC brands are motivated by the same issues of side-effects and poor cycle control[37]. Those who switch are most

Table 4 Percentage of women replying 'yes' or 'possibly' to questions about the disadvantages and advantages of oral contraceptives in Great Britain, Germany, Italy and Sweden

	Great Britain 1992[10]	Germany 1992[11]	Italy 1993[12]	Sweden 1994[13]
Regular periods	86	80	81	72
Less painful periods	84	72	69	75
Less heavy periods	84	75	57	78
Relief of skin disorders	28	55	52	11
Cancer prevention	19	29	27	20
Easy to obtain	92	95	84	97
Cardiovascular disease	45	40	36	59
Cancer risk	41	25	30	41
Weight gain	73	60	75	62
Depression	44	32	37	47
Headache	45	30	33	27
Painful tense breasts	35	36	43	40
Nausea	30	23	37	23

often short-term users whereas those who stop have used OCs for a longer period of time. Women who start using OCs are followed by the prescribing physician, who monitors for the occurrence of side-effects and the satisfaction of the client. Dissatisfaction often leads to changes in OC brand, in order to see if another preparation is better tolerated, which is in accordance with guidelines on OC prescription[38]. However, those who turn out to be dissatisfied in the middle-to-long term may 'drop out', i.e. stop using OCs without medical advice[37]. This is perhaps a consequence of prescribers being alert to problems only during the first months of OC use. Continuing this alertness and case-finding (opportunistically identifying 'drop-outs' among women who consult for other reasons) could make the difference between discontinuation (which often leads to use of less effective methods) and switching to another OC formulation or other effective method of contraception. The switching rates among short-term users suggest that many dissatisfied OC users can be helped to find a brand that they tolerate better.

One may wonder why so many women use OCs when they have doubts about the impact of OCs on their health. According to psychological theories, these doubts might be balanced by perceptions of the advantages of OCs, as well as advice to use OCs received from social referents including physicians, and beliefs about the inability to use another method correctly and consistently[39]. Indeed, many studies from the US indicate that these balancing mechanisms determine whether or not women use OCs. Evidence from Western Europe, however, is sparse and relates only to teenagers.

We have incorporated measurements of these issues in representative population surveys on contraception that were carried out in Great Britain ($n = 967$) and Germany ($n = 1064$), after a pilot study indicated that it was possible to study the relationship between these determinants and contraceptive use within the constraints of a population-based survey[39]. Similar results were obtained when studying British and German respondents. Women who recognized more advantages of OCs than disadvantages or gave greater weight to the advantages with respect to their personal situation were more likely to use the pill than another method. OC users had also more often been advised (predominantly by their physician) to use this method than other women. In terms of the contraceptive choice, i.e. the choice between the various methods, it was found that the attitudes towards medically prescribed methods (OCs and sterilization, and, to a lesser extent, intrauterine devices) played an important role in decisions to use a medical method or, alternatively, in case of a more negative attitude, to abstain from these methods and use condoms, rhythm, withdrawal or no method instead. The use of these latter methods was related both to perceptions about the advantages of these methods, and the disadvantages of medical methods (whereas the use of medical methods was, to a much lesser extent, related to a negative attitude towards the non-medical methods).

The principal determinant of the contraceptive choice was whether or not women had been advised by their physician to use OCs. In the subgroup who reported such advice, OC use rose to 75% (as compared to 52% in the total sample). Use of condoms, rhythm and withdrawal/no method was highest (i.e. 40%, 16% and 13%, respectively) in the subgroup of women who had less often than average been stimulated to use OCs, who had a below median score for the attitude towards OCs and who had less often received advice on intrauterine devices. The analyses showed that, for most, the woman's attitude and reported advice predicted adoption of the method rather than that use of the method lead to a more positive attitude or resulted in a greater tendency to report being advised to use the method. Perceptions about the ability to use a particular method correctly and consistently had less impact on contraceptive decisions than social influences or perceptions about advantages and disadvantages of each method.

These observations have several implications. First, they show that (negative) perceptions about OCs have an impact on most contraceptive use decisions including those relating to other methods, and must therefore be taken seriously. In this respect they confirm the findings of smaller US studies. Given the prevalence of these perceptions, the value of identifying women who are particularly concerned about the safety of OCs cannot be overestimated. Second, health-care professionals do influence a woman's contraceptive use, by simple advice and probably by the act of prescribing itself. If the behavior of an expert implicitly expresses confidence in the health safety of OCs (either by advising OC use or prescribing them), this confidence is conveyed to the woman concerned who may begin to feel that OCs are not as dangerous as she originally thought. Third, the use of less effective methods is often the result of a basic dislike/distrust of medical contraceptive methods, and not just an explicit choice in favor of less effective methods (statements such as a wish to use 'a more natural method' also point in this direction).

We have also looked at the demographic determinants of contraceptive use. A clear pattern emerged which can be broadly summarized as follows. When you are young you use OCs, and when you get older you change to an intrauterine device, sterilization or sometimes condoms, rhythm, withdrawal or no method. The change from OCs was related to beliefs that intrauterine devices and sterilization were easier to use, but also to perceptions that one should not use the pill for too long. These latter perceptions were among the primary motives for women who changed to non-prescription methods, although, in the case of withdrawal and no method, beliefs

Table 5 Percentages of current oral contraceptive users who reported missed pills during the 12 months preceding the interview, by number of tablets missed. Previously unpublished findings from references 10–13

	0	*1–3*	*4–6*	*>6*
Great Britain, 1992	53	28	10	10
Germany, 1992	54	28	12	6
Italy, 1993	66	25	7	2
Sweden, 1994	34	40	14	13

about declining fecundability ('contraception no longer necessary') also played a role. This pattern of a 'contraceptive career' rather than a contraceptive choice confirms again that perceptions about the characteristics of the pill play a predominant role in decisions about which contraceptive method to use.

As mentioned, perceptions about the ability to use a method correctly and consistently were not found to play a significant role in decisions about contraceptive choice. In the case of OC use, these perceptions relate to compliance (forgetting pills). Most women, users and non-users, apparently feel capable of remembering to take the pills. In practice, however, reality may be very different: studies have shown that at least 20–30% of individuals miss a pill every month[40]. The difference between the typical failure rate of OCs (3.8% among women aged 15–44, amounting to 18.1% among adolescent subpopulations who are prone to imperfect use[2]) and the failure rate with perfect use (0.1%) is attributed to non-compliance. In the British and German surveys, as well as in later surveys carried out in Sweden and Italy, 47%, 46%, 34% and 66%, respectively *admitted* to having forgotten at least one pill over the 12 months preceding the interview (Table 5). The true number of pills, however, forgotten was probably much higher. Among those who admitted missing pills, 52%, 37%, 24% and 36%, respectively reported at least one incident at which no specific action was taken ('keeping your fingers crossed'). Most episodes of forgotten pills were not brought to the attention of prescribers. These findings suggest that compliance problems partly originate from the fact that women believe that they will not forget to take their pills, even though in practice they do. This discrepancy calls for extensive counselling of OC users and case-finding: women need to know how to manage missed pills particularly when they do not anticipate such an event.

CONCLUSION

In this paper, I have drawn attention to a number of issues that act as a barrier towards effective utilization of family planning within our West European communities. These notably concern accessibility problems among young women, negative perceptions about OCs and pill non-compliance. It is important to note that providers will not actually see women experiencing these difficulties, since the women concerned do not attend the services (accessibility), use other than prescription methods (negative OC perceptions) or do often not share their experiences with their prescriber (non-compliance).

Recognition of these problems may change our views of what we see as the tasks of family planning providers. On the one hand, providers need to take care of contraception users in the more medical sense, i.e. undertake eligibility screening (for example, checking for contraindications), monitor for adverse side-effects and follow-up client satisfaction with the method. Traditionally, these are often viewed as 'the' responsibilities of providers. On the other hand, data on the determinants of contraceptive use indicate that providers also need to be psychologically involved in family planning use, giving advice, answering questions and making their clients feel confident about the chosen method. In this respect, it must be kept in mind that no contraceptive method is perfect and that contraceptive choices constitute compromises about the risks and benefits related to each method, compromises which are not always easy to adhere to in the long term. In my opinion, the psychological role of providers as advisers may ultimately prove to be more relevant than the provision of purely 'medical' care. This applies across the entire range of contraceptive methods. With respect to the proposal that OCs be made available without medical prescription, I support the need to limit initial and follow-up medical checks to the absolute minimum, but feel that providers have an important advisory role. The absence or a reduction of this facility will leave many women – except perhaps the most assertive – alone with their doubts and contraceptive problems. The high use of less effective methods among British and German women who were less likely to receive contraception advice or who had negative perceptions of OCs emphasizes the point. Rather than abandon medical input into OC provision, I would suggest that contraceptive 'prescription services' increasingly become 'advisory services', no so much part of health care but of daily social life.

REFERENCES

1. Shah, I.H. (1994). The advance of the contraceptive revolution. *World Health Stat. Q.*, **47**, 9–15
2. Harlap, S., Kost, K. and Forrest, J.D. (1991). *Preventing Pregnancy, Protecting Health; A New Look at Birth Control Choices in the United States.* (New York: The Alan Guttmacher Institute)
3. Trussell, J., Stewart, F., Potts, M., Guest, F. and Ellertson, C. (1993). Should oral contraceptives be available without prescription? *Am. J. Public Health*, **83**, 1094–9
4. Anonymous (editorial) (1993). OCs o-t-c? *Lancet*, **342**, 565–6
5. Riphagen, F.E. and Lehert, P. (1989). A survey of contraception in five West European countries. *J. Biosoc. Sci.*, **21**, 23–46
6. Vityska-Binstorfer, E., Huber, J.C. and Riphagen, F.E. (1990). Kontrazeption in Österreich. *Wien Med. Wochenschr.*, **140**, 357–60
7. Osler, M. and Riphagen, F.E. (1990). Contraception survey: Denmark 1988. *Contraception*, **42**, 507–21
8. Toulemon, L. and Leridon, H. (1991). Vingt années de contraception en France: 1968–1988. *Population*, **4**, 777–812
9. Vennix, P. (1990). *De pil en haar alternatieven; ervaringen van Nederlandse vrouwen met de pil en andere vormen van anticonceptie.* (NISSO Studies No 6). (Delft: Eburon)
10. Oddens, B.J., Visser, A.P., Vemer, H.M., Everaerd, W.T.A.M. and Lehert, Ph. (1994). Contraceptive use and attitudes in Great Britain. *Contraception*, **49**, 73–86
11. Oddens, B.J., Visser, A.P., Vemer, H.M. and Everaerd, W.T.A.M. (1994). Contraceptive use and attitudes in reunified Germany. *Eur. J. Obstet. Gynecol. Reprod. Biol.*, **57**, 201–8

12. Oddens, B.J. (1996). Contraceptive use and attitudes in Italy 1993. *Hum. Reprod.*, in press

13. Oddens, B.J. and Milsom, I. (1996). Contraceptive practice and attitudes in Sweden 1994. *Acta Gynecol. Obstet. Scand.*, in press

14. David, H.P. (1992). Abortion in Europe, 1920–91: a public health perspective. *Stud. Fam. Plann.*, **23**, 1–22

15. Ketting, E. (1990). Family planning in Western Europe: an overview of major issues. In Ketting, E. (ed.) *Contraception in Western Europe: A Current Appraisal*, pp. 1–7. (Carnforth: Parthenon Publishing)

16. Henshaw, S.K. and Morrow, E. (1990). *Induced Abortion; A World Review*. 1990 Supplement. (New York: The Alan Guttmacher Institute)

17. Oddens, B. (1994). Contraceptive use in developed countries. In Senanayake, P. (ed.) *The Reproductive Revolution: The Role of Contraception and Education in Population and Development*, pp. 38–55. (Carnforth: Parthenon Publishing)

18. Dillner, L. (1991). Promoting teenage friendly contraception. *Br. Med. J.*, **303**, 1355

19. Pearson, V.A.H., Owen, M.R., Phillips, D.R., Pereira Gray, D.J. and Marshall, M.N. (1995). Family planning services in Devon, UK: awareness, experience and attitudes of pregnant teenagers. *Br. J. Fam. Plann.*, **21**, 45–9

20. Seamark, C.J. and Pereira Gray, D.J. (1995). Do teenagers consult general practitioners for contraceptive advice? *Br. J. Fam. Plann.*, **21**, 50–1

21. Hughes, M.E., Furstenberg, F.F. and Teitler, J.O. (1995). The impact of an increase in family planning services on the teenage population of Philadelphia. *Fam. Plann. Perspect.*, **27**, 60–5, 78

22. Persson, E., Gustafsson, B. and van Rooijen, M. (1994). Subsidising contraception for young people in Sweden. *Plann. Parenth. Eur.*, **23**, 1: 2–4

23. Allaby, M.A.K. (1995). Contraceptive services for teenagers: do we need family planning clinics? *Br. Med. J.*, **310**, 1641–3

24. Wellings, K., Wadsworth, J., Johnson, A.M., Field, J., Whitaker, L. and Field, B. (1995). Provision of sex education and early sexual experience: the relation examined. *Br. Med. J.*, **311**, 417–20

25. Rademakers, J. (1991). *Anticonceptie en interactie; de preventie van ongewenste zwangerschap door jongeren in Nederland* (thesis with a summary in English). University of Utrecht

26. Oddens, B.J. (1996). *Determinants of contraceptive use; national population-based studies in several West European countries* (thesis). University of Nijmegen, in press

27. Kirby, D. (1995). Sex and HIV/AIDS education in schools; have a modest but important impact on sexual behaviour. *Br. Med. J.*, **311**, 403

28. Visser, A.P. and Van Bilsen, P. (1994). Effectiveness of sex education provided to adolescents. *Pat. Educ. Counsel.*, **23**, 147–60

29. Mellanby, A.R., Phelps, F.A., Crichton, N.J. and Tripp, J.H. (1995). School sex education: an experimental programme with educational and medical benefit. *Br. Med. J.*, **311**, 414–17

30. Donovan, P. (1992). Delaying pelvic exams to encourage contraceptive use. *Fam. Plann. Perspect.*, **24**, 136–44

31. Van Bergen, J.E.A.M. (1995). Preventie van seksueel overdraagbare infecties. *Medisch. Contact*, **51**, 84–8

32. Bromham, D.R. and Cartmill, R.S.V. (1993). Are current sources of contraceptive advice adequate to meet changes in contraceptive practice? A study of patients requesting termination of pregnancy. *Br. J. Fam. Plann.*, **19**, 179–83

33. Rimpelä, A.H., Rimpelä, M.K. and Kosunen, E.A.L. (1992). Use of oral contraceptives by adolescents and its consequences in Finland 1981–1991. *Br. Med. J.*, **305**, 1053–7

34. Van Lunsen, R.H.W., Arnolds, H.Th. and Louwen, F. (1992). Contraceptive behaviour in the Netherlands in 1989 and 1990; first results of a cohort analysis. In Bezemer, W., Cohen-Kettenis, P., Slob, K. and Van Son-Schoones, N. (eds.) *Sex Matters*. International Congress Series 983, pp. 111–13. (Amsterdam: Excerpta Medica)

35. Russell, M.L. and Love, E.J. (1991). Contraceptive prescription: physician beliefs, attitudes and socio-demographic characteristics. *Can. J. Public Health*, **82**, 259–63

36. Riphagen, F.E., Lehert, P., Boulet, M., Lebrun, T. and Sailly, J.C. (1988). Etude des opinions des gynécologues et généralistes français concernant la contraception. *Contracept. Fertil. Sexualité*, **16**, 385–91

37. Oddens, B.J., Arnolds, H.Th., Van Maris, M.G.M. and Van Lunsen, H.W. (1994). The dynamics of oral contraceptive use in the Netherlands 1991–1993. *Adv. Contracept.*, **10**, 167–74

38. Guillebaud, J. (1989). Practical prescribing of the combined oral contraceptive pill. In Filshie, M. and Guillebaud, J. (eds.) *Contraception: Science and Practice*, pp. 69–93. (London: Butterworths)

39. Oddens, B.J., Potting, M.A.C.J., Visser, A.Ph., Oostveen, T. and Everaerd, W.Th.A.M. (1995). Attitude, social influences and self-efficacy as determinants of contraceptive use among West-German women aged 15–45: a pilot survey. *Int. J. Health Sci.*, **6**, 25–32

40. Adams Hillard, P.J. (1992). Oral contraception noncompliance: the extent of the problem. *Adv. Contracept.*, **8** (Suppl. 1), 13–20

4

Ethics and problems with screening

J.S. McCormick

INTRODUCTION

Screening is the presymptomatic diagnosis of disease but has been extended, often unhappily and unwittingly, to the presymptomatic identification of 'risk markers'.

It is almost 25 years since Cochrane and Holland published their paper on the validation of screening procedures[1]. In that paper they wrote: 'We believe that there is an ethical difference between everyday medical practice and screening. If a patient asks a medical practitioner for help, the doctor does the best he can. He is not responsible for defects in medical knowledge. If, however, the practitioner initiates screening procedures, he is in a very different situation. He should, in our view, have conclusive evidence that screening can alter the natural history of disease in a significant proportion of those screened.' The ethical imperative, which has never, so far as I am aware, been challenged, has, alas, often been neglected.

THE FIRST ETHICAL QUESTION

This brings me to the first of my ethical questions. Is screening for risk markers in contraceptive pill takers likely to do more harm than good? The justification for such screening rests on three assumptions:

firstly, there is good evidence that the marker is associated with altered risk, secondly, that the marker can be validly and reliably identified and, lastly, that the alteration of risk is large enough to be important to the individual.

Are the markers associated with altered risk?

We now know, largely as a result of the work of Clifford Kay, that some markers are associated with increased risk, for example, the risk of vascular disease in older pill takers who smoke. Others are more uncertain, for instance, the presence of varicose veins in pill users[2].

Can the markers be reliably and validly identified?

Some markers can only be identified by asking questions. It is well recognized that smokers tend to answer questions about their habit dishonestly. Some other markers, the presence of hypertension or varicose veins, for example, are extremely subjective. The measurement of blood pressure, the commonest investigation in general practice, is appallingly badly executed.

Is the alteration of risk large enough to be important for the individual?

The failure of the public health establishment, and some doctors, to emphasize the difference between absolute and relative risk has led to an unquantifiable but large growth in unnecessary and pointless anxiety and is ethically indefensible. The increased absolute risks associated with 'risk markers' are often extremely small and even the relative risk increases are modest. The relative risk of an airline pilot being killed in an air crash must be some 100-fold more than most other people's, yet few of us would be distressed if our children took up commercial flying as a career.

The doctor who refuses a 35-year-old woman, who smokes ten cigarettes a day and who has a diastolic pressure of 95 mmHg on casual measurement, a prescription for the pill, and who fails to suggest an alternative efficient method of contraception, may be responsible for her subsequent unwanted 'high-risk' pregnancy.

If all contraindications to pill taking were ignored, the consequent increase in serious morbidity and mortality would, in absolute terms, be extremely small.

THE SECOND ETHICAL QUESTION

My second ethical question is this: Is denying women a prescription for the pill an unjustified erosion of their legitimate autonomy? Whose risk is it anyway?

The four pillars of medical ethics are beneficence, non-maleficence, justice or equity, and autonomy. Of these autonomy has, until recently, been the most neglected. Medical paternalism has had a sometimes unjustified bad press. Unjustified because those who are ill regress towards childlike dependence and need someone in whom they can place their unconditional trust. Father figures are, at times, necessary and human plumbers may fail to meet the needs of the sick[3]. On the other hand, those who seek a prescription for the contraceptive pill are not, and do not perceive themselves as, ill.

In so much that access to most medicines of value is restricted by the necessity of physician approval, medical paternalism is enshrined in law. This restriction is only ethically defensible if open access might lead to seriously damaging consequences for either individuals or for society at large. The risks to the individual of misuse of paracetamol, aspirin or cimetidine, all of which are available 'over the counter', are greater than the risks associated with the pill. Contraceptive pill packs are accompanied by information leaflets which indicate those circumstances when it might be wise to access medical advice. Bought 'over the counter' such information would be available to women and would leave their autonomy intact.

The ethics of economics

It can easily be argued that replacing prescription by over the counter availability would produce savings in doctors' time and possibly in unjustified investigation. The 'opportunity cost' sacrificed by undertaking that which is not cost-effective has an ethical dimension. By comparison with the questions already raised the economic argument is weak but, nonetheless, tenable.

CONCLUSION

The thesis that the contraceptive pill should only be available upon a doctor's prescription is ethically dubious on two major counts. First, screening for risk markers may lead to inappropriate advice, mainly because of the reluctance of doctors to distinguish between relative and absolute risk. Being on the safe side is a cause of iatrogenic harm. Second, restricting availability to a doctor's prescription can be viewed as an unjustifiable erosion of reasonable and legitimate autonomy. Such medical paternalism may be regarded as ethically indefensible.

REFERENCES

1. Cochrane, A.L. and Holland, W.W. (1971). Validation of screening procedures. *Br. Med. Bull.*, **21**, 3–8
2. Campbell, B. (1996). Thrombosis, phlebitis and varicose veins. *Br. Med. J.*, **312**, 198
3. McCormick, J.S. (1978). *The Doctor: Father Figure or Plumber.* (London: Croom Helm)

Section 2

Vascular disease and the pill

5

Oral contraceptives and risk of arterial disease: epidemiological evidence on acute and long-term effects

L. Chasan-Taber and M.J. Stampfer

INTRODUCTION

Early epidemiological studies of high-dose oral contraceptives (OCs) found significantly increased risks of cardiovascular disease among OC users but the formulations of combination oral contraceptives have changed dramatically over the past 30 years. Modern OCs have a third to a quarter of the estrogen dose and a tenth of the progestogen. To minimize the associated androgenic side-effects, new synthetic progestogens have been introduced. The newest progestogens (desogestrel, gestodene and norgestimate) are always found in combination with not more than 35 µg ethinylestradiol. Hence, the findings of early epidemiological studies may not be fully generalizable to today's preparations. The population of OC users has also changed. Women are beginning to use OCs earlier and for longer durations. A current user may now be in her forties or older, an age of use unheard of previously. While serious cardiovascular disease is quite uncommon among women in their twenties or thirties, it is not rare among women in this age group, especially among those who smoke.

49

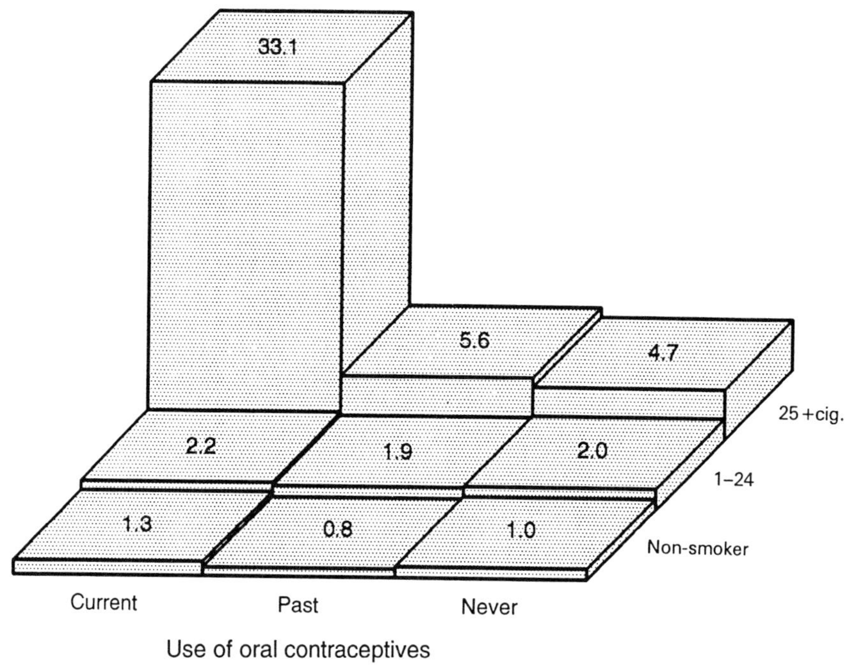

Figure 1 Relative risks of myocardial infarction by cigarette smoking and use of oral contraceptives. Adapted from reference 2

ORAL CONTRACETIVE USE AND MYOCARDIAL INFARCTION

For more than a decade it has been considered established that current use of OCs increases the risk of myocardial infarction. Most of the excess risk, however, is attributable to the striking interaction between OCs and cigarette smoking. In 1979, Shapiro and colleagues reported a relative risk of 39 among women who smoked 25 or more cigarettes per day and used OCs compared to women who did neither[1]. Similarly, Rosenberg and colleagues found that current OC users who smoked more than one pack per day had a 30-fold excess risk compared to non-smokers who had never used OCs (Figure 1)[2]. These extreme relative risks contrast with the four- to eight-fold excess risks associated with smoking, and the far lower risks among

OC users who do not smoke. Hence, studies of OCs and risk of myocardial infarction which do not consider smoking are of limited value. Even those which adjust for smoking may not yield reliable estimates because of the interaction. It is therefore instructive to assess the findings among smokers and non-smokers separately.

Taken together, case–control and cohort studies prior to 1980 suggested little or no increase in risk of myocardial infarction among current OC users under age 40 who do not smoke[1–7]. The more recent studies tend to find even smaller relative risks for current OC use (regardless of smoking) than did the earlier studies. Any increased risk in OC users appears to be confined to women with additional risk factors for cardiovascular disease such as hypertension, diabetes, hyperlipidemia and smoking. Case–control studies with data collection after 1980[8–13] did not report any statistically significant increased risk of myocardial infarction among OC users (Table 1). Due to small numbers of cases, several of these studies were unable to stratify by smoking status.

The cohort studies with the most recent experience have also observed lower relative risks: no cases in the Group Health Co-operative[14,15], a relative risk of 0.2 (95% CI 0.05–0.7) in the Finnish study[16], and 1.1 (95% CI 0.5–2.5) in the Copenhagen City Heart Study[17]. In the Royal College of General Practitioners' (RCGP) study, current users of OCs who did not smoke had no increased risk of myocardial infarction (Table 2).

Several factors may be responsible for the decline in the absolute and relative risks of myocardial infarction associated with OC use. Increased knowledge among health professionals of the effects of OCs has led to better selection of potential OC users on the basis of medical history and better supervision of users during follow-up. OCs containing the new progestogens may not carry the same risk as earlier forms, although their effect on incidence of myocardial infarction or stroke has not yet been fully examined. Interim results from an ongoing case–control study based on 153 cases of myocardial infarction show an odds ratio of 0.36 (95% CI 0.1–1.2) for use of third- as compared with second-generation OC use[18]. This analysis, however, was based on six cases exposed to third-generation OCs and 23 cases exposed to second-generation products.

Table 1 Relative risks of myocardial infarction in current oral contraceptive users who do not smoke

Reference	Years of study	Number of cases using OCs	RR	95% CI
Data collection prior to 1980				
Mann *et al.*, 1975[3]	1968–1972	3	2.0	0.5–8.5
Jick *et al.*, 1978[22]	1975–1978	2	not available	
Petitti *et al.*, 1979[4]	1969–1976	0	0	
Shapiro *et al.*, 1979[1]	1976–1978	4	4.5	1.4–14.1
Rosenberg *et al.*, 1980[5]	up to 1976	5	1.9	0.7–5.2
Krueger, 1980	1/74–6/75	6	2.2	0.6–7.3
Adam *et al.*, 1981[8]	1978	(5)*	1.4[†]	0.8–2.4
Salonen, 1982[6]	1972	0	0	
Porter *et al.*, 1987[15]	1977–1981	0	0	
Croft *et al.*, 1989[7]	1968–1987	5	0.9	0.3–2.7
Data collection post 1980				
WHO, 1989[10]	1979–1984	3[†]	0.4	0.1–1.6
Rosenberg *et al.*, 1990[11]	1985–1988	2[‡]	<1.1	
Hirvonen and Idänpään-Heikkilä, 1990[16]	1980–1984	2[†]	0.2	0.05–0.7
Jensen *et al.*, 1991[17]	1976–1983	0	0	
Thorogood *et al.*, 1991[12]	1986–1988	4	1.1[§]	0.3–3.8
D'Avanzo *et al.*, 1994[13]	1983–1992	7[¶]	2.0	0.6–6.7

RR, relative risk; CI, confidence interval
*Estimated number, based on 24 total cases, of whom 80% smoked
[†]Smokers and non-smokers were combined
[‡]These 'non-smokers' could not be distinguished from subjects smoking up to 24 cigarettes/day
[§]Relative risk based on current and past OC use combined; smokers and non-smokers were included, and adjustment was made for smoking
[¶]Smokers and non-smokers were combined and smoking was included in the model

PAST ORAL CONTRACEPTIVE USE AND CORONARY HEART DISEASE

Because OC use can have adverse effects on risk factors for coronary disease, considerable concern was expressed over whether women in their fifties and sixties would suffer the delayed effects of OCs as they reached the age when clinical coronary disease is more common. Data are quite consistent in demonstrating no increased risk associated with past use.

Table 2 Findings from the Royal College of General Practitioners' study of oral contraceptives use and myocardial infarction and stroke, according to smoking status

	Oral contraceptive use		
Cigarette smoking	*Never*	*Former*	*Current*
Myocardial infarction			
Never	1.0	1.1	0.9
		(0.6–2.2)	(0.3–2.7)
1–14/day	2.0	1.3	3.5
	(1.0–3.9)	(0.6–2.8)	(1.3–9.5)
≥15/day	3.3	4.3	20.8
	(1.6–6.7)	(2.3–8.0)	(5.2–83.1)
All stroke			
Non-smoker	1.0	0.9	2.4
	referent	(0.6–1.5)	(1.3–4.7)
Smoker	1.0	1.8	2.9
	referent	(1.1–2.8)	(1.5–5.7)
Fatal stroke			
Non-smoker	1.0	1.2	0.3
	referent	(0.4–3.5)	(0.0–3.0)
Smoker	1.0	5.0	7.1
	referent	(1.8–14.0)	(1.5–33.0)

Adapted from references 7 and 37

Stampfer and co-workers conducted a meta-analysis of the 10 studies of past use of OCs and myocardial infarction risk[1,3,4,5,7,8,20–23], which yielded an estimated relative risk of 1.01 (95% CI 0.91–1.13)[24]. Only one study, by Jick and colleagues, found an elevated (although not significant) relative risk of 3.6, based on only four cases[22]. When the analysis was limited to the prospective cohort studies[4,7,25] the relative risk was 0.85 (95% CI 0.69–1.05).

PATHOPHYSIOLOGY

The interaction of OCs and smoking, and the lack of an increased risk in past, users suggest that the pathophysiology of myocardial infarction among OC users in earlier studies was an acute effect, probably thrombosis. If the mechanism was increased atherosclerosis, one might expect an elevated risk after discontinuation of OCs and an increase in risk with increasing length of use. Corroborating evidence comes from angiographic and anatomical studies of young women with myocardial infarction which tend to show an absence of atherosclerosis in cases associated with OC use[26–28]. In studies of monkeys fed an atherogenic diet, OCs markedly decreased the extent of atherosclerosis compared with placebo, suggesting that perhaps the estrogenic component in OCs may have a direct protective effect on the wall of the coronary vessels[29,30].

Estrogen tends to increase factors II, VII, VIII, IX, X and fibrinogen and decreases antithrombin III, with a possible resultant thrombogenic tendency[31]. Ernst reviewed the evidence that OCs may contribute to cardiovascular risk partly by elevating fibrinogen levels[32]. Prospective studies demonstrated a significant rise in fibrinogen levels within 1–3 months of use (average increments of 7–25% after six cycles), particularly for OCs with high doses of estrogen. Upon cessation, fibrinogen returned to normal within 3 months. Even though the average increment is quantitatively small, other procoagulant factors are raised in parallel, possibly raising the fibrinogen level into a range where cardiovascular risk is increased (3 g/l). Presumably, these effects are amplified in the presence of smoking[33,34].

Current data on the effect of new progestogens on coagulation and antithrombotic factors are fragmentary and based on diverse laboratory techniques. However, in a review of 21 published reports, Speroff and colleagues observed relatively minor effects on the levels of selected clotting factors and natural anticoagulant proteins. As a rule, a 10–20% increase in fibrinogen was observed in these studies along with variable effects on levels of factor VII[35]. Fibrinolytic activity was also mildly increased. The natural anticoagulant proteins antithrombin III and protein C were unchanged, whereas levels of protein S were reduced by 10–20%.

ORAL CONTRACEPTIVE USE AND RISK OF STROKE

Even a small effect of OCs on the risk of stroke would have important public health implications. Unlike the studies conducted before the modern, low-dose OC came into widespread use, most recent cohort studies have not demonstrated an increase in risk among either past or ever users.

One meta-analysis combined the results of 47 case–control and cohort studies and found a relative risk among OC users of 1.8 (95% CI 1.6–2.0) for stroke of all types combined[36]. However, the studies included both low- and high-dose formulations. The RCGP performed a nested case–control study of 253 women who had a first ever stroke between 1968 and 1990, age matched to three controls[37]. Current users had an elevated relative risk for all stroke even among non-smokers (RR = 2.4, 95% CI 1.3–4.7) (Table 2). However, the relative risk among current users of OCs containing <50 μg estrogen was 0.6 (95% CI 0.1–2.9) as compared to OCs with 50+ μg estrogen. Risk for past users was increased only among smokers (RR = 1.8, 95% CI 1.1–2.8). The Nurses' Health Study found no statistically significant increase in risk of stroke among past OC users (ischemic and subarachnoid were combined)[25]. Provisional results from the WHO case–control study show no substantial difference in risk of stroke when comparing the new progestogens to other low-dose preparations when combined with low-dose estrogen[38].

In many studies of ischemic stroke, only a small number of cases were observed; more recent data are sparse. The Oxford study observed no ischemic strokes in 9100 person-years of observation among current users of OCs with less than 50 μg of estrogen[39]. Hirvonen and Idänpään-Heikkilä reported no fatal ischemic strokes in 1 585 000 person-years of OC use in Finland from 1975 to 1984[16]. Similarly, among current users in the Group Health Co-operative enrolled between 1980 and 1982, only one stroke of any kind was observed in 37 807 person-years of follow-up, for a relative risk of 0.9 (95% CI 0.1–6.4)[11]. There is no evidence to support an increased risk of ischemic stroke among past OC users.

OC use appears to be associated with little or no increase in the risk of fatal subarachnoid hemorrhage. Several studies performed prior to 1980 observed an increased risk for subarachnoid hemorrhage among past OC users, but were based on a small number of cases[4,39–44]. Recent data for the modern preparations are sparse. The Finnish study, assessing cerebral hemorrhage and subarachnoid hemorrhage together in 1980, 1982 and 1984, observed nine exposed cases in 485 000 person-years of use[16]. Current OC users had a relative risk of 0.7 (95% CI 0.2–0.9) as compared to never users. Thorogood and colleagues examined the association between OCs and fatal stroke in a matched case–control study of 296 cases of subarachnoid hemorrhage and 21 cases of occlusive stroke occurring between 1986 and 1988 among women aged under 40 years[45]. The adjusted relative risk for subarachnoid hemorrhage was 1.1 (95% CI 0.6–1.9) for current use and 1.3 (95% CI 0.9–1.8) for ever use.

Previous studies of OCs and risk of cerebral thromboembolic attacks have been limited by the small number of cases and typically did not discriminate between hemorrhagic and thromboembolitic stroke, nor between users of high- and low-dose estrogen. Lidegaard performed a case–control study in Denmark among 794 cases of cerebral thromboembolitic attack occurring between 1985 and 1989, and 1588 age-matched controls[46]. Current users of combined or sequential OCs containing 30–40 µg estrogen had a multivariate relative risk of 1.8 (95% CI 1.1–2.9), as compared to never users. This relative risk was one-third of the risk associated with preparations containing 50 µg estrogen. Progestin-only OCs did not increase the risk of cerebral thromboembolitic attack. Former users of OCs were at 50% decreased risk as compared with never users (95% CI 0.4–0.7). While use of OCs among the controls was assessed in 1990, use among cases was recorded at some point during 1985–1989. (The authors accounted for this by including a time trend covariate in their analyses which reflected the change in the distribution of OCs with different hormonal contents from 1985 to 1989.) Thorogood and co-workers found a non-significant increased risk of 4.4 (95% CI 0.8–24.4) for fatal occlusive disease among ever users (analysis based on 21 case–control sets)[45]. Because the number of case–control sets was too limited (11 sets), it was not possible to estimate a relative risk associated with current use. Overall, occlusive stroke is very rare in young women, and fatal occlusive stroke is so rare that any attributable risk of death from occlusive stroke associated with the use of OCs remains very small.

SUMMARY AND CONCLUSIONS

Current use of contemporary OC preparations among non-smokers does not appear to increase risk of myocardial infarction. Even among smokers, the benefits of OCs may outweigh their risks. However, every effort should be made to encourage smoking cessation among potential OC users. The pathogenic role of smoking in OC users is still unclear. Perhaps women with an inherited abnormality such as factor V Leiden mutation are most susceptible. Atherosclerosis does not appear to be an important mechanism for myocardial infarction in women who use OCs and lack of an adverse effect of past use is now well documented.

Current information is insufficient to permit a definitive statement about the risk of stroke in women who use the modern, low-dose OCs, but a large increase in risk can be excluded. Again, recent investigations do not demonstrate an increase in risk among past users.

OCs containing the newest progestogens are less androgenic, have less impact on carbohydrate and lipid metabolism, and may be associated with stronger suppression of ovarian activity. However, their effect on risk of myocardial infarction and stroke remains to be fully explored.

REFERENCES

1. Shapiro, S., Slone, D., Rosenberg, L., Kaufman, DW., Stolley, P.D. and Miettinen, O.S. (1979). Oral-contraceptive use in relation to myocardial infarction. *Lancet*, **1**, 743–7
2. Rosenberg, L., Kaufman, D.W., Helmrich, S.P., Miller, D.R., Stolley, P.D. and Shapiro, S. (1985). Myocardial infarction and cigarette smoking in women younger than 50 years of age. *J. Am. Med. Assoc.*, **253**, 2965–9
3. Mann, J.I., Vessey, M.O., Thorogood, M. and Doll, R. (1975). Myocardial infarction in young women with special reference to oral contraceptive practice. *Br. Med. J.*, **2**, 241–5
4. Petitti, D.B., Wingerd, J., Pellegrin, F. and Ramcharan, S. (1979). Risk of vascular disease in women. Smoking, oral contraceptives, noncontraceptive estrogens, and other factors. *J. Am. Med. Assoc.*, **242**, 1150–4
5. Rosenberg, L., Hennekens, C.H., Rosner, B., Belanger, C., Rothman, K.J. and Speizer, F.E. (1980). Oral contraceptive use in relation to nonfatal myocardial infarction. *Am. J. Epidemiol.*, **111**, 59–66

6. Salonen, J.T. (1982). Oral contraceptives, smoking and risk of myocardial infarction in young women. *Acta Med. Scand.*, **212**, 141–4

7. Croft, P. and Hannaford, P.C. (1989). Risk factors for acute myocardial infarction in women: evidence from the Royal College of General Practitioners' oral contraception study. *Br. Med. J.*, **298**, 165–8

8. Adam, S.A., Thorogood, M. and Mann, K.I. (1981). Oral contraception and myocardial infarction revisited: the effects of new preparations and prescribing patterns. *Br. J. Obstet. Gynaecol.*, **88**, 838–45

9. LaVecchia, C., Franceschi, S., Decarli, A., Pampallona, S. and Tognoni, G. (1987). Risk factors for myocardial infarction in young women. *Am. J. Epidemiol.*, **125**, 823–43

10. WHO Collaborative Study (1989). Cardiovascular disease and use of oral contraceptives. *Bull. WHO*, **67**, 417–23

11. Rosenberg, L., Palmer, J.R., Lesko, S.M. and Shapiro, S. (1990). Oral contraceptive use and the risk of myocardial infarction. *Am. J. Epidemiol.*, **131**, 1009–16

12. Thorogood, M., Mann, J., Murphy, M. and Vessey, M. (1991). Is oral contraceptive use still associated with an increased risk of myocardial infarction? Report of a case–control study. *Br. J. Obstet. Gynaecol.*, **98**, 1245–53

13. D'Avanzo, B., LaVecchia, C., Negri, E., Parazzini, F. and Franceschi, S. (1994). Oral contraceptive use and risk of myocardial infarction: an Italian case–control study. *J. Epidemiol. Comm. Hlth.*, **48**(3), 324–5

14. Porter, J.B., Hunter, J.R., Jick, H. and Stergachis, A. (1985). Oral contraceptives and nonfatal vascular disease. *Obstet. Gynecol.*, **66**, 1–4

15. Porter, J.B., Jick, H. and Walker, S.M. (1987). Mortality among oral contraceptive users. *Obstet. Gynecol.*, **70**, 29–32

16. Hirvonen, E. and Idänpään-Heikkilä, J. (1990). Cardiovascular death among women under 40 years of age using low-estrogen oral contraceptives and intrauterine devices in Finland from 1975 to 1984. *Am. J. Obstet. Gynecol.*, **163**, 281–4

17. Jensen, G., Nyboe, J., Appleyard, M. and Schnohr, P. (1991). Risk factors for acute myocardial infarction in Copenhagen II: Smoking, alcohol intake, physical activity, obesity, oral contraception, diabetes, lipids, and blood pressure. *Eur. Heart J.*, **12**, 298–308

18. Lewis, M.A., Spitzer, W.O., Heinemann, L.A., MacRae, K.D., Bruppacher, R. and Thorogood, M. (1996). Third generatiion oral contraceptives and risk of myocardial infarction: an international case–control study. *Br. Med. J.*, **312**, 88–90

19. Krueger, D.E., Ellenberg, S.S., Bloom, S. *et al.* (1980). Fatal myocardial infarction and the role of oral contraceptives. *Am. J. Epidemiol.*, **111**, 655–74

20. Mann, J.I. and Inman, W.H.W. (1975). Oral contraceptives and death from myocardial infarction. *Br. Med. J.*, **2**, 245–8

21. Mann, J.I., Inman, W.H.W. and Thorogood, M. (1976). Oral contraceptive use in older women and fatal myocardial infarction. *Br. Med. J.*, **2**, 445–7

22. Jick, H., Dinan, B. and Rothman, K.J. (1978). Oral contraceptives and nonfatal myocardial infarction. *J. Am. Med. Assoc.*, **239**, 1403–6

23. Layde, P.M., Ory, H.W. and Schlesselman, J.J. (1982). The risk of myocardial infarction in former users of oral contraceptives. *Fam. Plan. Perspect.*, **14**, 78–80

24. Stampfer M.J., Willett, W.C., Colditz, G.A., Speizer, F.E. and Hennekens, C.H. (1990). Past use of oral contraceptives and cardiovascular disease: a meta-analysis in the context of the Nurses' Health Study. *Am. J. Obstet. Gynecol.*, **163**, 285–91

25. Stampfer, M.J., Willett, W.C., Colditz, G.A., Speizer, F.E. and Hennekens, C.H. (1988). A prospective study of past use of oral contraceptive agents and risk of cardiovascular disease. *N. Engl. J. Med.*, **319**, 1313–17

26. Engel, H.J., Engel, E. and Lichtlen, P.R. (1983). Coronary atherosclerosis and myocardial infarction in young women – role of oral contraceptives. *Eur. Heart J.*, **4**, 1–8

27. Engel, H.J., Hundeshagen, H. and Lichtlen, P. (1983). Transmural myocardial infarction in young women taking oral contraceptives. Evidence of reduced regional coronary flow in spite of normal coronary arteries. *Br. Heart J.*, **39**, 477–84

28. Jugdutt, B.I., Stevens, G.F., Zacks, D.J., Lee, S.J.K. and Taylor, R.F. (1983). Myocardial infarction, oral contraception, cigarette smoking, and coronary artery spasm in young women. *Am. Heart J.*, **106**, 757–61

29. Adams, M.B., Clarkson, T.B., Koritnik, D.R. and Nash, H.A. (1987). Contraceptive steroids and coronary artery atherosclerosis in cynomolgus macaques. *Fertil. Steril.*, **47**, 1010–18

30. Clarkson, T.B., Shively, C.A., Morgan, T.M., Koritnik, D.R., Adams, M.R. and Kaplan, J.R. (1990). Oral contraceptives and coronary artery atherosclerosis of cynomolgus monkeys. *Obstet. Gynecol.*, **75**, 217–22

31. Fotherby, K. and Caldwell, A.D.S. (1994). New progestogens in oral contraception. *Contraception*, **49**, 1–32

32. Ernst, E. (1992). Oral contraceptives, fibrinogen and cardiovascular risk. *Atherosclerosis*, **93**, 1–5

33. Fruzzetti, F., Ricci, C. and Fioretti, P. (1994). Haemostasis profile in smoking and nonsmoking women taking low-dose oral contraceptives. *Contraception*, **49**, 579–92

34. Basdevant, A., Conard, J., Pelissier, C., Guyene, T.-T., Lapousterle, C., Mayer, M., Guy-Grand, B. and Degrelle, H. (1993). Hemostatic and

metabolic effects of lowering the ethinylestradiol dose from 30 mcg to 20 mcg in oral contraceptives containing desogestrel. *Contraception*, **48**, 193–204

35. Speroff, L., DeCherney, A. and The Advisory Board for the New Progestin (1993). Evaluation of a new generation of oral contraceptives. *Obstet. Gynecol.*, **81**, 1034–47

36. Katerndahl, D.A., Realini, J.P. and Cohen, P.A. (1992). Oral contraceptive use and cardiovascular disease: is the relationship real or due to study bias? *J. Fam. Pract.*, **35**, 147–57

37. Hannaford, P.C., Croft, P.R. and Kay, C.R. (1994). Oral contraception and stroke: evidence from the Royal College of General Practitioners' Oral Contraception Study. *Stroke*, **25**, 935–42

38. WHO Collaborative Study of Cardiovascular Disease and Steroid Hormone Contraception (1995). Effect of different progestagens in low oestrogen oral contraceptives on venous thromboembolic disease. *Lancet*, **346**, 1582–8

39. Vessey, M.P., Lawless, M. and Yeates, D. (1984). Oral contraceptives and stroke: findings in a large prospective study. *Br. Med. J.*, **289**, 530–1

40. Petitti, D.B. and Wingerd, J. (1978). Use of oral contraceptives, cigarette smoking, and risk of subarachnoid hemorrhage. *Lancet*, **2**, 234–6

41. Inman, W.H.W. (1979). Oral contraceptives and fatal subarachnoid hemorrhage. *Br. Med. J.*, **2**, 1468–70

42. Royal College of General Practitioners' Oral Contraception Study (1981). Further analyses of mortality in oral contraceptive users. *Lancet*, **1**, 541–50

43. Collaborative Group for the Study of Stroke in Young Women (1973). Oral contraception and increased risk of cerebral ischemia or thrombosis. *N. Engl. J. Med.*, **288**, 871–8

44. Collaborative Group for the Study of Stroke in Young Women (1975). Oral contraceptives and stroke in young women. Associated risk factors. *J. Am. Med. Assoc.*, **231**, 718–22

45. Thorogood, M., Mann, J., Murphy, M. and Vessey, M. (1992). Fatal stroke and use of oral contraceptives: findings from a case–control study. *Am. J. Epidemiol.*, **136**, 35–45

46. Lidegaard, O. (1993). Oral contraception and risk of a cerebral thromboembolic attack: results of a case–control study. *Br. Med. J.*, **306**, 956–63

6

Evidence that currently available pills are associated with vascular disease: venous disease

K.W.M. Bloemenkamp, F.R. Rosendaal, F.M. Helmerhorst and J.P. Vandenbroucke

THIRTY YEARS OF EPIDEMIOLOGICAL RESEARCH

From the early days of the use of combined oral contraceptives (OCs), reports have emerged associating use of OCs with the development of venous thromboembolism. After the report of Jordan[1], numerous case–control[2–10] and cohort[11–16] studies followed. In an attempt to assess the thrombogenic potiential of new preparations introduced during the last decade through the assessment of surrogate end-points, young healthy volunteers have been recruited to randomized trials in which the effect of the new OC on variables in (anti)-coagulation, fibrinolysis and lipid metabolism were investigated, mostly in comparison with an older preparation. Several authors, however, have expressed doubts about the clinical relevance of this type of study, or whether they can reasonably be expected to reflect the risk of thrombosis during actual, large-scale use of a new type of OC[17,18].

Observational case–control and cohort studies have to be criticized. Not every study has been able to adjust for the influence of putative confounders or effect modifiers, like smoking, family history of venous thrombosis, history of varicose veins, body mass

61

index, duration of OC use, parity, age, blood group. Furthermore, some observational studies were not specifically designed to look at the side-effects of OCs. Other problems affecting comparability of data between studies include some authors reporting on fatal, and others on non-fatal, venous thromboembolism; and some authors differentiating between types of thrombosis, such as superficial, deep venous thrombosis or pulmonary embolism. In some studies, objective investigations for the diagnosis (such as venography, ultrasound, impedance plethysmography, ventilation-perfusion scans, postmortem examinations) were missing. Randomized studies with clinical end-points overcome other flaws of observational studies, such as selection, diagnostic, referral, recall and prescription bias. However, the low incidence of venous thrombosis during OC use, ethical and financial reasons prevent us from studying this association by a randomized trial. Consequently, we have to draw our conclusions from observational and laboratory studies.

For some time there has been (near) consensus that there is an association between OC use and venous thrombosis. Reports from various case–control and cohort studies attribute this risk to the estrogen content of the OCs, an effect which has not consistently been shown to be related to dose[19,20] and unrelated to duration of pill use[4,5,21]. The risk disappears once the OC is stopped; there is no elevated risk among past users. Women with blood group non-O appear to have higher risks than women with blood group O[22,23]. Smoking does not appear to be a risk factor for venous thrombosis[4,7,11,12,24]; obesity[4,25] and varicose veins[11] are at most weak risk factors. Prescribers, therefore, cannot readily identify women at risk.

The estimated relative risk of developing thromboembolism during OC use has been reported to be between 2 and 11. Case–control studies have usually yielded a higher relative risk than cohort studies. The risk estimates have been larger when associated with idiopathic events than when other risk factors were also involved[3,4]. Furthermore, the more certain the diagnosis[4,5,13,21,25] or the more severe[11,13] the venous thromboembolic events, the larger the estimated relative risks. Even though every study is likely to be affected by at least one bias, nearly all have reported elevated risk estimates, increasing the plausibility of a relationship between current OC use and venous thrombosis. Finally, it is a characteristic of true association that this shows up whatever the shortcomings of studies set up to investigate it (although an important flaw common to all studies can still produce erroneous conclusions).

In an attempt to lower the cardiovascular side-effects of OCs, newer generations of pills, containing lower doses of ethinylestradiol and lower doses, and new types, of progestogens, were introduced. The decrease in the amount of ethinylestradiol from 50 μg to 35 μg, 30 μg and even 20 μg was expected by some to result in a reduced risk of venous thrombosis[11,13,25,26]. Since most studies were conducted in the 1960s and 1970s, there is little information about clinical end-points for these newer preparations. Two case–control studies[9,10] and one cohort study[16] using clinical end-points were conducted in the late 1980s or early 1990s, when the newer preparations were on the OC market. These studies compared current users with non-users and reported relative risks of 2.1 (95% confidence interval (CI) 0.8–5.2) for fatal venous thromboembolism and pulmonary embolism[10], 3.8 (95% CI 2.4–6.0) for non-fatal deep vein thrombosis (age-adjusted risk 6.0 (95% CI 3.4–10.6))[9] and 2.7 (95% CI 1.8–4.2) for superficial venous thrombosis, deep vein thrombosis, pulmonary embolism, and venous thrombosis[16]. These data suggest that OCs with less than 50 μg ethinylestradiol may still have a thrombo-embolic risk.

INHERITABLE CLOTTING DEFECTS

One of the studies provided a new insight into the relation between OC use and thromboembolism[9]. An interaction between a newly discovered inheritable coagulation disorder[27] and OC use was described. Factor V Leiden mutation, which leads to resistance to activated protein C and which is commonly found among patients with venous thrombosis (up to 20% of patients with deep vein thrombosis are carriers)[28], displays a strong interaction with use of OCs. In non-carriers who use OCs, the risk of venous thrombosis is increased four-fold, in carrier non-users the risk is increased eightfold, but in users of OCs who also carry the factor V Leiden mutation the risk rises 30–50-fold[9]. Other inheritable clotting factors, protein C, protein S and antithrombin deficiency, which are themselves risk factors of venous thrombosis, also appeared synergistically to lead to an excess risk of venous thrombosis among OC users[29]. The prevalence of factor V Leiden in the Caucasian population is estimated to be between 3 and 5%, with much lower levels for the other inheritable clotting abnormalities[30–33].

SCREENING

It is questionable if the routine screening for genetic clotting disorders before starting OCs is useful or feasible[34]. Part of the problem is the lack of evidence concerning this issue. In general, however, family history is a strong risk factor for thromboembolism in healthy young people. It *may* be useful, therefore, to screen potiential users when there is a family history of inherited thrombophilia in a first-degree relative. On the other hand, it is not yet clear whether it is helpful to screen women with a positive family, or even personal, history of thrombosis. A major problem is that venous thrombosis is relatively common when viewed over the history of a life-time. Thus, many people have a positive history without having a genetic defect[35].

THE EFFECTS OF SOME NEWER PROGESTOGENS

In October 1995, the Committee on Safety of Medicines in the United Kingdom warned, in a letter to all doctors[36], of a differential risk between OC types. Based on at the time unpublished data, the Committee advised that several of the so-called third-generation preparations had a greater risk of venous thrombosis than older preparations. In December 1995 and January 1996, four studies were published which showed that women using OCs containing desogestrel and gestodene had, on average, twice the risk of developing venous thrombosis than users of older levonorgestrel-containing preparations[37–41]. Previous to these unexpected results, only two epidemiological studies had reported on the effects of the type and dose of progestogens used in OCs[11,19]. Other studies which examined surrogate and intermediate end-points distinguished between combined or progestogen-only oral contraceptives, different preparations, dose of ethinylestradiol or mestranol used, and type and dose of progestogen used[18]. However, as already stated, this type of study has now been discredited since results about surrogate endpoints have proved irrelevant when predicting future risk of venous thrombosis.

THE FOUR STUDIES

The different studies by the World Health Organization (WHO), Jick and colleagues, Bloemenkamp and co-workers and Spitzer and colleagues will now be briefly discussed (Tables 1 and 2).

WORLD HEALTH ORGANIZATION STUDY

The WHO conducted a case–control study in 21 hospitals in 17 countries[37]. Some 1143 women aged between 22 and 44 years with a history of idiopathic venous thromboembolism were recruited as cases. The control group consisted of 2998 age-matched women. In the European countries, use of the pill was associated with an overall relative risk of 4.15 (95% CI 3.09–5.57); in non-European countries the relative risk was 3.25 (95% CI 2.59–4.08). The risk estimates were generally higher for deep vein thrombosis than for pulmonary embolism, but no consistent trend was found for certainty of diagnosis (definite, probable, possible). An increased risk was apparent within 4 months of starting OCs, was unaffected by duration of current episode of OC use, and had disappeared within 3 months of stopping the pill. The relative risks were not related to age, history of hypertension (except during pregnancy) or smoking. A body mass index (BMI) of more than $25\,\text{kg/m}^2$ appeared a weak risk factor. In a subgroup analysis on OC type, the risk was found to be highest among users of OCs containing desogestrel and gestodene. This prompted a more detailed analysis of the WHO data which included all women for which these preparations had been prescribed during the study period[38]. A total of 769 cases were compared with 1979 age-matched hospital controls, and, in one center, with 246

Table 1 The characteristics of the studies examining the association between oral contraceptive use and venous thrombosis, which compared newer with older types of progestogen contained in the preparation

Database	First author	Type of study	Source data	Period	Countries	Age (years)	Event
WHO	Farley[38]	case–control	hospital	1989–93	nine	20–44	DVT, PE, F, NF
GPRD	Jick[39]	cohort + case–control	hospital	1991–94	UK	<40	case–control: DVT, PE, NF
LETS	Bloemenkamp[40]	case–control	anticoagulation clinics	1988–92	NL	15–49	DVT, NF
TRANS	Spitzer[41]	case–control	hospital	1993–95	UK, GER	16–44	DVT, PE, F, NF

WHO, World Health Organization; GPRD, General Practice Research Database; LETS, Leiden Thrombophilia Study; TRANS, Transnational Study
UK, United Kingdom; NL, The Netherlands; GER, Germany
DVT, deep venous thrombosis; PE, pulmonary embolism; SVT, superficial venous thrombosis; F, fatal; NF, non-fatal

Table 2 Relative risks (95% CI) for venous thrombosis according to type of oral contraceptive

Database	First author	OCs vs. non-use	DSG vs. LNG	GSD vs. LNG	Remarks
WHO	Farley[38]	4.1 (3.3–5.1)	2.6 (1.4–4.8)	2.6 (1.4–4.8)	adjusted for BMI respectively: 4.0 (all), 2.2 (DSG) and 3.0 (GSD)
GPRD	Jick[39]	—	2.2 (1.1–4.4)*	2.1 (1.0–4.4)*	non-fatal venous thromboembolism
LETS	Bloemenkamp[40]	6.0 (3.4–10.6)[†]	2.2 (0.9–5.4)[†]	—	DSG vs. all others: 2.5 (1.2–5.2)[†]
TRANS	Spitzer[41]	4.0 (3.1–5.3)[‡]	1.5 (1.1–2.2)[‡]	1.5 (1.0–2.2)[‡]	DSG and GSD were compared to second-generation products as defined in their study

WHO, World Health Organization; GPRD, General Practice Research Database; LETS, Leiden Thrombophilia Study; TRANS, Transnational Study
DSG, desogestrel-containing oral contraceptives; GSD, gestodene-containing oral contraceptives; LNG, levonorgestrel-containing oral contraceptives; BMI, body mass index
*Adjusted for smoking and BMI; [†]adjusted for age; [‡]adjusted for age, smoking, alcohol use, study center, BMI, and duration of exposure to oral contraceptives used before current oral contraceptive

community controls matched on age and general practice. Compared with non-users, those using OCs containing levonorgestrel had a three-fold elevated risk of thrombosis (odds ratio (OR) 3.5 (95% CI 2.6–4.7)) and those using desogestrel- or gestodene-containing pills a nine-fold risk (OR 9.1 (95% CI 4.9–17.0) and OR 9.1 (95% CI 4.9–16.7), respectively). After adjustment for BMI, the ORs were 3.4, 7.3 and 10.2, respectively. Direct comparison of desogestrel- and gestodene-containing oral contraceptives with levonorgestrel-containing preparations revealed risk estimates of 2.2 and 3.0, respectively (adjusted for body mass index).

GPRD (GENERAL PRACTICE RESEARCH DATABASE) STUDY

Jick and colleagues[39] presented data from 238 130 women derived from 365 general practices in a study on the risk on non-fatal thromboembolism. In the non-users group, 3.8 cases of non-fatal thromboembolism per 100 000 women-years were observed. In the OC users group, the rate in users of levonorgestrel-containing pills was 16.1 per 100 000 women-years, in the desogestrel group 29.3 per 100 000 women-years, and in the gestodene group 28.1 per 100 000 women-years. Thus, the relative risk associated with gestodene and desogestrel pills was approximately twice that of levonorgestrel preparations. In a nested case–control analysis, the adjusted matched relative risk estimates were 2.2 (95% CI 1.1–4.4) and 2.1 (95% CI 1.0–4.4) for desogestrel and gestodene users, respectively, compared with users of levonorgestrel. The excess risk for non-fatal venous thromboembolism associated with the oral contraceptives containing desogestrel or gestodene compared with levonorgestrel was estimated to be 16 per 100 000 women-years.

LETS (LEIDEN THROMBOPHILIA STUDY)

Using data from a previously published case–control study (Leiden Thrombophilia Study)[40], we compared 126 women, aged 15–49 years, with an objective diagnosis of deep venous thrombosis with

159 control subjects. Compared with non-use, the highest age-adjusted relative risk was found among current users of desogestrel pills (OR 8.7 (95% CI 3.9–19.3)). The numbers of gestodene and norgestimate-containing oral contraceptives were too small to arrive at meaningful conclusions. The relative risks of levonorgestrel-, lynestrenol- and norethisterone-containing oral contraceptives ranged between 2.2 and 3.8. In a direct comparison, users of desogestrel-containing oral contraceptives had a 2.5-fold higher risk (95% CI 1.2–5.2) than users of all other OC types combined. The relative risk for the desogestrel-containing OC was similar among women with and without a family history of venous thrombosis. The excess risk could also not be explained by previous pregnancy, and it was highest in the youngest age categories, where we could expect most new users. The age-adjusted relative risk for the desogestrel-containing OC was 9.2 (95% CI 3.9–21.4) among non-carriers of the factor V Leiden mutation and 6.0 (95% CI 1.9–19.0) among carriers of the mutation. This latter risk is superimposed on the eight-fold increased risk of venous thrombosis for carriers of the factor V Leiden mutation. The risk of carriers using the desogestrel-containing OC as compared with non-carrier non-users may therefore be increased almost 50-fold.

TRANSNATIONAL STUDY

After the publication of results of a pharmacokinetic study in Germany suggesting that gestodene may increase the risk of vascular events[42,43] (results which were not subsequently confirmed by other researchers[44–49]), an international study was started: the Transnational Study of Oral Contraceptives and the Health of Young Women[41]. In this case–control study, 471 cases were compared with 1772 control subjects, matched for hospital and age. The adjusted odds ratio for venous thromboembolism for use of any oral contraceptive versus no use was 4.0 (95% CI 3.1–5.3). The authors made a different subdivision between first-, second-, and third-generation preparations to that used in the other studies. The adjusted odds ratio for desogestrel- and gestodene-containing OCs versus second-generation OCs was 1.5 (95% CI 1.1–2.1) for both preparations.

REACTIONS TO THE INVESTIGATIONS

Authorities, the public, industry and researchers in several countries have reacted differently to these findings[50–58] and the scientific discussion is still developing. Among the comments so far are remarks that none of the studies have been able to adjust for all possible confounders, that a mainly Caucasian population was studied, that no distinction was made between monophasic, biphasic and triphasic preparations, that different studies had different criteria for defining first-, second- and third-generation progestogens, and that selective prescribing, healthy user effects, and differential referral bias could have contributed to the observations. Even so, as Weiss and McPherson point out[56,57], these theoretical objections may not matter given that all studies point in the same direction.

CONCLUSIONS

It can be concluded that there is still an association between OC use and venous thromboembolism, a relationship which also may be dependent on the type of progestogen. Women using desogestrel- and gestodene-containing OCs appear to have a higher risk of developing venous thrombosis compared to users of the other types of low-dose pill. These higher risks have not been completely explained (i.e. are not limited to subgroups defined) by age, duration of use, family history of thrombosis, parity, body mass index, varicose veins or factor V Leiden mutation. To our knowledge, no study has succeeded in overcoming the bias of selective diagnosis and referral; for many preparations the numbers of exposed cases have been too small to provide reliable estimates and an answer to extremely relevant clinical questions of what is the recurrence rate when continuing to use oral contraceptives after a first thrombosis is still lacking[59].

The higher relative risks of desogestrel- and gestodene-containing OCs have to be balanced against possible benefits of these OCs compared with the older preparations. It has to be emphasized, however, that until now these benefits have been much discussed, but not demonstrated except in intermediate end-point studies. Other effects of OC use, like the risk of arterial thrombosis and protection against endometrial and ovarian cancer, have still to be investigated for the newer preparations.

The absolute risk of fatal thromboembolism in women using oral contraceptives is small. Indeed, all serious diseases are rare in the young. Even so, when they occur they can have a serious impact. The chronic sequel of non-fatal venous thrombosis may place a heavier burden on young and active women than on the elderly, and may afflict their lives for many more years. When safety issues between different types of oral contraceptives are discussed, it is inappropriate to compare the risks to those experienced in other situations, such as pregnancy or puerperium, since these are not the alternatives under discussion (unless fears about safety lead to non-use of any contraceptive and subsequently result in pregnancy). The only useful comparison is between types of OCs, and the only logical choice is for the safest compatible with patient acceptance and tolerance.

THE FUTURE

The story of the third-generation OCs and venous thrombosis provides an example for studies of the side-effects of other drugs. Clinical end-points should be investigated instead of intermediate end-points.

Although many new insights into the relationship between venous thrombosis and OCs have been reported during the past years, much remains unknown and several problems are still to be solved.

REFERENCES

1. Jordan, W.M. (1961). Pulmonary embolism. *Lancet*, **2**, 1146–7
2. Records Unit and Research Advisory Service of the Royal College of General Practitioners (1967). Oral contraception and thrombo-embolic disease. *J. R. Coll. Gen. Pract.*, **13**, 267–79
3. Inman, W.H.W. and Vessey, M.P. (1968). Investigation of deaths from pulmonary, coronary, and cerebral thrombosis and embolism in women of child-bearing age. *Br. Med. J.*, **2**, 193–9

4. Vessey, M.P. and Doll, R. (1969). Investigation of relation between use of oral contraceptives and thromboembolic disease. A further report. *Br. Med. J.*, **2**, 651–7

5. Sartwell, P.E., Masi, A.T., Arthes, F.G., Greene, G.R. and Smith, H.E. (1969). Thromboembolism and oral contraceptives: an epidemiologic case-control study. *Am. J. Epidemiol.*, **90**, 365–80

6. Boston Collaborative Drug Surveillance Programme (1973). Oral contraceptives and venous thromboembolic disease, surgically confirmed gall-bladder disease, and breast tumours. *Lancet*, **1**, 1399–404

7. Maguire, M.G., Tonascia, J., Sartwell, P.E., Stolley, P.D. and Tockman, D.S. (1979). Increased risk of thrombosis due to oral contraceptives: a further report. *Am. J. Epidemiol.*, **110**, 188–95

8. Helmrich, S.P., Rosenberg, L., Kaufman, D.W., Strom, B. and Shapiro, S. (1987). Venous thromboembolism in relation to oral contraceptive use. *Obstet. Gynecol.*, **69**, 91–5

9. Vandenbroucke, J.P., Koster, T., Briët, E., Reitsma, P.H., Bertina, R.M. and Rosendaal, F.R. (1994). Increased risk of venous thrombosis in oral-contraceptive users who are carriers of factor V Leiden mutation. *Lancet*, **344**, 1453–7

10. Thorogood, M., Mann, J., Murphy, M. and Vessey, M. (1992). Risk factors for fatal venous thromboembolism in young women; a case–control study. *Int. J. Epidemiol.*, **21**, 48–52

11. Royal College of General Practitioners' Oral Contraception Study (1978). Oral contraceptives, venous thrombosis and varicose veins. *J. R. Coll. Gen. Pract.*, **28**, 393–9

12. Petitti, D.B., Wingerd, J., Pellegrin, F. and Ramcharan, S. (1978). Oral contraceptives, smoking, and other factors in relation to risk of venous thromboembolic disease. *Am. J. Epidemiol.*, **108**, 480–5

13. Vessey, M., Mant, D., Smith, A. and Yeates, D. (1986). Oral contraceptives and venous thromboembolism: findings in a large prospective study. *Br. Med. J.*, **292**, 526

14. Porter, J.B., Hunter, J.R., Danielson, D.A., Jick, H. and Stergachis, A. (1982). Oral contraceptives and nonfatal vascular disease – recent experience. *Obstet. Gynecol.*, **59**, 299–302

15. Porter, J.B., Hunter, J.R., Jick, H. and Stergachis, A. (1985). Oral contraceptives and nonfatal vascular disease. *Obstet. Gynecol.*, **66**, 1–4

16. Farmer, R.T. and Preston, T.D. (1995). The risk of venous thromboembolism associated with low oestrogen oral contraceptives. *J. Obstet. Gynaecol.*, **15**, 195–200

17. Speroff, L., DeCherney, A. and The Advisory Board for the New Progestins (1993). Evaluation of a new generation of oral contraceptives. *Obstet. Gynecol.*, **81**, 1034–47

18. Robinson, G.E. (1994). Low-dose combined oral contraceptives. *Br. J. Obstet. Gynaecol.*, **101**, 1036–42

19. Inman, W.H.W., Vessey, M.P., Westerholm, B. and Engelund, A. (1970). Thromboembolic disease and the steroidal content of oral contraceptives. A report to the Committee on Safety of Drugs. *Br. Med. J.*, **2**, 203–9

20. Böttiger, L.E., Boman, G., Eklund, G. and Westerholm, B. (1980). Oral contraceptives and thromboembolic disease: effects of lowering oestrogen content. *Lancet*, **1**, 1097–101

21. Vessey, M.P. and Doll, R. (1968). Investigation of relation between use of oral contraceptives and thromboembolic disease. *Br. Med. J.*, **2**, 199–205

22. Jick, H., Slone, D., Westerholm, B. *et al.* (1969). Venous thromboembolic disease and ABO blood type. *Lancet*, **1**, 539–42

23. Böttiger, L.E. and Westerholm, B. (1971). Oral contraceptives and thromboembolic disease. *Acta Med. Scand.*, **190**, 455–63

24. Sartwell, P.E. (1971). Oral contraceptives and thromboembolism: a further report. *Am. J. Epidemiol.*, **94**, 192–201

25. Stolley, P.D., Tonascia, J.A., Tockman, M.S., Sartwell, P.E., Rutledge, A.H. and Jacobs, M.P. (1975). Thrombosis with low-estrogen oral contraceptives. *Am. J. Epidemiol.*, **102**, 197–208

26. Gerstman, B.B., Piper, J.M., Tomita, D.K., Ferguson, W.J., Stadel, B.V. and Lundin, F.E. (1991). Oral contraceptive estrogen dose and the risk of deep venous thromboembolic disease. *Am. J. Epidemiol.*, **133**, 32–7

27. Bertina, R.M., Koeleman, R.P.C., Koster, T., Rosendaal, F.R., Dirven, R.J., de Ronde, H., van der Velden, P.A. and Reitsma, P.H. (1994). Mutation in blood coagulation factor V associated with resistance to activated protein C. *Nature (London)*, **369**, 64–7

28. Koster, T., Rosendaal, F.R., Ronde, H. de, Briët, E., Vandenbroucke, J.P. and Bertina, R.M. (1993). Venous thrombosis due to poor anticoagulant response to activated protein C: Leiden Thrombophilia Study. *Lancet*, **342**, 1503–6

29. Pabinger, I., Schneider, B. and the GTH Study Group on Natural Inhibitors (1994). Thrombotic risk of women with hereditary Antithrombin III-, Protein C- and Protein S- deficiency taking oral contraceptive medication. *Thromb. Haemost.*, **71**, 548–52

30. Allaart, C.F. and Briët, E. (1994). Familial venous thrombophilia. In Bloom, A.L., Forbes, C.D., Thomas, D.P and Tuddenham, E.G.D. (eds.) *Haemostasis and Thrombosis*, 3rd edn., pp. 1349–60. (New York: Churchill-Livingstone)

31. Svensson, P.J. and Dahlbäck, B. (1994). Resistance to activated protein C as a basis for venous thrombosis. *N. Engl. J. Med.*, **330**, 517–22

32. Rees, D.C., Cox, M. and Clegg, J.B. (1995). World distribution of factor V Leiden. *Lancet*, **346**, 1133–4

33. Ridker, P.M., Hennekens, C.H., Lindpainter, K., Stampfer, M.J., Eisenberg, P.R. and Miletich, J.P. (1995). Mutation in the gene coding for coagulation factor V and the risk of myocardial infarction, stroke, and venous thrombosis in apparently healthy men. *N. Engl. J. Med.*, **332**, 912–7

34. Rosendaal, F.R. (1996). Oral contraceptives and screening for factor V Leiden. *Thromb. Haemost.*, **75**, 524–5

35. Briët, E., van der Meer, F.J., Rosendaal, F.R., Houwing-Duistermaat, J.J. and van Houwelingen, H.C. (1994). The family history and inherited thrombophilia. *Br. J. Haematol.*, **87**, 348–52

36. Committee on Safety of Medicines (1995). *Combined Oral Contraceptives and Thromboembolism.* (London: CSM)

37. World Health Organization Collaborative Study of Cardiovascular Disease and Steroid Hormone Contraception (1995). Venous thromboembolic disease and combined oral contraceptives: results of international multicentre case–control study. *Lancet*, **346**, 1575–82

38. World Health Organization Collaborative Study of Cardiovascular Disease and Steroid Hormone Contraception (1995). Effect of different progestagens in low oestrogen oral contraceptives on venous thromboembolic disease. *Lancet*, **346**, 1582–8

39. Jick, H., Jick, S.S., Gurewich, V., Myers, M.W. and Vasilakis, C. (1995). Risk of idiopathic cardiovascular death and non-fatal venous thromboembolism in women using oral contraceptives with differing progestagen components. *Lancet*, **346**, 1589–93

40. Bloemenkamp, K.W.M., Rosendaal, F.R., Helmerhorst, F.M., Büller, H.R. and Vandenbroucke, J.P. (1995). Enhancement by factor V Leiden mutation of risk of deep-vein thrombosis associated with oral contraceptives containing third-generation progestagen. *Lancet*, **346**, 1593–6

41. Spitzer, W.O., Lewis, M.A., Heinemann, L.A.J., Thorogood, M. and MacRae, K.D. on behalf of Transnational Research Group on Oral Contraceptives and the Health of Young Women (1996). Third generation of oral contraceptives and risk of venous thromboembolic disorders: an international case–control study. *Br. Med. J.*, **312**, 83–8

42. Kuhl, H., Jung-Hoffman, C. and Heidt, F. (1988). Alterations in the serum levels of gestodene and SHBG during 12 cycles of treatment with 30 micrograms ethinylestradiol and 75 micrograms gestodene. *Contraception*, **38**, 477–86

43. Jung-Hoffman, C. and Kuhl, H. (1989). Interaction with the pharmacokinetics of ethinylestradiol and progestogens contained in OCs. *Contraception*, **40**, 299–312

44. Hümpel, M., Tauber, U., Kuhnz, W., Pfeffer, M., Brill, K., Heithecker, R., Louton, T. and Steinberg, B. (1990). Comparisons of serum ethinyl estradiol, sex-hormone-binding globulin, corticoid-binding globulin and cortisol levels in women using two low-dose combined oral contraceptives. *Horm. Res.*, **33**, 35–9

45. Kuhnz, W., Hümpel, M., Schütt, B., Louton, T., Steinberg, B. and Garsan, C. (1990). Relative bioavailability of ethinyl estradiol from two different oral contraceptive formulations after single oral administration to 18 women in an intraindividual cross-over design. *Horm. Res.*, **33**, 40–44

46. Dibbet, L., Knupper, R., Jutting, G., Heimann, S., Klipping, C.O. and Parikka-Olexik, H. (1991). Group comparison of serum ethinylestradiol, SHBG and CBG levels in 83 women using two low-dose combination oral contraceptives. *Contraception*, **43**, 1–21

47. Orme, M., Back, D.J., Wash, S. and Green, S. (1991). The pharmacokinetics of ethinylestradiol in the presence and absence of gestodene and desogestrel. *Contraception*, **43**, 305–16

48. Kuhnz, W., Back, D., Power, J., Schütt, B. and Louton, T. (1991). Concentration of ethinylestradiol in the serum of 31 young women following a treatment period of 3 months with two low-dose oral contraceptives in an intraindividual cross-over design. *Horm. Res.*, **36**, 63–9

49. Hammerstein, J., Daume, E., Simon, A., Winkler, U.H., Schindler, A.E., Back, D.J., Ward, S. and Neiss, A. (1993). Influence of gestodene and desogestrel as components of low-dose oral contraceptives on pharmacokinetics of ethinylestradiol (EE_2), on serum CBG and on urinary cortisol and 6β-hydroxycortisol. *Contraception*, **47**, 263–81

50. Clinical and Scientific Committee of the Faculty of Family Planning and Reproductive Health Care of the Royal College of Obstetricians and Gynaecologists. (1995). *Statement on Combined Oral Contraceptive Pills and Risk of Venous Thromboembolism.* (London: FFPRHC)

51. European Agency for the Evaluation of Medicinal Products (1995). *Position Statement of the CPMP on Oral Contraceptives Containing Gestodene and Desogestrel.* (London: European Agency for the Evaluation of Medicinal Products)

52. Carnall, D. (1995). Controversy rages over new contraceptive data. *Br. Med. J.*, **311**, 1117–18

53. Guillebaud, J. (1995). Advising women on which pill to take. *Br. Med. J.*, **311**, 1111–12

54. Bundesinstitut für Arzneimittel und Medizinprodukte (1995). Anwendungsbeschränkungen für orale Kontrazeptiva angeordnet. *Pressemitteilung*, 6 November

55. Editorial (1995). Sensible alerts. *Lancet*, **346**, 1569
56. Weiss, N. (1995). Third-generation oral contraceptives: how risky? (commentary). *Lancet*, **346**, 1570
57. Editorial (1996). Third generation oral contraception and venous thromboembolism. *Br. Med. J.*, **312**, 68–9
58. Mills, A.M., Wilkinson, C.L., Bromham, D.R., Elias, J., Fotherby, K., Guillebaud, J., Kubba, A. and Wade, A. (1996). Guidelines for prescribing combined oral contraceptives. *Br. Med. J.*, **312**, 121–2
59. Koster, T., Small, R.A., Rosendaal, F.R. and Helmerhorst, F.M. (1995). Oral contraceptives and venous thromboembolism; a quantitative discussion of the uncertainties. *J. Intern. Med.*, **238**, 31–7

7

Oral contraceptives and blood pressure

N.R. Poulter

Currently available data suggest that oral contraceptives (OCs), even the most modern low-dose preparations, increase blood pressure. The answers to several associated questions are, however, less clear. Namely, by how much does blood pressure rise; is the rise important; does the impact vary with OC composition, dosage or duration of use; are specific subgroups of users at increased risk; what mechanisms are involved; is the effect reversible; and what are the implications for screening OC users? This review attempts to summarize and evaluate the evidence relating to these questions.

BACKGROUND AND LIMITATIONS OF THE DATA

Shortly after the introduction of OCs, case reports linking OC use with marked increases in blood pressure were published[1]. These reports were followed by large numbers of mainly observational studies investigating the OC/blood pressure association. Most of these data arose from cross-sectional studies, based either in family planning clinics or in the community, in which women using OCs were compared with those using other methods or no contraception. Additional information has been acquired from prospective studies, most of which have been of relatively short duration and included small numbers of participants. There are several difficulties associated with the evaluation of contraceptive methods – the investigator is often

77

unable to randomize women, use placebos, or blinding techniques. Evidence from double-blind, randomized controlled trials therefore has been limited. In addition, many studies have failed to standardize the blood pressure measurement, even though problems of accurate measurement are well documented. Thus, it is not surprising that although extensive, much of the available data are of poor quality and the results conflicting.

ARE SMALL CHANGES IN BLOOD PRESSURE IMPORTANT?

Prospective data demonstrate a strong dose–response relationship between systolic or diastolic blood pressure and increasing risk of coronary heart disease and stroke, even at low-normal levels of blood pressure[2]. For example, it is clear in Figure 1 than an increase of 7 mmHg in diastolic blood pressure approximately doubles the risk of stroke, whether the 7 mmHg increase is from 84 to 91 mmHg or 98 to 105 mmHg. It is also established that the majority of adverse cardiovascular events attributable to elevated blood pressure do not occur in the hypertensive range (>160 mmHg systolic and/or >100 mmHg diastolic blood pressure) but instead occur at lower blood pressure levels frequently described as normal[3]. Consequently it appears that relatively modest increases in blood pressure even when they occur well within the normal blood pressure range, could be expected to induce increased relative risks of cardiovascular events. It should be stressed, however, that the absolute level of risk of cardiovascular disease in healthy young women is 'vanishingly small'[4] and consequently the attributable risk resulting from a doubling or trebling of such risk due to OC use remains very small.

Prentice assumed that OCs induce an average increase in blood pressure of 5/2 mmHg, and estimated the impact of this level of blood pressure elevation on cardiovascular end-points[5]. Having adjusted the data for regression dilution bias and the fact that the average blood pressure increase underestimates the impact of individual responses, he calculated that an increase of 5/2 mmHg was likely to be associated with an odds ratio of stroke of approximately 2. He concluded that 'blood pressure elevations may provide an explanation… for an important part of the elevated stroke risk among current users.'

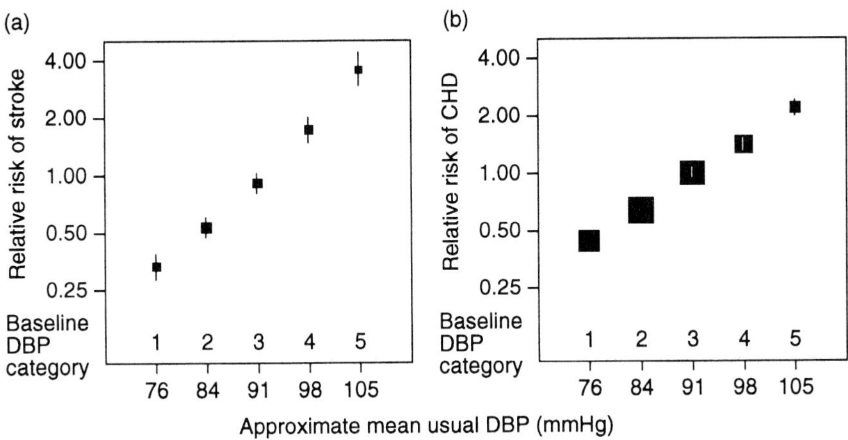

Figure 1 Relative risks of stroke (a) and of coronary heart disease (CHD) (b), estimated from combined results. Estimates of the usual diastolic blood pressure (DBP) category are taken from mean DBP values 4-years post-baseline in the Framingham study: solid squares represent disease risks in each category relative to risk in the whole study population; sizes of squares are proportional to number of events in each DBP category; and 95% CIs for estimates of relative risk are denoted by vertical lines. (a) Stroke and usual DBP (in five categories defined by baseline DBP) seven prospective observational studies: 843 events. (b) Coronary heart disease and usual DBP (in five categories defined by baseline DBP) nine prospective observational studies: 4856 events

In summary, although the absolute risk of cardiovascular disease among young women remains small, blood pressure increases are important in determining the level of risk among OC users. This conclusion is supported by data from case–control and cohort studies in which a history of hypertension increases the OC-associated risk of strokes[6,7] and acute myocardial infarction[8,9].

THE SIZE OF BLOOD PRESSURE CHANGES: BY COMPOSITION AND DOSE OF OCs

The reported size of OC-induced blood pressure changes has varied dramatically and many of the relevant studies have been comprehensively reviewed elsewhere[10].

One of the few early large controlled and standardized studies was carried out in 11 centers from around the world[11]. Blood pressure changes among 704 women who began to use OCs were monitored and compared with those among 703 women who started to use intra-uterine devices. Although results varied across centers, after 1 year of follow-up those taking OCs had mean blood pressure levels which were 5.0/2.7 mmHg higher than those using intrauterine devices. The OCs used in this WHO study contained 50 μg ethinylestradiol (EE) and 250 μg levonorgestrel. Other smaller studies with a similar design and type of OC (i.e. higher dose of estrogen) demonstrated blood pressure increases relative to controls of 13/7 after 3 years of follow up[12].

In a subsequent study of 14 women who had become hypertensive on combined OCs containing 50 μg EE, the effect of estrogen dose on blood pressure changes was investigated by rechallenging them with OCs containing 30 μg EE and the same dose and type of progestogen[13]. Although blood pressures rose significantly after using the lower dose formulations, they did not rise as high as when higher dose OCs had been used. In contrast after 1 year of follow-up in the WHO randomized controlled trial of low dose (EE 50 μg + 250 μg levonorgestrel) versus higher dose OCs (EE 30 μg + 250 μg levonorgestrel), blood pressures did not differ significantly between groups[14]. The results of this study were interpreted to imply that the progestogen component of combined OCs may be the major determinant of OC-associated blood pressure changes. Although not all studies were consistent[12], several other studies support this hypothesis[15,16] even though studies of progestogen-only preparations[17–19] consistently demonstrated no increases in blood pressure. The role of progestogens in inducing blood pressure increases is further complicated by the results of part of one of Weir's studies[13] in which six women who had become hypertensive using combined OCs were rechallenged with a progestogen-only preparation and their mean blood pressure rose by 12/12 mmHg (Figure 2).

The evidence relating to biphasic and triphasic preparations is limited[10] but it seems reasonable to assume, and compatible with available data, that the blood pressure changes they induce are similar to those produced by monophasic preparations of equivalent

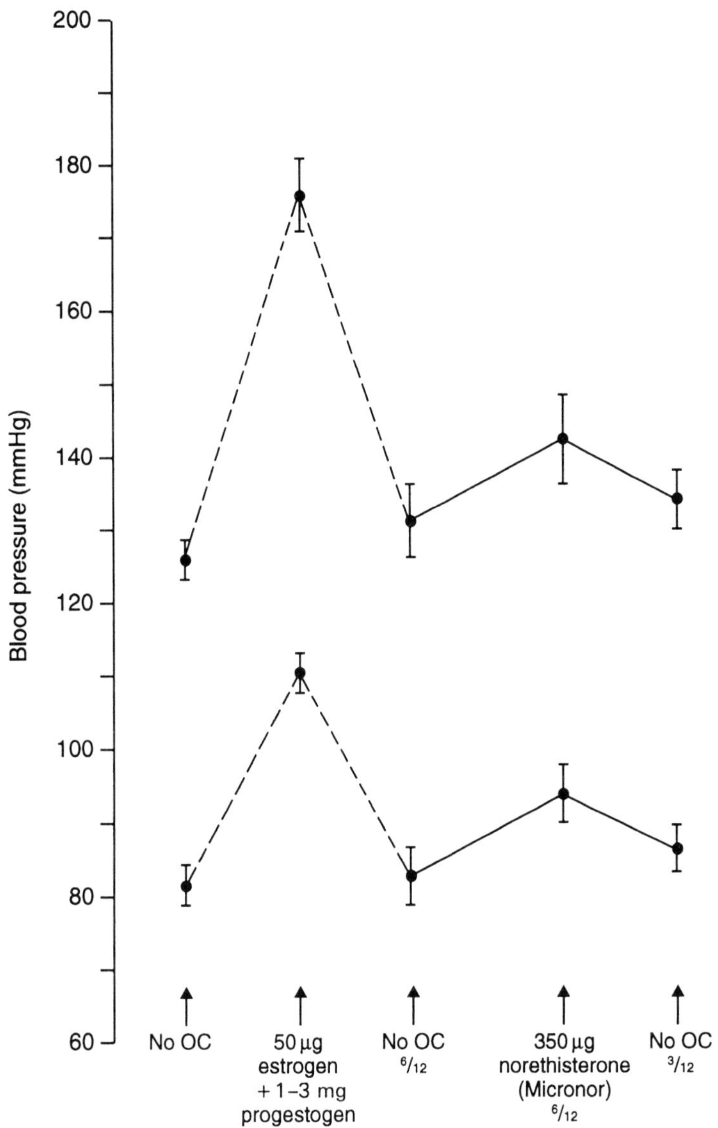

Figure 2 Reversibility of OC-induced hypertension and the impact of a progestogen-only preparation challenge (adapted from reference 13)

Table 1 Low-dose combined OCs and blood pressure changes: a randomized controlled trial on OCs containing 30 μg ethinylestradiol

OC type – ethinylestradiol plus	n	Increase in blood pressure from baseline after 6 months (mmHg)	
		Systolic	*Diastolic*
Norethisterone acetate (1000 μg)	30	4.8	3.1
Levonorgestrel (150 μg)	23	9.1	5.2
Desogestrel (150 μg)	30	4.4	4.2
Gestodene (75 μg)	32	5.7	4.0
Total	115	5.8	4.1

dosage. One recent small randomized controlled trial compared the effects on blood pressure of four different progestogens, each in combination with 30 μg EE[20]. The results of this study show that overall blood pressure increases of approximately 6/4 mmHg were observed after 6 months use (Table 1). No statistically significant differences were apparent among different OC brands, but this study had limited power to evaluate the question effectively.

In summary, it seems likely that the most modern currently available combined OCs do induce modest increases in blood pressure and that the dose of estrogen does affect the size of blood pressure increase. Progestogen-only preparations, at least among normotensive women, do not affect blood pressure levels, although the progestogen included in combined OCs may interact with the estrogen component to influence blood pressure changes.

THE IMPACT OF DURATION AND CESSATION OF OC USE

Studies are largely consistent in demonstrating that blood pressure levels increase with prolonged duration of OC use[11,12,20]. However, on average, most of the blood pressure increases occur during the first 6 months of use.

Table 2 OCs and blood pressure elevation: possible mechanisms

Body weight
Plasma volume, stroke volume and cardiac output
Sodium balance
Viscosity
Renin–angiotensin–aldosterone axis
Cortisol elevation
Sympathetic activity
Insulin resistance

OC-induced blood pressure changes are mainly reversible even among those with large increases (Figure 2). The reduction in blood pressure following OC cessation usually occurs within a few months but in some women takes up to 1 year. In the randomized controlled trial of four progestogens described above[20], OCs were stopped after 6 months and blood pressures were re-measured 2 months later. Although not statistically significant, blood pressures were still 2.6/2.2 mmHg higher than at baseline, suggesting full resolution of blood pressure increases had not yet occurred.

In a report of 34 consecutive cases of malignant hypertension in young women, 11 had been taking OCs, of whom three were taking low-dose OCs[21]. After stopping their OCs, blood pressure did not return to normal in any of these 11 women although they subsequently required less medication than the other 23 women and they had a greater 5- and 10-year survival rate.

MECHANISMS AND THOSE AT GREATER RISK

Table 2 lists some of the many mechanisms which have been postulated as explanations for OC-induced blood pressure increases. The data relating to each of these are conflicting[10] and are currently insufficient to allow any of them to be regarded as causative. It is unlikely that any single mechanism is responsible.

Efforts to identify those at particularly high risk of developing elevated pressure following OC use have failed. It has been proposed that those groups who are at higher risk of developing hypertension

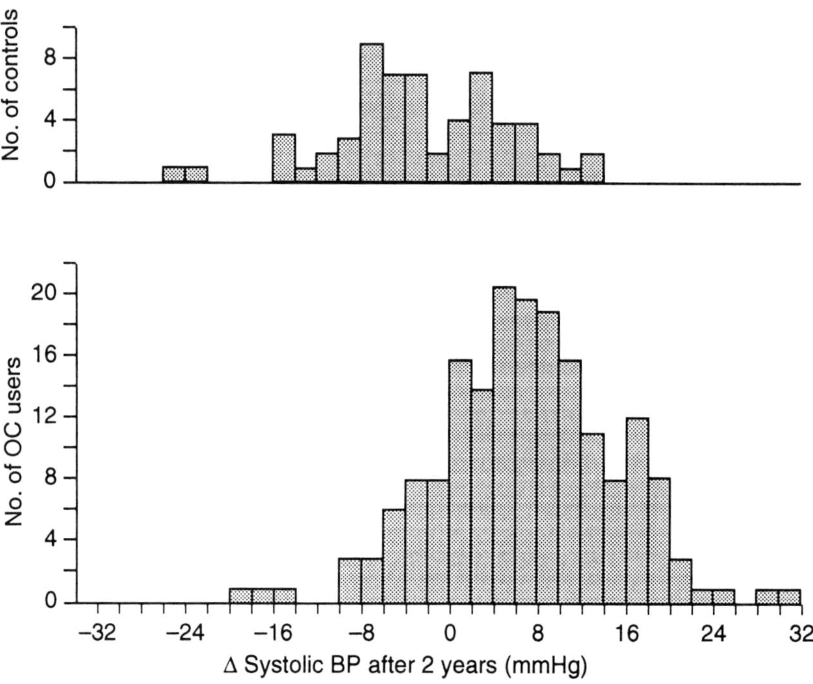

Figure 3 Changes in systolic blood pressure (BP) in controls (*n* = 60, mean Δ –1.2 mmHg) and in women taking combined OCs (*n* = 186, mean Δ +7.7 mmHg), adapted from reference 12

anyway are more prone to OC-induced increases in blood pressure. Studies do not consistently demonstrate, however, any increased propensity among women who are older, black, overweight or of lower socioeconomic status. Furthermore, those with a strong family history of cardiovascular disease or a personal history of pregnancy-associated hypertension do not appear to be any more susceptible to OC-induced blood pressure rises.

The data in Figure 3 demonstrate that OC-induced blood pressure increases do not appear to be peculiar to any particular subgroup of susceptible users. It is clear from this study that the blood pressures of the whole population of OC users were shifted upwards[12], and in this particular study 88% of women showed an increase in systolic and 81% an increase in diastolic blood pressure. Within this apparently generalized effect, however, some large individual increases in blood pressure occurred, for reasons and by mechanisms which are as yet unexplained.

IMPLICATIONS FOR OC USE

The evidence strongly supports the recommendation that blood pressure levels should be measured prior to OC use in all women. Thereafter a conservative approach based on no specific published data would be to measure blood pressure again after 1–3 months and then on a 6-monthly basis. It could be argued that after the initial 1 or 2 years of use annual blood pressure checks would suffice, but the following considerations support the admittedly conservative recommendation to continue 6-monthly check-ups:

(1)   The idiosyncratic rise in blood pressure in some women does not necessarily occur in the first 6 months of OC use;

(2)   The most severe rises observed in some women are usually *not* reversible – presumably some type of irreversible renal damage occurs[21]; and

(3)   Measuring blood pressure is cheap (relatively) and stroke is a devastating disorder.

If baseline blood pressure levels before OC use are in the high–normal range and/or blood pressure has increased during combined OC use, it is probably prudent to re-measure blood pressure before a further 6 months has passed. Unless it can be avoided, OCs (except progestogen-only preparations) should probably not be supplied to women whose blood pressures are above 140 mmHg systolic and 90 mmHg diastolic. If a woman's blood pressure increases above these levels during OC use, a management algorithm based on one originally produced by Weir[10] might usefully guide the clinician (Figure 4).

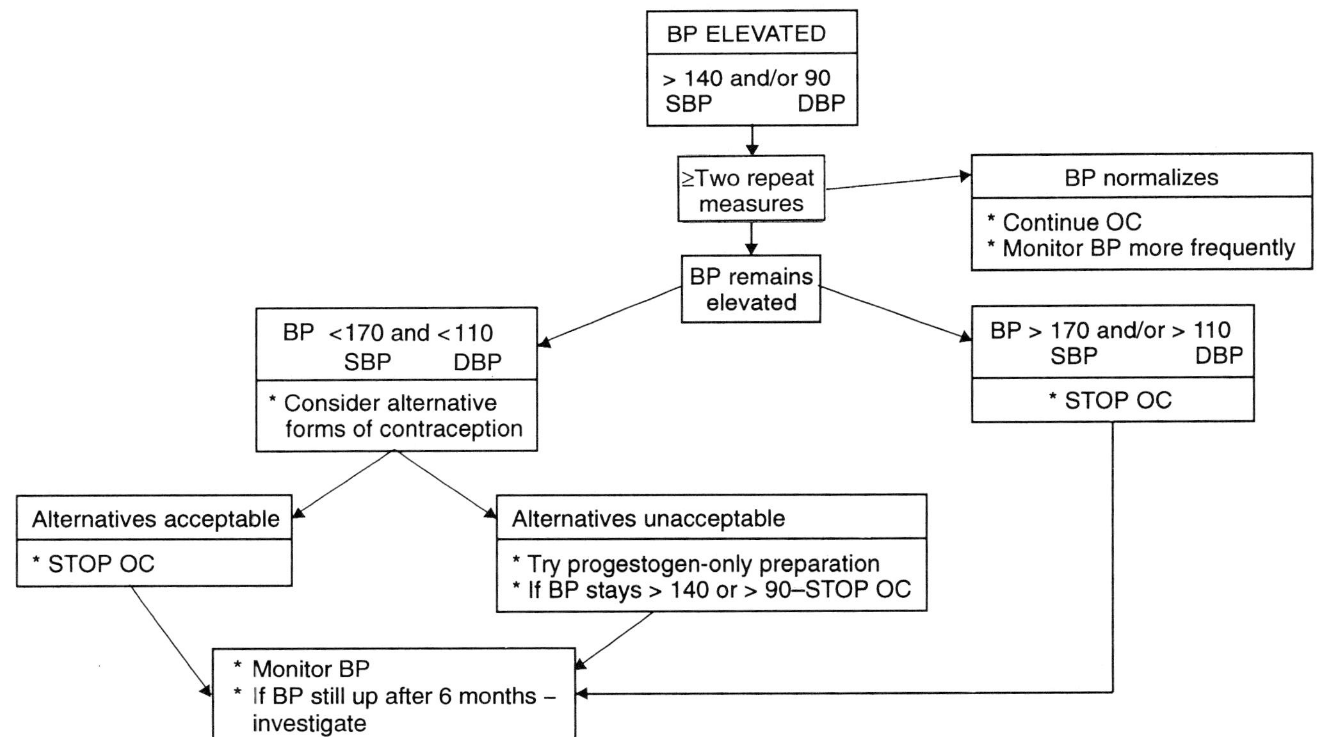

Figure 4 Management of oral contraceptive (OC)-induced raised blood pressure (BP, measured in mmHg)

REFERENCES

1. Brownrigg, G.M. (1962). Toxaemia in hormone-induced pseudo-pregnancy. *Can. Med. Assoc. J.*, **87**, 408–9

2. MacMahon, S., Peto, R., Cutler, J. *et al.* (1990). Blood pressure, stroke and coronary heart disease: Part 1, prolonged differences in blood pressure: prospective observational studies corrected for the regression dilution bias. *Lancet,* **335**, 765–74

3. Rutan, G.H., Kuller, L.H., Neaton, J.D., Wentworth, D.N., McDonald, R.H. and McFate Smith, W. (1988). Mortality associated with diastolic hypertension and isolated systolic hypertension among men screened for the Multiple Risk Factor Intervention Trial. *Circulation,* **77**, 504–14

4. Thorogood, M. (1993). Oral contraceptives and cardiovascular disease: an epidemiologic overview. *Pharmacoepidemiol. Drug Safety,* **2**, 3–16

5. Prentice, R.L. (1988). On the ability of blood pressure effects to explain the relation between oral contraceptives and cardiovascular disease. *Am. J. Epidemiol.,* **127** (2), 213–19

6. Collaborative Group for the Study of Stroke in Young Women (1975). Oral contraceptives and stroke in young women. *J. Am. Med. Assoc.,* **231**, 718–22

7. World Health Organization Collaborative Study of Cardiovascular Disease and Steroid Hormone Contraception (1996). Haemorrhagic stroke and combined oral contraceptives: results of an international multicentre case–control study. *Lancet,* in press

8. Stadel, B.V. (1981). Oral contraceptives and cardiovascular disease. *N. Engl. J. Med.,* **12**, 672–7

9. Croft, P. and Hannaford, P.C. (1989). Risk factors for acute myocardial infarction in women: evidence from the Royal College of General Practitioners' oral contraception study. *Br. Med. J.,* **298**, 165–8

10. Weir, R.J. (1994). Oral contraceptives, hormone replacement therapy and hypertension. In Swales, J.D. (ed.) *Textbook of Hypertension,* pp. 904–22. (Oxford: Blackwell Scientific Publications)

11. World Health Organization (1989). The WHO multicentre trial of the vasopressor effects of combined oral contraceptives: 1. Comparisons with IUD. *Contraception,* **40** (2), 129–45

12. Weir, R.J., Briggs, E., Mack, A., Naismith, L., Taylor, L. and Wilson, E. (1974). Blood pressure in women taking oral contraceptives. *Br. Med. J.,* **1**, 533–5

13. Weir, R.J. (1982). Effect on blood pressure of changing from high to low dose steroid preparations in women with oral contraceptive induced hypertension. *Scott. Med. J.,* **27**, 212–15

14. World Health Organization (1989). The WHO multicentre trial of the vasopressor effects of combined oral contraceptives: 2. Lack of effect of estrogen. *Contraception*, **40**(2), 147–56

15. Royal College of General Practitioners (1974). *Oral Contraceptives and Health*, pp. 37–42. (New York: Pitman)

16. Khaw, K.T. and Peart, W.S. (1982). Blood pressure and contraceptive use. *Br. Med. J.*, **285**, 403–7

17. Hawkins, D.F. and Benster, B. (1977). A comparative study of three low dose progestagens, chlormadinone acetate, megestrol acetate and norethisterone, as oral contraceptives. *Br. J. Obstet. Gynaecol.*, **84**, 708–13

18. Hall, W.D., Douglas, M.B., Blumenstein, B.A. and Hatcher, R.A. (1980). Blood pressure and oral progestational agents. A prospective study of 119 black women. *Am. J. Obstet. Gynecol.*, **136**, 344–8

19. Wilson, E.S.B., Cruikshank, J., McMaster, M. and Weir, R.J. (1984). A prospective controlled study of the effect on blood pressure of contraceptive preparations containing different types and dosages of progestagen. *Br. J. Obstet. Gynaecol.*, **91**, 1254–60

20. Nichols, M., Robinson, G., Bounds, W., Newman, B. and Guillebaud, J. (1993). Effect of four combined oral contraceptives on blood pressure in the pill-free interval. *Contraception*, **47**, 367–76

21. Lim, K.G., Isles, C.G., Hodsman, G.P., Lever, A.F. and Robertson, J.W.K. (1987). Malignant hypertension in women of childbearing age and its relation to the contraceptive pill. *Br. Med. J.*, **294**, 1057–9

8

Role of screening for vascular disease in pill users: lipids and lipoproteins

D. Crook

BACKGROUND

Combined oral contraceptives (OCs) influence diverse areas such as lipoprotein and insulin metabolism and hemostasis, leading to concern over their effect on cardiovascular disease[1,2]. An increased incidence of coronary heart disease in OC users has been demonstrated in some studies[3,4], although the epidemiological evidence for such an association remains controversial.

The Royal College of General Practitioners' (RCGP) study clearly linked OC progestogen dose to the incidence of arterial disease[5]. In parallel with this development, studies in the USA[6] and UK[7] linked OC composition to serum levels of the protective high density lipoprotein (HDL) fraction. Oral estrogen tends to increase HDL levels, an effect opposed (in a dose-dependent manner) by progestogens such as levonorgestrel and norethindrone. The RCGP study linked those OC formulations which induced the greatest falls in HDL levels with an excess of arterial disease. This led to a process of OC reformulation, culminating in the development of 'third-generation' OCs containing low (20–35 µg) doses of ethinylestradiol combined with desogestrel, gestodene or norgestimate progestogens.

Such formulations tend to increase HDL levels[8,9] and so would be expected to reduce the risk of arterial disease associated with older formulations. Preliminary data from at least one international trial[4] indicate that this may be so, although the influence of these formulations on venous thromboembolism remains to be resolved[10].

ROLE OF LIPID SCREENING

Because the different OC formulations in current use may have different effects on the risk of cardiovascular diseases (coronary heart disease, venous thromboembolism and stroke), three possibilities are being addressed at this workshop:

(1)   That women requesting contraceptive advice could be screened for their risk of cardiovascular disease in order to assess whether or not it would be appropriate to prescribe OCs, and, if so, which formulations should be used;

(2)   That such women could be given a brief trial of OCs to quantify their metabolic response to these steroids; and

(3)   That current users could be screened so that any metabolic abnormality (which may or may not be OC-related) could be detected. Such women could then be switched to other formulations, or away from OCs altogether, so as to prevent any progression to symptomatic disease.

In the case of serum lipids and lipoproteins (Table 1), there is little evidence to support screening as part of a strategy to improve OC safety, either in women requesting OCs for the first time or in established users. Lipoprotein profiling is mandatory in women with symptomatic cardiovascular disease or multiple risk markers (hypertension, obesity, diabetes mellitus, cigarette smoking or a family history of premature cardiovascular disease)[11], but is more difficult to justify in healthy women. In particular, the routine measurement of serum lipids and lipoproteins fails a basic criterion for a screening program: the need to have proved *beyond doubt* the existence of an association between a given lipoprotein profile and OC-induced

Table 1 Lipid and lipoprotein abnormalities which may increase the risk of coronary heart disease

Low density lipoprotein (LDL) levels
Small dense LDL particles
Oxidized LDL
Lipoprotein(a)*
High density lipoproteins
Fasting triglycerides
Postprandial lipemia

*But only if LDL levels are also high

cardiovascular disease, such as the association between the factor V Leiden mutation and venous thrombosis[12].

Elevated serum total cholesterol levels

An elevated total cholesterol level due to high levels of low density lipoproteins (LDL) only weakly predicts coronary heart disease in asymptomatic young women, and so the screening and treatment of this condition are unlikely to be cost-effective[13] (Figure 1). In contrast, hypercholesterolemic women with established coronary heart disease will benefit from lipid-lowering therapy[14], but, even if their hypercholesterolemia is successfully treated, combined OCs carry the risk of initiating thrombosis in an already damaged vasculature and are clearly contraindicated[15].

In the case of *asymptomatic* hypercholesterolemic women, non-steroidal methods of contraception would be preferable, even though there is as yet no evidence that OCs would increase their risk of cardiovascular disease. An argument can be made for the use of OCs in such women if they do not smoke, have no family history of premature cardiovascular disease and carry no other risk factors[16]. In such women, 'third-generation' OCs might avoid the increased risk of myocardial infarction seen with other OCs[4], but the risk of inducing an episode of venous thromboembolism must be a concern. The desogestrel formulation containing 20 μg ethinylestradiol would, in theory, carry the least risk of initiating an episode of cardiovascular

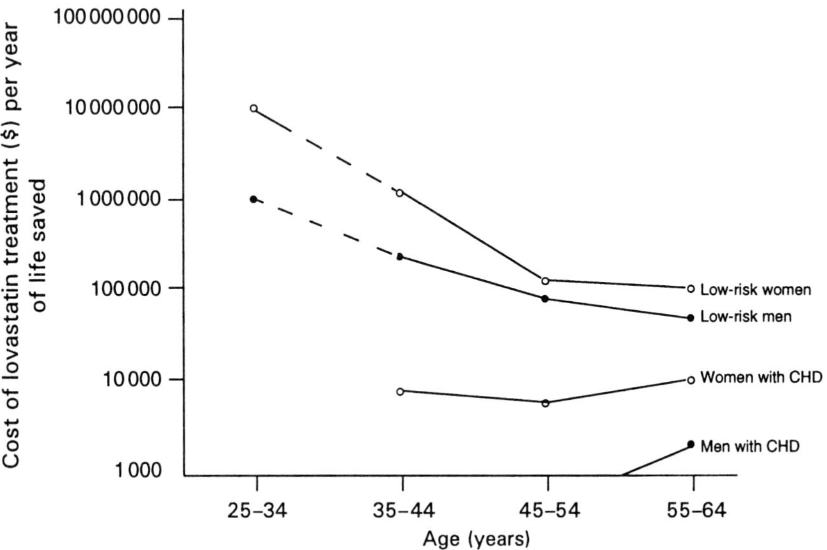

Figure 1 Cost effectiveness of treating high plasma cholesterol levels with lovastatin (20 mg/day). Dotted lines are extrapolations. The models assume only favorable effects on mortality and do not include the costs of screening. High plasma cholesterol is defined as levels ≥8.0 mmol/l for primary prevention ('low risk men and women') and ≥6.5 mmol/l for secondary prevention in those with prior coronary heart disease ('men and women with CHD'). Source: reference 13

disease, but a recent study[17] indicates a paradoxically increased risk of cardiovascular deaths in comparison with women using the equivalent 30 μg ethinylestradiol formulation, presumably reflecting prescription and other biases.

Low levels of serum high density lipoproteins

Elevated HDL levels protect against coronary heart disease, especially in women[18], consistent with the anti-atherogenic properties of this lipoprotein. Transgenic mice with elevated HDL levels, achieved by engineering them to express the gene for human apolipoprotein A-I, are protected not only from diet-induced arterial disease but

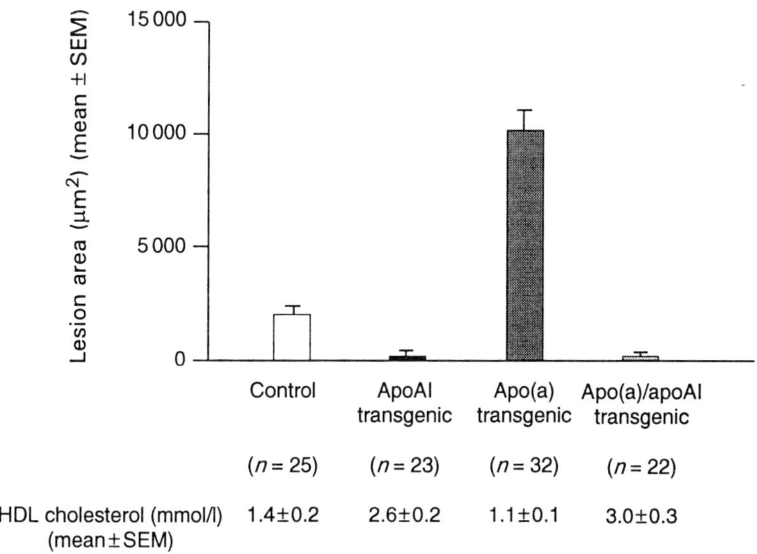

Figure 2 Protective effect of increasing high density lipoprotein (HDL) levels in mice fed an atherogenic diet. Transgenic mice expressing the gene for human apolipoprotein (apo) A-I have elevated HDL levels and are resistant to diet-induced disease, even in the face of an additional atherogenic stimulus, elevated serum levels of apo(a). Source: reference 18

from the double insult of an atherogenic diet and genetically engineered elevated serum levels of apolipoprotein(a)[19] (Figure 2). Additional anti-atherogenic properties for HDL continue to emerge, such as a role as a carrier for paraoxonase[20], an enzyme capable of hydrolyzing lipid peroxides and thus reducing oxidative damage to the arterial wall.

Nevertheless, screening HDL cholesterol levels in OC users would not be justified until it has been proven beyond reasonable doubt that those OC users who develop coronary heart disease have low HDL levels. Furthermore, the laboratory assessment of low HDL levels may not be sufficiently robust to serve for screening purposes. Substantial interlaboratory biases have recently been described in the UK[21] (Figure 3). According to this survey, a sample with a true HDL cholesterol level of 1.0 mmol/l would be reported as between 0.8 and 1.3 mmol/l, depending on the laboratory used. Additional

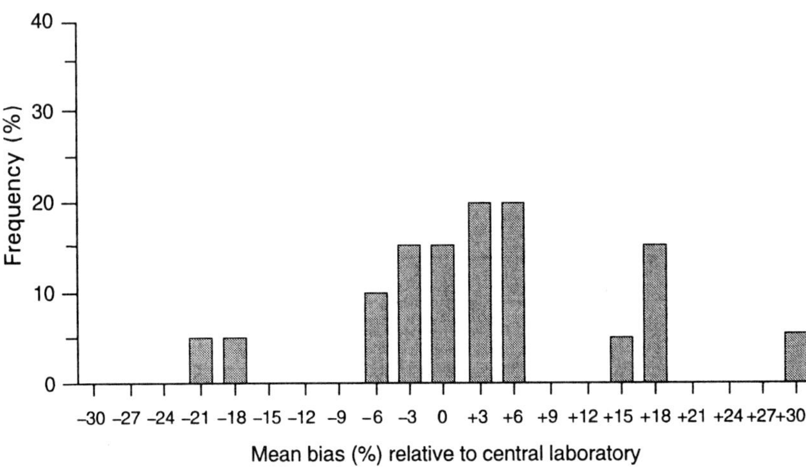

Figure 3 Frequency distribution of the mean biases in the assay of high density lipoprotein (HDL) cholesterol in 633 plasma samples analyzed in 20 individual hospital laboratories in the UK. Biases are calculated from split samples analyzed in a central laboratory (Wynn Division of Metabolic Medicine, London). Each bar represents a 3% cut of the distribution of biases; thus the central bar indicates laboratories with biases between –1.5 and +1.5%, the bar to the immediate right indicates biases between +1.5 and +4.5%, and so on. Reproduced from reference 21, with permission

limitations to the use of HDL cholesterol to screen OC users include the intraindividual variability in HDL levels, problems with assay cost and standardization and sample handling requirements.

Elevated serum triglyceride levels

Reports[22,23] of gross hypertriglyceridemia in OC users, associated with massive and life-threatening pancreatitis, appear to be due to the unmasking of covert hypertriglyceridemia. The rationale for screening triglyceride levels would, therefore, seem to be stronger than for LDL or HDL, but such cases are rare and so this policy is unlikely to be cost-effective. Furthermore, these extreme responses occur within months of starting OCs, and so the screening of established users is unlikely to be of benefit.

Epidemiological studies have linked elevated fasting serum triglyceride levels to female coronary heart disease[24], but screening for triglycerides suffers from many of the problems that beset screening for HDL: lack of agreement as to the definition of normality, intraindividual variation and inter-laboratory differences. Postprandial triglyceride levels may be more predictive of coronary heart disease than are fasting levels[25], but the measurement of postprandial responses requires a standardized protocol which is at present unsuitable for routine screening purposes. Most importantly, any link between elevated fasting (or postprandial) triglyceride levels and coronary heart disease in OC users remains theoretical and has yet to be proven beyond reasonable doubt.

Hypertriglyceridemia has been linked to increases in prothrombotic factors and decreases in fibrinolytic capacity[26]. 'Third-generation' OCs tend to induce higher fasting serum triglyceride levels than do the older formulations, raising the possibility that OC-induced increases in triglyceride levels may interfere with hemostasis and so contribute to the increased incidence of venous thrombosis linked to these OCs. Such interrelationships need further study before the potential for screening triglycerides can be evaluated in this context. A related hypothesis, that fasting triglyceride levels provide an inexpensive marker of OC-induced hepatic dysfunction and thus disturbances in the hemostatic system, has recently been raised by de Lignieres[27] but is as yet untested.

CONCLUSIONS

An ideal oral contraceptive would be one that only affected cardiovascular disease risk markers in directions perceived as reducing risk. Depending on the doses and types of the component steroids, the oral contraceptives in current use induce a variety of changes in serum lipids and lipoproteins and other risk markers for cardiovascular disease. Some of these changes are in a direction which would decrease the risk of cardiovascular risk and some may be associated with an increase in risk. Recent developments support the development of new formulations which increase HDL levels. Despite the associations between serum lipid and lipoprotein levels and cardiovascular disease, there is at present little justification for screening serum lipid and lipoprotein levels as part of a strategy to improve oral contraceptive safety.

REFERENCES

1. Wynn, V., Doar, J.W.H. and Mills, G.L. (1966). Some effects of oral contraceptives on serum-lipid and lipoprotein levels. *Lancet*, **ii**, 720–3
2. Godsland, I.F. and Crook, D. (1994). Update on the metabolic effects of steroidal contraceptives and their relationship to cardiovascular disease risk. *Am. J. Obstet. Gynecol.*, **170**, 1528–36
3. Wynn, V. (1991). Oral contraceptives and coronary heart disease. *J. Reprod. Med.*, **36**, 219–25
4. Lewis, M.A., Spitzer, W.O., Heinemann, L.A.J., MacRae, K.D., Bruppacher, R. and Thorogood, M. (1996). Third generation oral contraceptives and risk of myocardial infarction: an international case–control study. *Br. Med. J.*, **312**, 88–90
5. Kay, C.R. (1982). Progestogens and arterial disease – Evidence from the Royal College of General Practitioners' study. *Am. J. Obstet. Gynecol.*, **142**, 762–5
6. Bradley, D.D., Wingerd, J., Pettiti, D.B., Krauss, R.M. and Ramcharan, S. (1978). Serum high-density-lipoprotein cholesterol in women using oral contraceptives, estrogens and progestins. *N. Engl. J. Med.*, **299**, 17–20
7. Wynn, V. and Niththyananthan, R. (1982). The effects of progestins in combined oral contraceptives on serum lipids with special reference to high-density lipoproteins. *Am. J. Obstet. Gynecol.*, **142**, 766–72
8. Speroff, L., DeCherney, A., Burkman, R.T., Carr, B.R., Comp, P.C., Crook, D., Darney, P.D., Godsland, I.F., Grimes, D.A., Jones, K.P., Kafrissen, M.E., Knopp, R.H., LaRosa, J.C., Stubblefield, P.G. and Whitehead, M.I. (1993). Evaluation of a new generation of oral contraceptives. *Obstet. Gynecol.*, **81**, 1034–47
9. Godsland, I.F., Crook, D., Simpson, R., Proudler, T., Felton, C., Lees, B., Anyaoku, V., Devenport, M. and Wynn, V. (1990). The effects of different formulations of oral contraceptive agents on lipid and carbohydrate metabolism. *N. Engl. J. Med.*, **323**, 1375–81
10. Crook D. (1996). Oral contraceptives and the risk of cardiovascular disease. *Br. J. Obstet. Gynaecol.*, in press

11. Crook, D. and Stevenson, J.C. (1996). CHD in women – are lipids and lipoproteins important? In Betteridge, J. (ed.) *Difficult Concepts in Lipidology*. (London: Martin Dunitz), in press

12. Vandenbroucke, J.P., Koster, T., Brit, E., Reitsma, P.H., Bertina, R.M. and Rosendaal, F.R. (1994). Increased risk of venous thrombosis in oral contraceptive users who are carriers of the factor V Leiden mutation. *Lancet*, **344**, 1453–7

13. Hulley, S.B., Newman, T.B., Grady, D., Garber, D., Baron, R.B. and Browner, W.S. (1993). Should we be measuring blood cholesterol levels in young adults? *J. Am. Med. Assoc.*, **269**, 1416–9

14. Walsh, J.M.E. and Grady, D. (1995). Treatment of hyperlipidemia in women. *J. Am. Med. Assoc.*, **274**, 1152–8

15. Crook, D., Hampton, N. and Godsland, I.F. (1996). Oral contraception and heart disease. In Julian, D.G and Wenger, N.K. (eds.) *Women and Heart Disease*. (London: Martin Dunitz), in press

16. Knopp, R.H., LaRosa, J.C. and Burkman, R.T. (1993). Contraception and dyslipidemia. *Am. J. Obstet. Gynecol.*, **168**, 1994–2005

17. Jick, H., Jick, S.S., Gurewich, V., Myers, M.W. and Vasilakis, C. (1995). Risk of idiopathic cardiovascular death and nonfatal venous thromboembolism in women using oral contraceptives with differing progestogen components. *Lancet*, **346**, 1589–93

18. Jacobs, D.R., Mebane, I.L., Bangdiwala, S.I., Criqui, M.H. and Tyroler, H.A. (1990). High density lipoprotein cholesterol as a predictor of cardiovascular disease mortality in men and women: the follow-up study of the Lipid Research Clinics prevalence study. *Am. J. Epidemiol.*, **131**, 32–47

19. Liu, A.C., Lawn, R.M., Verstuyft, J.G. and Rubin, E.M. (1994). Human apolipoprotein A-I prevents atherosclerosis associated with apolipoprotein(a) in transgenic mice. *J. Lipid Res.*, **35**, 2263–7

20. Mackness, M.I., Arrol, S. and Durrington, P.N. (1991). Paraoxonase prevents accumulation of lipoperoxides in low-density lipoprotein. *FEBS Lett.*, **286**, 152–4

21. Crook, D. (1996). A survey of biases in the measurement of plasma lipid and lipoprotein concentrations in 32 Lipid Clinics in the UK. *Ann. Clin. Biochem.*, **33**, 82–3

22. Banks, S. and Marks, I.N. (1970). Hyperlipaemic pancreatitis and the pill. *Postgrad. Med. J.*, **46**, 576–8

23. Davidoff, F., Tishler, S. and Chester, R. (1973). Marked hyperlipidemia and pancreatitis associated with oral contraceptives. *N. Engl. J. Med.*, **289**, 552–5

24. NIH Consensus Development Panel on Triglyceride, High-Density Lipoprotein, and Coronary Heart Disease (1993). Triglyceride, high

density lipoprotein, and coronary heart disease. *J. Am. Med. Assoc.*, **269**, 505–10

25. Patsch, J.R., Miesenbock, G., Hopferweiser, T., Muhlberger, A., Knapp, E. and Dunn, J.K. (1993). Relation of triglyceride metabolism and coronary artery disease. Studies in the postprandial state. *Arterioscler. Thromb.*, **12**, 1336–45

26. Miller, G.J. (1993). Hyperlipidemia and hypercoagulability. *Prog. Lipid. Res.*, **32**, 61– 9

27. de Lignieres, B. (1996). Safety of combined oral contraceptive pills. *Lancet*, **347**, 548–9

9

Screening for disturbances in glucose metabolism: can it prevent cardiovascular disease in pill users?

S.O. Skouby, K.R. Petersen and J. Jespersen

INTRODUCTION

Ever since the first reports of altered glucose metabolism during the use of combined oral contraceptives (COCs) appeared more than 30 years ago[1,2], discussions have taken place about the clinical relevance of such changes in non-diabetic women. Many of the vast number of studies on this matter have described a decrease in glucose tolerance and a hyperinsulinemic response to a glucose load during OC use (reviewed in reference 3). These changes are recognized risk factors for the development of cardiovascular disease in the general population[4,5]. Furthermore, a growing awareness that the many metabolic effects of OCs may be related to their influence on the metabolism and action of insulin suggests that more detailed assessments of carbohydrate metabolism, including estimates of insulin sensitivity, in normal women are highly relevant[6]. Such studies, however, may be more of scientific than direct clinical importance and the clinical significance of potential adverse effects of OCs on carbohydrate metabolism may be more relevant in women with pre-existing disturbances. In this short review, we try to evaluate the available evidence for the need for screening of disturbances in carbohydrate metabolism in normal women. Based on our own studies, we also try to suggest some guidelines for safe prescription and metabolic screening of women with insulin-dependent diabetes mellitus (IDDM) and previous gestational diabetes (GDP) before and during use of OCs.

NON-DIABETIC WOMEN

The finding of decreased glucose tolerance in non-diabetic women using OCs is believed to reflect resistance to the insulin-mediated glucose disposal in peripheral tissues[3]. Insulin resistance, which is associated with increased risk of vascular disease and non-insulin-dependent diabetes mellitus, has been demonstrated in cross-sectional studies of non-diabetic pill users[6], but the clinical significance of this has not yet been settled. Thus, it is not known if the pill-induced fluctuations in insulin resistance or other variables within the carbohydrate metabolism *per se* are associated with a risk of vascular disease in normoglycemic young women. Certainly, OC use does not seem to induce overt diabetes[7,8]. There is, therefore, no evidence that screening for changes in carbohydrate metabolism in non-diabetic women is beneficial.

WOMEN WITH IDDM

Diabetic pregnancy carries an appreciable risk of maternal and fetal complications. Strict glucose regulation at the time of conception and in the first trimester, however, is able to reduce the complication rate to that of the background population[9–11]. Planning of pregnancy therefore is imperative in women with IDDM and the possible interactions between the available reversible contraceptive methods and the diabetic state should be recognized by the physician caring for these women.

As the metabolic effects of OCs may be linked to an increased risk of cardiovascular complications[12], concern has been expressed that OCs may add to the already raised risk of such disorders in diabetic women. Moreover, it was thought that OCs may reduce glycemic control, thereby exposing diabetic women to an increased risk of developing the characteristic microvascular complications of IDDM[13,14]. Indeed, serious atherothrombotic complications have been reported to be more frequent in diabetic women taking OCs than in women of similar diabetic status using non-hormonal contraception[13,14]. Rapid progression of proliferative retinopathy has also been described in diabetic women on the pill[14]. These observations contributed towards a widespread scepticism about the extended use of the pill in women with IDDM. The finding of excess cardiovascular complications in women with IDDM taking OCs has not been confirmed in later studies, and recent findings suggest that OCs influence the risk of cerebral thromboembolism to the same degree in diabetic and non-diabetic women[15]. The development of retinopathy has not been studied longitudinally during OC use, but in a cross-sectional study Klein and colleagues found a similar incidence of non-proliferative as well as proliferative retinopathy in women who had used the pill for 5 years or more as in never-users[16]. The study also failed to support the assumption that OC use may be associated with an increased risk of hypertension in diabetic women. In order to evaluate the possible risk of OC use in women with IDDM, we have studied the influence of OCS on the variables within glycometabolic control, lipid metabolism and endothelial function, which are recognized as risk factors for the development of vascular disease.

GLYCOMETABOLIC CONTROL

A number of different types of OCs including compounds containing the third generation of progestogens were included in this evaluation[17,18]. As seen from Table 1, none of the preparations induced significant changes in fasting plasma glucose, hemoglobin A_{1c}, insulin requirement or plasma levels of free fatty acids. Thus, in these patients, all of whom were in stable glycemic control, below 35 years of age and free of vascular complications, the investigated preparations were neutral with respect to glycometabolic control.

Table 1 Effects of different oral contraceptives on glycometabolic control and lipoproteins. Values expressed as percentage change of pretreatment mean values

Variable	*30 μg EE + 75 μg GST* (*n* = 11)	*35 μg EE + 500 μg NET* (*n* = 10)	*Triphasic EE + LNG** (*n* = 9)
Fasting glucose	+7	0	–23
Insulin requirement/24 h	–4	0	0
Hemoglobin A_{1c}	0	0	0
Total cholesterol	–5	+14	0
Low density lipoprotein cholesterol	–24[†]	+11	0
High density lipoprotein cholesterol	–7	+7	0
Very low density lipoprotein cholesterol	+42	+50	–7
Triglycerides	+42	+50	–10

*Day 1–6, 30 μg ethinylestradiol (EE) + 50 μg levonorgestrel (LNG); day 7–11, 40 μg ethinylestradiol + 75 μg levonorgestrel; day 12–21, 30 μg ethinylestradiol + 125 μg levonorgestrel
[†]Changes from pretreatment values where $p < 0.05$
NET, norethindrone; GST, gestodene

LIPID METABOLISM

Since individuals with IDDM are prone to the development of atherosclerosis, we also evaluated whether the different hormonal formulations induced the changes in lipoproteins and lipids thought to promote this condition. As Table 1 shows, only a few statistically significant changes were noted. The observed changes were small and not different from those frequently observed in non-diabetic women during the use of similar compounds[19,20], indicating that the effect of exogenous sex steroids on the mechanisms regulating serum lipid and lipoprotein concentrations is not different in diabetic women. Our findings suggest that OCs do not induce adverse changes in serum lipid or lipoprotein levels in women with IDDM. It must be remembered, however, that qualitative alterations in the biological properties of the lipoproteins caused by the diabetic state itself, changes which cannot be measured with conventional laboratory assays, may be present in these women[21,22].

ENDOTHELIAL FUNCTION

OCs influence the endothelial functions which are involved in the development of macro- as well as microvascular complications of IDDM[23,24]. In an assessment of variables reflecting the status of the endothelium (including the endothelium-related processes of coagulation and fibrinolysis), we have found an enhanced activity of the coagulation system as indicated by increased plasma levels of thrombin–antithrombin III (TAT) complexes, during use of a monophasic combination of ethinylestradiol and gestodene[25] (Table 2). Decreased antigen levels of tissue plasminogen activator (t-PA) and plasminogen activator inhibitor type 1 (PAI-1) antigen were also observed. The activities of t-PA and PAI, however, were unchanged and the levels of the fibrin degradation product D-dimer increased, indicating an increased efficacy of the fibrinolytic system. The increases in TAT complexes and D-dimer were of similar proportion, and the ratio between them was unchanged, so the balance between fibrin formation and removal seems to be maintained during pill usage. It is not known if the absence of increased systemic t-PA activity reflects a compromised fibrinolytic response to the increased activity of the coagulation system. If so, this could be of clinical significance.

None of the participating women developed microalbuminuria (nocturnal renal albumin excretion rate >30 µg/min) during pill use, so there was no evidence of a direct effect on the glomerular endothelium.

These metabolic changes have not previously been evaluated in diabetic women taking OCs.

Table 2 Effects of a monophasic combination of 30 µg ethinylestradiol and 75 µg gestodene on variables of coagulation and fibrinolysis in women with IDDM (*n* = 11). Values expressed as percentage change of pretreatment mean values

Variable	% change
Thrombin–antithrombin III (TAT) complexes	+33*
Tissue plasminogen activator (t-PA) antigen	–51*
Tissue plasminogen activator (t-PA) activity	+11
Type 1 plasminogen activator inhibitor (PAI-1) antigen	–72*
Plasminogen activator inhibitor (PAI-1) activity	–34
D-dimer	+78*
TAT-complexes/fibrin degradation product	+25

*Changes from pretreatment values where $p < 0.05$

WOMEN WITH PREVIOUS GESTATIONAL DIABETES

The inability to increase insulin secretion sufficiently to maintain euglycemia in response to the insulin resistance of pregnancy may lead to gestational diabetes mellitus (GDM). The limited β-cell reserve of women with previous GDM exposes them to increased risk of subsequently developing diabetes[26]. This process seems to be accelerated by another pregnancy and it is, therefore, possible that episodes of increased insulin resistance promote the decline in β-cell function in susceptible individuals[27]. Since OCs have been shown to cause insulin resistance when assessed by both the euglycemic hyperinsulinemic clamp technique and the minimal model of glucose disappearance, they may theoretically promote diabetes in women with previous GDM[6,28]. This possibility is supported by our finding that women with previous GDM develop a more pronounced state of insulin insensitivity when taking OCs than a comparable group of controls[28]. In this study, we also found evidence of compromised insulin secretion in the GDM women during OC use. No studies in women with previous GDM have assessed insulin sensitivity during treatment with OCs containing the new progestogens (desogestrel, gestodene and norgestimate). In normal women, preparations with desogestrel impair insulin sensitivity to the same degree as compounds with levonorgestrel and norethindrone[6]. The newer compounds therefore may not have a reduced effect on insulin sensitivity in women with previous GDM. Indeed relative insulin insensitivity may be affected through the estrogen component of the OCs[6]. It is not known if OCs influence the risk of developing clinical diabetes in this high-risk group, but our findings stress the need for such a study.

The serum lipid levels of women with previous GDM do not differ from those found in control subjects[29], and the effects of OCs do not seem to be substantially different from those observed in women without such a history[30,31].

The effects of OCs on coagulation, fibrinolysis and measures of endothelial function have not been evaluated in women with previous GDM. Such studies are greatly needed, considering the interrelated metabolic disturbances observed in individuals with insulin resistance[6].

CONCLUSION

OCs may induce adverse changes in carbohydrate metabolism, but there is no evidence that they have clinical consequences in normal women. Screening for such changes therefore does not seem rational in healthy women not predisposed to vascular disease or diabetes.

The available evidence suggests that women with IDDM, below the age of 35, who are in stable glycemic control and free of vascular complications, can use low-dose OC combinations of ethinylestradiol and levonorgestrel, norethisterone or gestodene without impairing their diabetic control or adversely affecting their lipoprotein metabolism. The more detailed metabolic evaluation of only one ethinylestradiol/gestodene preparation suggests that the fibrinolytic response to an increased activity of the coagulation system may be compromised. The clinical significance of these observations has not been determined. There was no evidence of impaired renal function but it is not presently known whether OCs may in the long term influence the renal and vascular status of diabetic women. Until further information is available, we believe that OCs may be used in younger women with uncomplicated IDDM if thorough clinical and metabolic control, for example, by screening for micro-albuminuria, is performed. The main concern about OC use in women with previous GDM is the possible exaggeration of an already increased risk of developing frank diabetes. By itself, this risk is of sufficient magnitude to justify regular screening whether or not OCs are used. A possible suggestion might be biennial oral glucose tolerance testing in order to detect a progression to frank diabetes at an early stage. It is not known if this screening should be intensified during OC use.

REFERENCES

1. Waine, H., Frieden, E.H., Caplan, H.I. and Colt, T. (1963). Metabolic effects of enovid in rheumatoid patients. *Arthritis Rheum.*, **6**, 796–7
2. Wynn, W. and Doar, J.W.H. (1966). Some effects of oral contraceptives on carbohydrate metabolism. *Lancet*, **2**, 715–19
3. Gaspard, U.J. and Lefebvre, P.J. (1990). Clinical aspects of the relationship between oral contraceptives, abnormalities in carbohydrate metabolism and the development of cardiovascular disease. *Am. J. Obstet. Gynecol.*, **163**, 334–43
4. Ducimetieri, P., Eschwege, E., Papoz, L., Richard, J.L., Claude, J.R. and Rosselin, G. (1980). Relationship of plasma insulin to the incidence of myocardial infarction and coronary heart disease mortality in middle-aged population. *Diabetologia*, **19**, 205–10
5. Pyorala, K. (1979). Relationship of glucose tolerance and plasma insulin to the incidence of coronary heart disease. Results from two population studies in Finland. *Diabetes Care*, **2**, 154–60
6. Godsland, I.F. and Crook, D. (1994). Update on the metabolic effects of steroidal contraceptives and their relationship to cardiovascular disease risk. *Am. J. Obstet. Gynecol.*, **170**, 1528–36
7. Rimm, E.B., Manson, J.E., Stampfer, M.J., Colditz, G.A., Willett, W.C., Rosner, B., Hennekens, C.H. and Speizer, F.E. (1992). Oral contraceptive use and the risk of type 2 (non-insulin-dependent) diabetes mellitus in a large prospective study of women. *Diabetologia*, **35**, 967–72
8. Wingrave, S.J., Kay, C.R. and Vessey, M.P. (1979). Oral contraceptives and diabetes mellitus. *Br. Med. J.*, **1**, 23

9. Oats, J.N. (1991). Obstetrical management of diabetic pregnancy. *Baillière's Clin. Obstet. Gynecol.*, **5**, 395–413

10. Hanson, U., Persson, B. and Thunell, S. (1990). Relation between hemoglobin A1c in early type 1 (insulin dependent) diabetic pregnancy and the occurrence of spontaneous abortions and fetal malformation in Sweden. *Diabetologia*, **33**, 100–4

11. Mills, J.L., Simpson, J.L., Driscoll, S.G. Jovanovic-Peterson, L., van Allen, M., Aarous, J.H. *et al.* (1988). Incidence of spontaneous abortion among normal women and insulin dependent diabetic women whose pregnancies were identified within 21 days of conception. *N. Engl. J. Med.*, **319**, 1617–23

12. Consensus development meeting (1990). Metabolic aspects of oral contraceptives relevant for cardiovascular disease. *Am. J. Obstet. Gynecol.*, **162**, 1335–7

13. Steele, J.M. and Duncan, L.J.P. (1980). Contraception for insulin dependent diabetic women: the view from one clinic. *Diabetes Care*, **3**, 557–60

14. Steele, J.M. and Duncan, L.J.P. (1978). Serious complications of oral contraception in insulin dependent diabetes. *Contraception*, **17**, 291–5

15. Lidegaard, Ø. (1995). Oral contraceptives, pregnancy and the risk of cerebral thromboembolism: the influence of diabetes, hypertension, migraine and previous thrombotic disease. *Br. J. Obstet. Gynaecol.*, **102**, 153–9

16. Klein, B.E., Moss, S.E. and Klein, R. (1990). Oral contraception in women with diabetes. *Diabetes Care*, **13**, 8895–8

17. Skouby, S.O., Mølsted-Pedersen, L., Kuhl, C. and Bennet, P. (1986). Oral contraceptives in diabetic women: metabolic effects of four compounds with different estrogen/progestogen profiles. *Fertil. Steril.*, **46**, 858–64

18. Petersen, K.R., Skouby, S.O., Sidelmann, J., Mølsted-Pedersen, L. and Jespersen, J. (1994). Effects of contraceptive steroids on cardiovascular risk factors in women with insulin dependent diabetes mellitus. *Am. J. Obstet. Gynecol.*, **171**, 400–5

19. Petersen, K.R., Skouby, S.O. and Pedersen, R.G. (1991). Desogestrel and gestodene in oral contraceptives: 12 months assessment of glucose and lipoprotein metabolism. *Obstet. Gynecol.*, **78**, 666–72

20. Godsland, I.F., Crook, D., Simpson, R., Proudler, T., Felton, C., Lees, B., Anyaoku, V., Devenport, M. and Wynn, V. (1990). The effect of different formulations of oral contraceptive agents on lipid and carbohydrate metabolism. *N. Engl. J. Med.*, **323**, 1375–81

21. Witztum, J.L., Mahoney, E.M., Branks, M.J., Fisher, M., Elam, R. and Steinberg, D. (1982). Non enzymatic glycosylation of low-density lipoprotein alters its biological activity. *Diabetes*, **31**, 283–91

22. Duell, P.B., Oram, J.F. and Bierman, E.L. (1991). Non enzymatic glycosylation of HDL and impaired HDL receptor mediated cholesterol efflux. *Diabetes*, **40**, 377–84

23. Jensen, T., Bjerre Knudsen, J., Feldt-Rasmussen, B. and Deckert, T. (1989). Features of endothelial dysfunction in early diabetic nephropathy. *Lancet*, **1**, 461–3

24. Fuster, V., Badimon, L., Badimon, J.J. and Chesebro, J.H. (1992). The pathogenesis of coronary artery disease and the acute coronary syndromes. *N. Engl. J. Med.*, **326**, 310–18

25. Petersen, K.R., Skouby, S.O., Sidelmann, J. and Jespersen, J. (1994). Assessment of endothelial function in women with insulin dependent diabetes mellitus during oral contraception. *Metabolism*, **43**, 1379–83

26. Damm, P., Kuhl, C., Bertelsen, A. and Mølsted-Pedersen, L. (1992). Predictive factors for the development of diabetes in women with previous gestational diabetes mellitus. *Am. J. Obstet. Gynecol.*, **167**, 607–16

27. Peters, R.K., Kjos, S.L., Xiang, A. and Buchanan, T.A. (1996). Long term diabetogenic effect of a single pregnancy in women with previous gestational diabetes mellitus. *Lancet*, **347**, 227–30

28. Skouby, S.O., Andersen, O., Petersen, K.R., Mølsted-Pedersen, L. and Kuhl, C. (1990). Mechanism of action of oral contraceptives on carbohydrate on the cellular level. *Am. J. Obstet. Gynecol.*, **163**, 343–8

29. Kjos, S.L., Buchanan, T.A., Montoro, M., Coulson, A. and Mestman, J.H. (1991). Serum lipids within 36 months of delivery in women with recent diabetes mellitus. *Diabetes*, **40** (Suppl. 2), 142–6

30. Skouby, S.O., Kuhl, C., Mølsted-Pedersen, L., Petersen, K. and Sandvig Christensen, M. (1985). Triphasic oral contraceptives: metabolic effects in normal women and those with previous gestational diabetes. *Am. J. Obstet. Gynecol.*, **153**, 495–500

31. Kjos, S.L., Shoupe, D., Douyan, S., Friedman, R.L., Bernstein, G.S., Mestman, J.H. and Mishell (1990). Effect of low dose oral contraceptives on carbohydrate and lipid metabolism in women with recent gestational diabetes: results of a controlled, randomized, prospective trial. *Am. J. Obstet. Gynecol.*, **163**, 1822–7

10

Role of screening for vascular disease in pill users: the hemostatic system

U.H. Winkler

ORAL CONTRACEPTIVE-ASSOCIATED THROMBOEMBOLISM AND HEMOSTASIS

In their 'Guidelines for prescribing combined oral contraceptives', the Faculty of Family Planning and Reproductive Health Care of the Royal College of Obstetricians and Gynaecologists has summarized data from several recent epidemiological studies on the risk of thromboembolic diseases[1]. The incidence of non-fatal thrombosis in western Europe was estimated to be 1.4 per 10 000 women-years in users of combined oral contraceptives (OCs), a relative risk (RR) of 3–4 compared with non-users of hormonal contraceptive measures.

Two major studies have recently supported the notion that a considerable number of these thromboembolic complications occur in women carrying a congenital predisposition to thrombotic diseases[2,3]. While a congenital thrombophilia has been a well-known feature in antithrombin III (AT III), protein C and protein S deficiency, it was shown only recently that women suffering from such deficiencies (with the possible exception of protein S deficiency) are

---

This paper is dedicated to Prof. Dr. med. A.E. Schindler on the occasion of his 60th birthday, June 6th, 1996

109

at an enhanced risk while taking OCs (RRs up to 8-fold in AT III-deficient women)[2]. Recently, Koster and co-workers provided evidence from the Leiden Thrombophilia Study (LETS), a population-based case–control study of thromboembolic diseases in the northwestern parts of The Netherlands, that the risk of thrombotic disease is increased up to 8-fold in carriers of a single mutation in the genetic coding for the coagulation factor V[3]. This study has provided the largest database to assess the prevalance of coagulation abnormalities in patients with thrombosis and in the asymptomatic population. The factor V Leiden mutation has been shown markedly to slow down the proteolytic activity of activated protein C (APC) on factor V, i.e. to induce a resistance to APC[4]. While all carriers of the mutation were found to be APC-resistant[5], up to 20% of APC-resistant individuals may carry other genetic abnormalities[6], the thrombogenic potential of which has not yet been entirely elucidated. APC-resistant women with the mutation are at particular risk of thrombotic disease while taking the pill. Their risk was found to be more than 30 times that of non-users of hormonal contraceptives without the factor V Leiden mutation[7,8].

Thus, congenital thrombophilia may be caused by functional deficiencies in either of the two major anticoagulant pathways, the antithrombin III and protein C pathways. OC use does not simply add to, but multiplies, the risks of thrombotic disease in predisposed women. It is worth considering whether screening for thrombophilic disorders prior to prescribing the pill might help to prevent thromboembolic complications of OC use.

THROMBOPHILIA

The British Committee for Standards in Haematology has issued guidelines on the investigation of thrombophilia[9]. A modified summary of the relevant disorders is given in Table 1 (APC resistance and factor V Leiden have also been included). It is important to note that there are several disorders such as lupus anticoagulant and plasminogen deficiency that may be possible factors in pill-associated thromboses. These, however, were not considered to be proven congenital disorders and investigation for these abnormalities was recommended in symptomatic patients only.

Table 1 Thrombophilic disorders (modified after reference 9)

Inherited thrombophilia	Acquired thrombophilia	Disorders which may be associated with increased risk of thrombosis
Antithrombin III deficiency	lupus anticoagulant	plasminogen deficiency
Protein C deficiency	anticardiolipin	plasminogen activator
Protein S deficiency	antibodies	deficiency
Resistance to activated		increased concentrations
protein C		of fibrinolytic inhibitors
Factor V Leiden mutation		dysfibrinogenemia
		heparin co-factor II
		deficiency
		increased concentrations
		of histidine-rich
		glycoprotein
		factor XII deficiency
		homocystinuria

Methods

A prerequisite of any screening program is the availability of reliable assays. Both the precision and cost of the assay need to be considered.

Inhibitor deficiencies

Inhibitors have long been measured by immunological assays. A considerable number of functional (type II) deficiencies of coagulation inhibitors, however, have been found that were undetected by immunological measurement, suggesting that only some of the type I deficiencies are caused by mutations affecting the active center of the inhibitor. Functional measurements assessing the physiological activity of the molecule, therefore, are considered to be better screening instruments[9]. Plasma samples have to be sent to a specialized laboratory and there are concerns about a potential underestimation of the true activities due to *ex vivo* effects. Thus, if the test results suggest a deficiency syndrome (e.g. below 60% of normal values), a second assessment conducted by a specialized center should be considered. A complete set of all three assays (AT III, protein C and protein S activities) may be available for the cost of two packets of a modern low-dose OC.

OC use has been shown to influence coagulation inhibitors. In particular, protein S activity was found to be reduced by 15%, even in users of low-dose OCs[10,11]. Assessments of coagulation inhibitors, therefore, should not be performed in women using the pill.

APC resistance and factor V Leiden

APC resistance is determined as an APC sensitivity ratio comparing the native activated prothrombin time (aPTT) with the aPTT after preincubation with the activated inhibitor protein C. If the APC-induced prolongation of the aPTT does not exceed 100%, the sensitivity to APC is considered to be inadequate[12]. Homozygous individuals for the factor V Leiden mutation have been shown to have an extremely low sensitivity, suggesting that the APC resistance assay may also usefully differentiate between hetero- and homozygote carriers of the factor V Leiden mutation. Since the assay is based on the coagulometric assessment of clotting time, effects on other coagulation factors may have some impact on the measurement[13] and should be minimalized by an adequate assay technology (e.g. dilution of the plasma sample with factor V deficient plasma) whenever appropriate (e.g. in patients on heparin or coumarins)[14,15]. There are, however, no data yet on the performance of these improved assays in OC users. It has been demonstrated that OC-induced effects on protein S, factor VIII and X activities may interfere with older APC assessments, inducing an 'acquired APC resistance' in some women[16,17]. The thrombogenicity of this condition is unknown. Thus, if APC resistance is found in women on the pill, analysis of the factor V Leiden mutation may be required. For the time being, the interpretation of results in women off the pill is on much more solid ground.

The APC resistance assay requires only basic hemostaseological equipment (coagulometer) and limited laboratory experience. Costs depend on the frequency of calibration and the use of factor V deficient plasma, but will rarely exceed the price of 2 months' supply of OCs.

The factor V Leiden mutation must be identified by the polymerase chain reaction (PCR), rendering the accessibility of this assay rather low. While the precision of the test is unprecedented, current status of pill use being unimportant, the penetration of the phenotype appears to be rather low. Homogenicity for the factor V mutation, however, was shown markedly to improve the predictive value for thromboembolic disease in the LETS database[5]. The PCR determination of the factor V Leiden mutation is standardized and commercially available. The price, however, is about 4–10 times higher than an APC sensitivity test.

SCREENING

Screening for thrombophilia may improve public health by reducing the number of women who suffer from a pill-associated thromboembolism each year. Screening should also aid an individual pill user by helping her make her contraceptive choices easily and in a straightforward manner. A measure of the public health value is the sensitivity and specificity of the screening test, i.e. the ability to identify women at risk and the ability not to identify falsely women not at any risk. A measure of the value to the individual is the predictive value, i.e. the probability with which a positive test result indicates that a woman will suffer from a thromboembolic complication if she uses an OC.

Prevalence in the general population

Calculations of the validity of tests are based on the prevalence of abnormal findings in the asymptomatic and symptomatic populations. Several studies have reported the prevalence of AT III, protein C or protein S deficiencies in patients with thromboembolic conditions compared with asymptomatic controls[18–25]. The prevalence of all inhibitor deficiencies appears to be only about 0.5% in the asymptomatic population and about 10 times higher in an unselected cohort of patients with thrombosis (Table 2). Among patients with thrombosis who have a positive family history of thrombosis, the

Table 2 Prevalence of inhibitor deficiencies as well as resistance to activated protein C in a population sample, among thrombosis patients and among thrombosis patients giving a positive family history (cited after reference 5 and calculated from references 18–25)

Prevalence (%)	Population (asymptomatic)	Thrombosis (unselected)	Thrombosis (if positive family history)
Antithrombin III deficiency	0.1	1.2	4.2
Protein C deficiency	0.3	3.6	4.9
Protein S deficiency	0.1	2.4	5.1
APC resistance	5.7	28	46
Total	6.2	35.2	60.2

APC, activated protein C

prevalence is estimated to be about 15%[5]. APC resistance is found in 28% of unselected thrombosis patients and 46% of symptomatic patients with a positive family history[5]. The prevalence in the asymptomatic population, however, was found to be as high as 5.7% in one study[3].

Prevalence among pill users

There are only limited data on the prevalence of the inhibitor deficiencies among women experiencing a pill-associated thromboembolic event. Based on prospective studies of the OC-induced excess risk in affected families[2], it may be assumed that AT III-deficient women may be slightly overrepresented, while protein S-deficient women may be somewhat underrepresented, in this subgroup of patients. Nevertheless, in the absence of data, it is fair to state that the overall prevalence of inhibitor deficiencies in women suffering from pill-associated thromboembolic diseases will not exceed the highest estimates of the prevalence in unselected thrombosis patients, i.e. 7.2% (Table 2).

For the factor V Leiden mutation, prevalence data in pill users are available from the LETS database[7,8]; 3.6% of the asymptomatic and

Table 3 Sensitivity, specificity and positive predictive value of possible screening tests in 1 million pill users (based on data from references 5, 8, 18–25)

	Without thrombotic complications (n = 999 160)	*With thrombotic complications* (n = 140)	*Sensitivity* (%)	*Specificity* (%)	*Positive predictive value*
APC resistance	56 952 (5.7%)	39 (28%)	28	94.3	7×10^{-4}
Factor V Leiden mutation	35 970 (3.6%)	32 (23%)	23	96.4	9×10^{-4}
Inhibitor deficiencies	4 996 (0.5%)	10 (7.2%)	7.2	99.5	2×10^{-3}
Family history	144 878 (14.5%)	46 (32.5%)	32.5	85.5	3×10^{-4}

APC, activated protein C

23% of the symptomatic pill users were carriers of the factor V Leiden mutation. These figures compare well with the general prevalence in the LETS population[3]. Thus, it is reasonable to assume that the prevalence of APC resistance in pill users is also likely to resemble the situation in the general population. Recent work based on a rather small data base supports this assumption[16,17].

Validity of general hemostaseological screening

Assuming an incidence of thromboembolic disease of 1.4 per 10 000 women, the sensitivity and specificity of each test can be calculated (Table 3). While it is true that OC-associated thromboembolic diseases do not necessarily occur in the first year of OC use, there is evidence that the risk is highest during the first year[26]. None the less, the cumulative risk of thromboembolic disease may be somewhat higher over the life exposure to OCs. The potential underestimation of OC-associated cases, however, is balanced by the fact that there is a considerable risk of thromboembolic disease (0.4 per

10 000 women) in those not using the pill. Thus, if a potential user, as a consequence of screening, refrains from using hormonal contraception, she still has some increased risk of thrombotic disease. We can be confident, therefore, that the case estimate is balanced.

Among 1 million pill users, 140 will suffer from pill-associated thromboembolic problems. Of these, ten women will be found on screening to have an inhibitor deficiency, giving a sensitivity of 7.2%. Screening for the factor V Leiden mutation or the APC resistance would have detected another 32 or 39 women with coagulation abnormalities, respectively. As mentioned before, both assays detect approximately the same group of symptomatic as well as asymptomatic women. Among the asymptomatic women, however, up to 60 000 clotting abnormalities would have been detected in women who would not experience an OC-associated thromboembolic complication. Thus, in spite of the quite impressive specificity (ranging from 95 to 99%), the positive predictive value of these laboratory tests is poor (varying between 1 in 1000 and 1 in 19 000 (Table 3).

Thus, only 49 (35%) of the 140 patients at risk may be detected by a general screening protocol. Moreover, the probability of thrombosis during pill use may be less than 1/1000 for individuals presenting only with APC resistance or factor V Leiden mutation and 1/500 for an inhibitor deficiency. Considering the numerous non-contraceptive benefits of OC use, and the contraceptive and non-contraceptive risks of alternative contraceptive methods, it is reasonable to conclude that the value of general screening, both for the individual user as well as the general population, is rather limited.

Family history

Obviously, the low absolute risk of thromboembolic complications in pill users is the reason for the tremendous number of false-positive results, even though the specificity of the screening assays exceeds 90%. With the exception of a homozygous factor V Leiden mutation and the AT III deficiency, none of the findings may yield a predictive value in the order of 1 in 1000 or better (Table 3). There is only one feasible way of reducing the number of false-positive results of screening: perform the laboratory screening only after a pre-selection step, i.e. only in women with a positive family history.

In principle, the family history should be the ideal tool for pre-selecting for congenital thrombophilia. Given a cumulative thrombosis incidence of 70% in inhibitor-deficient individuals[21] and about 30% in APC-resistant individuals[8], it is tempting to speculate that almost all cases of congenital thrombophilia might be detectable by family history. One has to bear in mind, however, that age is probably the most important trigger for the presentation of a thrombotic episode. Since screening in OC users is likely to be performed in very young women, the probability of a positive family history is rather low. The likelihood of a positive family history, therefore, depends largely on the age of the index case and the number of pedigrees[27]. Moreover, given the fact that there are numerous other, mostly non-congenital disorders, that may cause thrombosis (Table 1), it is not surprising that even the strictest criterion (a case of thrombosis among first-degree relatives) will yield a considerable number of false-positive results (Table 3). In addition, because of the age dependency of the thrombotic phenotype, the sensitivity of screening such strict criteria is bound to be low.

Of the 140 cases of thrombosis among pill users, 49 may be prevented by general screening for APC resistance and inhibitor deficiencies. At least 30 of these (60.2%) will give a positive family history (Table 2). In clinical practice, family history is not restricted to first-degree relatives only and the reported cases will be evaluated as being 'expected', i.e. in association with typical trigger conditions or higher age, or 'unexpected'. While expanding the search to the second- and third-degree relatives will improve the sensitivity of family history, the evaluation of each report is likely to improve the specificity. Thus, it is reasonable to assume that, in clinical practice, the concept of pre-selection using family history and confirmation by laboratory screening may have only a marginally decreased sensitivity. The positive predictive value, however, will be markedly improved due to the fact that contraceptive decisions may then be based on at least two risk markers.

CONCLUSION

In conclusion, several highly specific hemostaseological assays are now available to identify women at risk of OC-associated thromboembolic complications. More than 50% of cases, however, cannot be predicted by these assays. Due to the very low absolute risk of thrombosis in OC users, the predictive value of these assays is low, thus limiting both the public as well as the individual benefit of a general screening protocol. After pre-selecting women by family history, targeted screening for AT III, protein C and S deficiency as well as APC resistance appears to be only slightly less sensitive but considerably more specific, suiting both the public and individual need for providing essential facts for informed contraceptive choices.

REFERENCES

1. Mills, A.M., Wilkinson, C.L., Bromham, D.R., Elias, J., Fotherby, K., Guillebaud, J., Kuhba, A. and Wade, A. (1996). Guidelines for prescribing combined oral contraceptives. *Br. Med. J.*, **312**, 121–2
2. Pabinger, I., Schneider, B. and the GTH Study Group on Natural Inhibitors (1994). Thrombotic risk of women with hereditary antithrombin III, protein C and protein S deficiency taking oral contraceptives. *Thromb. Haemostas.*, **71**, 548–52
3. Koster, T., Rosendaal, F.R., de Ronde, H., Briet, E., Vandenbroucke, J.P. and Bertina, R.M. (1993). Venous thrombosis due to poor anticoagulant response to activated protein C: Leiden thrombophilia study. *Lancet*, **342**, 1503–6
4. Bertina, R.M., Koeleman, B.P.C., Koster, T., Rosendaal, F.R., Dirven, R.J., de Ronde, H., van der Velden, P.A. and Reitsma, P.H. (1994). Mutation in blood coagulation factor V associated with resistance to activated protein C. *Nature (London)*, **369**, 64–7
5. Bertina, R.M., Reitsma, P.H., Rosendaal, F.R. and Vandenbroucke, J.P. (1995). Resistance to activated protein C and factor V Leiden as risk factors for venous thrombosis. *Thromb. Haemostas.*, **74**, 449–53
6. Zöller, B. and Dahlbäck, B. (1994). Linkage between inherited resistance to activated protein C and factor V gene mutation in venous thrombosis. *Lancet*, **343**, 1536–8
7. Vandenbroucke, J.P., Koster, T., Briet, E., Reitsma, P.H., Bertina, R.M. and Rosendaal, F.R. (1994). Increased risk of venous thrombosis in

oral-contraceptive users who are carriers of factor V Leiden mutation. *Lancet*, **344**, 1453–7

8. Bloemenkamp, K.W.M., Rosendaal, F.R., Helmerhorst, F.M., Büller, H.R. and Vandenbroucke, J.P. (1995). Enhancement by factor V Leiden mutation of risk of deep-vein thrombosis associated with oral contraceptives containing a third-generation progestogen. *Lancet*, **346**, 1593–6

9. The British Committee for Standards in Haematology (1990). Guidelines on the investigation and management of thrombophilia. *J. Clin. Pathol.*, **49**, 703–9

10. Winkler, U.H., Schindler, A.E., Endrikat, J., Müller, U. and Düsterberg, B. (1996). A comparative study of the effects on the hemostatic system of two monophasic gestodene oral contraceptives containing 20 μg and 30 μg ethinylestradiol. *Contraception*, **53**, 75–84

11. Winkler, U.H., Oberhoff, C., Bier, U. and Schindler, A.E. (1995). Hemostatic effects of two oral contraceptives containing low doses of ethinylestradiol and either gestodene or norgestimate: an open, randomized, parallel-group study. *Int. J. Fertil. Menopaus. Stud.*, **40**, 260–8

12. Dahlbäck, B., Carlsson, M. and Svensson, P.J. (1993). Familial thrombophilia due to a previous unrecognized mechanism characterized by poor anticoagulant response to activated protein C: prediction of a cofactor to activated protein C. *Proc. Natl. Acad. Sci. USA*, **90**, 1004–8

13. De Ronde, H. and Bertina, R.M. (1994). Laboratory diagnosis of APC-resistance: a critical evaluation of the test and the development of diagnostic criteria. *Thromb. Haemostas.*, **72**, 880–6

14. Colucci, M., Ciavarella, N., Giliberti, M.G. and Semeraro, N. (1994). Resistance to activated protein C (APC): influence of factor V levels. (Letter). *Thromb. Haemostas.*, **72**, 985–9

15. Denson, K.W.E., Reed, S.V. and Haddon, M.E. (1995). The modified APC-resistance test. *Thromb. Haemostas.*, **74**, 995

16. Österud, B., Robertsen, A., Asvang, G.B. and Thyssen, F. (1994). Resistance to activated protein C is reduced in women using oral contraceptives. *Blood Coag. Fibrin.*, **5**, 853–4

17. Hellgren, M., Svensson, P.J. and Dahlbäck, B. (1995). Resistance to activated protein C as a basis for venous thromboembolism associated with pregnancy and oral contraceptives. *Am. J. Obstet. Gynecol.*, **173**, 210–13

18. Ben Tal, O., Zivelin, A. and Seligsohn, U. (1989). The relative frequency of hereditary thrombotic disorders among 107 patients with thrombophilia in Israel. *Thromb. Haemostas.*, **61**, 50–4

19. Engesser, L., Broekmans, A.W., Briet, E., Brommer, E.J. and Bertina, R.M. (1987). Hereditary protein S deficiency: clinical manifestations. *Ann. Intern. Med.*, **106**, 677–82

20. Gladson, C.L., Scharrer, I., Hack, V., Beck, K.H. and Griffin, J.H. (1988). The frequency of type I heterozygous protein S and protein C deficiency in 141 unrelated young patients with venous thrombosis. *Thromb. Haemostas.*, **59**, 18–22

21. Heijboer, H., Brandjes, D.P.M., Büller, H.R., Sturk, A. and Ten Cate, J.W. (1990). Deficiencies of coagulation-inhibiting and fibrinolytic proteins in outpatients with deep-vein thrombosis. *N. Engl. J. Med.*, **323**, 1512–16

22. Malm, J., Laurell, M., Nilsson, I.M. and Dahlbäck, B. (1992). Thromboembolic disease – critical evaluation of laboratory investigation. *Thromb. Haemostas.*, **68**, 7–13

23. Miletich, J.P., Prescott, S.M., White, R., Majerus, P.W. and Bovill, E.G. (1993). Inherited predisposition to thrombosis. *Cell*, **72**, 477–80

24. Pabinger, I., Brücker, S., Kyrle, P.A., Scheider, B., Kominger, H.C., Niessner, H. and Lechner, K. (1992). Hereditary deficiency of antithrombin III, protein C and protein S: prevalence in patients with a history of venous thrombosis and criteria for rational patient screening. *Blood Coag. Fibrin.*, **3**, 547–53

25. Tabemero, M.D., Tomas, J.F., Alberca, I., Orfao, A., Lopez Borrasca, A. and Vicente, V. (1991). Incidence and clinical characteristics of hereditary disorders associated with venous thrombosis. *Am. J. Hematol.*, **136**, 249–54

26. Reijnen, H.B.M. and Atsma, W.J. (1995). Risk is highest during first months of use. Letter to the editor. *Br. Med. J.*, **311**, 1639

27. Briet, E., van der Meer, F.J.M., Rosendaal, F.R., Houwing-Duistermaat, J.J. and van Houwelingen, H.C. (1994). The family history and inherited thrombophilia. *Br. J. Haematol.*, **87**, 348–52

11

The Second European Consensus Development Meeting, Amsterdam 1995: Combined oral contraception and cardiovascular diseases – summary and main conclusions

*J. Jespersen for The Consensus Committee**

INTRODUCTION

The Second European Esbjerg Conference on Sex Steroids and Metabolism took place in Amsterdam, The Netherlands, on 9–10 November 1995, with 153 participants from 16 countries. As with the First European Esbjerg Conference in 1989, an interdisciplinary approach was used with particular reference to the relation between combined oral contraceptives (COCs) and cardiovascular diseases, i.e. heart disease, in particular ischemic heart disease (acute myocardial infarction), cerebrovascular disease and peripheral vascular disease, including venous disease, and pulmonary embolism. Up-to-date information was presented by invited speakers on epidemiological, pharmacological and pathogenetic aspects of relevance for the development of, and screening for, cardiovascular

---

*Committee members and members of the expert panels are listed at the end of this summary of the Consensus Statement, published in *Gynecol. Endocrinol.*, 1996; **10**, 1–5.

diseases. As for the first conference[1,2], these contributions provided a platform[3] for the development of a consensus statement[4].

CONSENSUS DEVELOPMENT MEETING 1995

The Consensus Statement was developed by three expert panels on epidemiology, pharmacology, and cardiovascular diseases (mechanism and screening), based on questions formulated by the Consensus Committee. These questions focused on, in addition to epidemiology, apparently relevant biochemistry, i.e. glucose metabolism, lipid and lipoprotein metabolism and hemostasis.

Since the statement has been published *in extenso*[4], only a brief summary of the questions/answers and recommendations will be given, with particular reference to the clinical recommendations.

Epidemiology

Do COCs increase the risk of cardiovascular diseases?

Summarizing the specific aspects:

(1)　Deep vein thrombosis and pulmonary embolism: there is an increased risk among current users. The relative risk is probably increased three- to six-fold.

(2)　Thrombotic strokes: there is an increased risk among current users. The relative risk is probably increased two- to four-fold.

(3)　Hemorrhagic strokes: the risk is more modest than thrombotic strokes, probably less than twofold for current users. There is limited evidence of an increased risk in past users.

(4)　Acute myocardial infarction: there is an increased risk in current users, perhaps two- to three-fold.

General aspects:

(1)　The relative risk associated with COCs is unaffected by age for stroke and deep vein thrombosis. There may be some increase in the relative risk of acute myocardial infarction with age.

(2)   The absolute risks are small, especially among young healthy women, and particularly for the more serious conditions – strokes, heart attacks and pulmonary emboli.

(3)   There is no relationship between the duration of use of COCs and the risk of any of these diseases.

(4)   There is no consistent evidence of an increased risk in past users.

(5)   Each of the diseases has a different set of risk factors and for some diseases new risk factors are just beginning to emerge.

(6)   The relative and absolute risks may be increased in the presence of other risk factors.

Can we identify the high-risk users, among whom prescription of COCs should be weighed carefully against potential benefits?

(1)   Deep vein thrombosis and pulmonary embolism: there is consistent evidence of an increased risk among women with certain genetic factors, i.e. certain variants of clotting genes. The evidence for varicose veins, obesity and smoking as risk factors is inconsistent.

(2)   Thrombotic stroke: the risk factors are diabetes, previous thrombosis, hypertension, migraine with neurological manifestations, and probably smoking.

(3)   Hemorrhagic strokes: the risk factor is hypertension.

(4)   Acute myocardial infarction: the risk factors are smoking, hypertension, diabetes, coagulopathies, severe hyperlipidemia.

Has the risk changed, and if yes, what is the reason?

(1)   There is evidence of a decreased risk of stroke and probably of acute myocardial infarction associated with the use of low-dose oral contraceptives (COCs with less than 50 µg estrogen – independent of progestogen type).

(2)   There is evidence that the risk of deep vein thrombosis has not fallen with use of low-dose pills.

What component in the COC is responsible for the possible risk?

There is some evidence that both the estrogen and progestogen components of the COC are associated with the increased risk.

Is there any evidence that pills with third-generation progestogens are safer?

There is no published epidemiological evidence of the cardiovascular risks of third-generation progestogens (desogestrel, gestodene and norgestimate).

Research priorities, inter alia

(1)   To explore the potential phenomenon of prescribing bias. This may require the examination of existing databases or new studies.

(2)   To consider overall morbidity and mortality associated with use of newer preparations.

(3)   To use existing data and databases in order to clarify the impact of third-generation pills.

(4)   In countries where third-generation progestogen pills are in use, new epidemiological studies should be conducted.

Pharmacology

General questions:

Are new formulations desirable, and if so, which requirements of COCs should be aimed at?

COCs are the most effective reversible form of contraception currently available. Minimizing risk and maximizing benefits should always be the main objective for future development.

*Is variability in pharmacodynamics mainly determined by
interindividual differences or by differences in COCs?*

Both are important. Variability is determined mainly by interindividual differences but also by differences in COCs.

Specific questions:

Do COCs cause changes in carbohydrate metabolism?

Yes, COCs cause changes in carbohydrate metabolism.

Which component of the COC formulation is responsible for these changes?

Both components of the COC formulation are involved in changes in carbohydrate metabolism. When changes do occur they are minor and do not affect all areas of carbohydrate metabolism.

Are these alterations dependent on dose?

Changes appear to be dose-dependent as far as the estrogen is concerned although there are only limited data in support of this.

Are these changes related to duration of use?

Yes, up to 1 year. No data are available beyond this time.

Lipid and lipoprotein metabolism

Do COCs induce change in lipid metabolism?

Yes, but the changes in lipids are difficult to interpret since the normal physiological regulating mechanism is altered.

Are these changes related to dose and composition?

Lipid changes are related to the dose of estrogen and progestogen, to the type of progestogen and to the ratio of the steroids.

Are these changes related to duration of use?

Changes may be duration-dependent up to 1 year but after that there is little information.

Hemostasis

Do COCs induce changes in hemostatic variables?

COCs induce changes in the concentrations of a large number of specific plasma components of the coagulation and fibrinolytic systems.

Are these changes related to dose/composition?

These changes seem to be estrogen-dependent, with progestogens exerting a modifying effect. There is insufficient information to show that these changes are related to estrogen dose but it would appear that changes are small for doses below 50 μg.

Are these changes related to duration?

Up to 1 year; beyond this period there is little information.

Research priorities, inter alia

(1)   Sex steroids are vasoactive substances which affect the vasculature of many systems; particular emphasis should now be directed towards the local interaction and metabolism at the vessel wall with special emphasis on the vein.

(2)   Hepatic effects of COCs are not well understood with respect to certain areas of carbohydrate and lipid metabolism and hemostatic factors.

(3)   Data on the relationship between blood levels of COCs and specific metabolic changes are important and may give insights into individual susceptibility. To elucidate this, further studies are necessary.

Cardiovascular disease – mechanisms and screening

Carbohydrate metabolism

General aspects of potential relevance for cardiovascular diseases:

(1) COCs cause deterioration in glucose tolerance and increased insulin concentrations.

(2) COCs cause insulin resistance to an extent which may largely depend on the estrogen content.

(3) Hyperinsulinemia in COC users accompanies this insulin resistance and is modulated by the progestogen type and dose. Modification of insulin sensitivity and elimination may contribute.

(4) Some but not all features of the insulin resistance syndrome may be apparent in COC users. The extent to which these appear together depends on COC formulation.

What is the clinical relevance of these findings?

(1) Evaluation of the clinical importance of these changes awaits further epidemiological studies of hyperinsulinemia and insulin resistance.

(2) There is no increased risk of clinical diabetes in COC users.

Which formulation of COCs should be aimed at?

Minimization of hyperinsulinemia and its associated metabolic changes would seem prudent in COC users.

What are the absolute contraindications for COC use related to overt diabetes?

Short-term COC use is not accompanied by a change in glycemic control in women with uncomplicated diabetes.

Lipid and lipoprotein metabolism

General aspects of potential relevance for cardiovascular disease:

(1) Changes in high-density lipoprotein (HDL) cholesterol (increases with COCs containing 'third-generation' progestogens).

(2) Fasting triglycerides are raised by most COCs, depending on the estrogen and progestogen content.

(3) There are only minor changes in total and low-density lipoprotein (LDL) cholesterol.

(4) LDL oxidation may be diminished by COCs.

Hemostasis

General aspects of potential relevance for cardiovascular disease:

(1) There are changes in the concentration of a large number of specific plasma components of the coagulation and fibrinolytic systems, although usually within the population range.

(2) There are changes in the concentration of molecular markers of coagulation and fibrinolysis indicative of increased activation of procoagulant factors, profibrinolytic factors and of fibrin turnover.

(3) There is a dose-dependent relationship with estrogen dose >50 µg although the progestogen might exert a modifying effect.

(4) These changes are still present in the new preparations (<50 µg), but are smaller.

What is the clinical relevance of these findings?

(1) Further assessment of the clinical importance of these changes is needed. Epidemiological studies should assess the degree of change in hemostatic variables associated with risk of arterial and venous thrombotic events in women.

(2) COCs can precipitate venous thrombosis in cases of familial thrombophilia and in cases with established coagulation defect(s). Coagulation defects with a potentially increased risk are factor V Leiden, antithrombin III deficiency, possibly protein C deficiency, and protein S deficiency. Combinations of

disorders and homozygous cases are most likely at further increased risk.

(3) The mechanisms by which COCs increase this risk are not known.

Is a documented genetic disorder and/or past history of cardiovascular diseases a contraindication for COC use?

The presence of thrombophilia may be a contraindication to COCs, subject to assessment of individual risk, including the increased risk of venous thrombosis during pregnancy.

Screening

How should COC users be screened, if at all?

(1) Familial thrombophilia at present.

(2) Routine laboratory screening to be evaluated (i.e. general screening).

(3) In women with thrombotic events during COC use, an assessment of underlying hemostatic and metabolic risk factors (e.g. thrombophilia) is appropriate not only for evaluation of future risk in the patient, but also to elucidate mechanisms of risk. In this and other studies, genotypes related to cardiovascular risk and involved in estrogen–progestogen response should be investigated.

Research priorities, inter alia

(1) Hemostatic factors may be expressed in the vessel wall to different degrees in different vascular compartments. The effects of oral contraceptives on vessel wall expression of these factors might provide new mechanisms and also account for different effects on arterial and venous thrombosis.

(2) The relationship between elevated triglyceride levels and hemostatic factors in women taking COCs should be studied.

(3)   The elevations in fibrinogen and factor VII are a matter of concern as regards thrombotic risk (risk predictors). In general, formulations with the least effects on these factors and on molecular markers are favored.

CONCLUDING REMARKS

The Conference and the Consensus Development meeting were planned in 1994 as a follow-up of the First Esbjerg Conference. We felt that a new conference was needed in order to update the clinicians and also to see whether the questions raised during the first conference had been answered, whether the recommendations were still valid, and whether new aspects, etc. had to be taken into account concerning the effects of COCs on the cardiovascular system.

The importance of this conference was emphasized by the renewed concern about some cardiovascular aspects of COCs[5–10]. At the time of the conference, the regulatory authorities in the UK and Germany announced that they had unpublished data which indicated a twofold excess of deep venous thrombosis among users of preparations containing gestodene or desogestrel compared with brands containing levonorgestrel. Unfortunately, a full evaluation of this evidence was not possible during the conference, but had to await publication of the data. These are now available and a matter of discussion in the scientific world[5–10]. At present we believe that, irrespective of this ongoing discussion, the present Consensus Statement[3] provides valuable and evidence-based guidelines for prescribing COCs in clinical practice. In particular, routine screening was again not recommended except for women with some predisposing factors within glucose metabolism (gestational diabetes or first-degree relatives with diabetes), lipid and lipoprotein metabolism (hyperlipidemia) and the hemostatic system (thrombophilia).

REFERENCES

1. First European Esbjerg Conference on Sex Steroids and Metabolism (1990). Oral contraceptives in the nineties: metabolic aspects – facts and fiction. *Am. J. Obstet. Gynecol.*, **163** (Suppl. 2), 273–446

2. Consensus Development Meeting (1990). Metabolic aspects of oral contraceptives of relevance for cardiovascular diseases. *Am. J. Obstet. Gynecol.*, **162**, 1335–7

3. The Consensus Committee (1996). Proceedings of the Second European Esbjerg Conference on Sex Steroids and Metabolism. *Gynecol. Endocrinol.*, in press

4. The Consensus Committee (1996). Consensus Development Meeting 1995: combined oral contraceptives and cardiovascular disease. *Gynecol. Endocrinol.*, **10**, 1–5

5. World Health Organization Collaboration Study of Cardiovascular Disease and Steroid Hormone Contraception. (1995). Venous thromboembolic disease and combined oral contraceptives: results of international multicentre case–control study. *Lancet*, **346**, 1575–82

6. World Health Organization Collaboration Study of Cardiovascular Disease and Steroid Hormone Contraception. (1995). Effect of different progestogens in low oestrogen oral contraceptives on venous thromboembolic disease. *Lancet*, **346**, 1582–8

7. Jick, H., Jick, S.S., Gurewich, V., Myers, M.W. and Vasilakis, C. (1995). Risk of idiopathic cardiovascular death and nonfatal venous thromboembolism in women using oral contraceptives with differing progestogen components. *Lancet*, **356**, 1589–93

8. Spitzer, W.O., Lewis, M.A., Heinemann, L.A.J., Thorogood, M. and MacRae, K.D. (1996). Third generation oral contraceptives and risk of venous thromboembolic disorders: an international case–control study. *Br. Med. J.*, **312**, 83–8

9. Lewis, M.A., Spitzer, W.O., Heinemann, L.A.J., MacRae, K.D., Bruppacher, R. and Thorogood, M. (1996). Third generation oral contraceptives and risk of myocardial infarction: an international case–control study. *Br. Med. J.*, **312**, 88–90

10. Bloemenkamp, K.W.M., Rosendaal, F.R., Helmerhorst, F.M., Büller, H.R. and Vandenbroucke, J.P. (1995). Enhancement by factor V Leiden mutation of risk of deep-vein thrombosis associated with oral contraceptives containing third-generation progestogen. *Lancet*, **346**, 1593–6

APPENDIX

Consensus committee:

K. Bloemenkamp (The Netherlands), F. Helmerhorst (The Netherlands), J. Jespersen (Denmark), C. Kluft (The Netherlands), S. Skouby (Chairperson, Denmark)

Expert panels

Epidemiology

D. Archer (United States), P. Hannaford (United Kingdom), F. Helmerhorst (The Netherlands), Ø. Lidegaard (Denmark), K. Lubsen (Switzerland), F. Rosendaal (The Netherlands), M. Thorogood (Chairperson, United Kingdom), J. Vandenbroucke (The Netherlands)

Pharmacology

D. Back (United Kingdom), P. Brakman (Chairperson, The Netherlands), K. Fotherby (United Kingdom), J. Gevers Leuven (The Netherlands), J. Hamerlynck (The Netherlands), J. Jespersen (Denmark), H. Kuhl (Germany), G. Samsioe (Sweden)

Cardiovascular disease: mechanisms and screening

H. Blom (The Netherlands), G. Creatsas (Greece), D. Crook (United Kingdom), J. Godsland (United Kingdom), J. Gram (Denmark), V. van Hinsbergh (The Netherlands), C. Kluft (The Netherlands), T. Kooistra (The Netherlands), G. Lowe (Chairperson, United Kingdom), L. Norris (United Kingdom), S. Skouby (Denmark), U. Winkler (Germany)

Section 3

Genital tract disease and the pill

12

Oral contraceptive use and risk of cancer of the ovary and corpus uteri

S. Franceschi

INTRODUCTION

Oral contraceptives (OCs) were first approved for marketing in the United States in November 1959 and soon became a very popular method of family planning. It is estimated that over 60 million women around the world are now using them[1]. One recurring concern about OCs has been, however, the possibility that they may increase the risk of neoplasia, particularly of hormone-dependent ones. This concern was mitigated by the unexpected finding that they reduced the risk of two important female tumors: cancers of the ovary and the endometrium.

Worldwide, cancers of the ovary and the endometrium are the sixth and the eighth most frequent cancers in women, accounting for approximately 160 000 and 140 000 new cases per year, respectively[2]. In terms of mortality burden, cancer of the ovary is estimated to cause, each year, over 100 000 deaths (i.e. approximately twice the number of those attributed to cancer of the endometrium)[3].

The present article will briefly review the available estimates of the reduction of ovarian and endometrial cancer risk following OC

This paper has ben reproduced by kind permission of the publishers from *Gynaecology Forum* use. Special attention will be paid to issues which could not be addressed in early studies on the topic, most notably, the persistence of protection after usage discontinuation and the effect of new OCs with lower hormonal content.

CANCER OF THE OVARY

Table 1 summarizes the results of 20 case–control[4–23] and four cohort studies[24–27] (see also reference 28) where the assessment of various indicators of OC use with respect to ovarian cancer risk was possible. As in Table 2, risk estimates adjusted for the most important confounding factors were displayed, whenever available from published material. Relative risk (RR) estimates for ever versus never OC users are presented; these were below 1 in 22 investigations. In seven of them, the 95% confidence interval (CI) did not include 1 (Table 1). The only two exceptions were represented by one study carried out in China[17], where OC users were a small and, probably, highly selected group, and by a North American study[16], where risk reduction was restricted to women below the age of 40 or those who had been taking OCs in the preceding year. In most investigations, prolonged OC use led to especially low ovarian cancer risk, e.g. approximately 0.4 for more than 5 years of use in pooled European[29] and United States studies[30].

Protection did not seem to be systematically restricted (or more marked) in any specific stratum of age, parity, etc. It also did not differ substantially according to whether hospital or community controls were used[30].

Some investigations[12,15,21,23] have been able to show persistence of a substantial protection up to 15–19 years since last OC use, with, however, some waning after 5–10 years[30]. Data are scanty and uncertain as concerns persistence after 20 or more years since last OC use[23]. Some, but not all[31], studies[12,23] also suggested that both higher-dose and the newer lower-dose preparations were protective. This may apply also to progestogen-only contraceptives. New types of formulations, such as the biphasics and triphasics, have not, however, yet been assessed sufficiently, on account of the still limited number of women-years of use. It is, finally, worth bearing in mind

Table 1 Relative risk estimates of cancer of the ovary in relation to oral contraceptive use

Study	Relative risk*	95% Confidence interval
Case–control studies		
Newhouse *et al.* (1977)[4]	0.6	0.3–1.1
Casagrande *et al.* (1979)[5]	0.7	0.4–1.1
Hildreth *et al.* (1981)[6]	0.5	0.2–1.7
Weiss *et al.* (1981)[7]	0.6	0.4–1.0
Cramer *et al.* (1982)[8]	0.4	0.2–1.0
Rosenberg *et al.* (1982)[9]	0.6	0.4–0.9
Tzonou *et al.* (1984)[10]	0.4	0.1–1.1
La Vecchia *et al.* (1986)[11]	0.6	0.4–1.0
CASH (1987)[12]	0.6	0.4–0.9
Harlow *et al.* (1988)[13]	0.4	0.2–0.9
Wu *et al.* (1988)[14]	0.7	0.5–1.1
Booth *et al.* (1989)[15]	0.5	0.3–0.9
Hartge *et al.* (1989)[16]	1.0	0.7–1.7
Shu *et al.* (1989)[17]	1.8	0.8–4.1
WHO (1989)[18]	0.8	0.6–1.0
Gwinn *et al.* (1990)[19]	0.5	0.5–0.7
Harlow *et al.* (1991)[20]	0.7	0.4–1.2
Parazzini *et al.* (1991)[21]	0.7	0.5–1.0
Risch *et al.* (1994)[22]	0.5	0.4–0.7
Rosenberg *et al.* (1994)[23]	0.8	0.6–1.0
Cohort studies		
Ramcharan *et al.* (1981)[24]	0.4	0.1–1.0
Willett *et al.* (1981)[25]	0.8	0.4–1.5
Beral *et al.* (1988)[26]	0.6	0.3–1.4
Vessey and Painter (1995)[27]	0.4	0.2–0.8

*Lifetime non-users were the reference category

that the vast majority of available data refers to invasive epithelial ovarian cancer. Some hints, however, exist that the risk of epithelial tumors of low malignant potential and of some non-epithelial ovarian cancers (i.e. stromal tumors) may also be reduced by OC use[32,33].

Table 2 Relative risk estimates of cancer of the endometrium in relation to oral contraceptive use

Study	Relative risk*	95% Confidence interval
Case–control studies		
Kaufman *et al.* (1980)[34]	0.4	0.2–0.8
Weiss and Sayvetz (1980)[35]	0.5	0.2–1.0
Hulka *et al.* (1982)[36]	0.4	0.2–1.2
Kelsey *et al.* (1982)[37]	0.6	0.2–1.5
Henderson *et al.* (1983)[38]	0.5	0.2–0.9
La Vecchia *et al.* (1986)[11]	0.6	0.2–1.3
CASH (1987)[39]	0.5	0.3–0.8
WHO (1988)[40]	0.5	0.2–1.1
Koumantakis *et al.* (1989)[41]	0.5	0.1–1.8
Levi *et al.* (1991)[42]	0.5	0.3–0.8
Shu *et al.* (1991)[43]	0.4	0.1–1.2
Jick *et al.* (1993)[44]	0.5	0.3–0.9
Stanford *et al.* (1993)[45]	0.4	0.3–0.7
Voight *et al.* (1994)[46]	0.4	0.2–0.6
Cohort studies		
Ramcharan *et al.* (1981)[24]	0.6	0.3–0.9
Trapido (1983)[47]	1.4	0.9–2.4
Beral *et al.* (1988)[26]	0.2	0.0–0.7
Vessey and Painter (1995)[27]	0.1	0.0–0.7

*Lifetime non-users were the reference category

CANCER OF THE ENDOMETRIUM

Table 2 summarizes the results of 14 case–control[11,34–46] and four cohort studies[24,26,27,47] which provided information on the effect of OC use on endometrial cancer risk (see also reference 28 for a review). Available data suggest that OC use diminishes cancer risk by about 50%, and long-term use confers about an 80% reduction in risk. The only exception was the positive association found by Trapido[47] in an early cohort investigation. It must, however, be borne in mind that, on account of the age distribution of endometrial cancer, relatively few postmenopausal women in these studies had the opportunity to use OCs in their reproductive years.

With respect to the duration of risk reduction, most recent work has shown that OC users remain at a somewhat lower risk than never users for at least 20 years following discontinuation of usage[42,45].

It has been suggested that other risk factors for endometrial cancer, most notably obesity[38], nulliparity[45], and long-term estrogen replacement therapy[45,46], may partly offset the benefit of OC use, but these findings are inconsistent between different studies and are possibly due to chance.

At variance with ovarian cancer, where the specific hormonal determinants are still obscure, it is clear that endometrial cancer results from an excess of estrogens accompanied by an inadequate cyclic exposure to progestins[11,38]. The progestational potency of OCs may, therefore, influence risk reduction.

Sequential oral contraceptives (SOCs), which have a very strong estrogenic component, were shown to increase the risk of endometrial cancer but on the basis of very few SOC users[38]. With respect to combined OCs, however, most studies did not find a substantial difference in the effect of long-term OC usage according to the progestin content[38,39,46,48]. This led to the conclusion that the amount of progestins contained in most OCs exceeded the threshold needed to reduce endometrial cancer risk. The effect of progestin content on the risk of endometrial cancer among short-term OC users remains unclear. It is, however, important to bear in mind that present classifications of OCs according to relative estrogenic and progestational activity are not satisfactory. Besides, the accuracy of OC classification is limited further by the inability of many women to recall correctly the brand(s) of OC used. Finally, as for cancer of the ovary, it is still impossible to assess the specific effect of the latest biphasic and triphasic formulations.

CONCLUSION

Data from many case–control studies and several cohort investigations, carried out in many different countries, show a consistent reduction of risk of cancers of the ovary and endometrium following use of oral contraceptives. The protection seems substantial (reduction of 40–50%), dependent upon duration of usage but not, as far as available evidence is concerned, oral contraceptive formulation. The protection appears also to be long-lasting (i.e. 15–20 years at least). Decreased risks from cancer of the ovary and endometrium (approximately 400 fewer cases for 100 000 women using oral contraceptives for 8 years) allow the net effect of oral contraceptives on cancer risk to be negligible, under the assumption of a modest increased risk for cancer of the breast and cervix uteri[49]. Studies in this area should, however, not be stopped in order to assess the impact of new patterns of oral contraceptive use, especially with respect to age at cessation of oral contraceptive use and modern low-dose pills.

ACKNOWLEDGEMENTS

This work was conducted within the framework of the CNR (Italian National Research Council) Applied Project 'Clinical Applications of Oncological Research' (Contract No. 94.01268.PF39) and with the contributions of the Italian Association for Research on Cancer. The author wishes to thank Mrs Anna Redivo for editorial assistance.

REFERENCES

1. WHO Scientific Group on Oral Contraceptives and Neoplasia (1992). *Oral Contraceptives and Neoplasia: Report of a WHO Scientific Group.* WHO technical report series n. 817. (Geneva: WHO)
2. Parkin, D.M., Pisani, P. and Ferlay, J. (1993). Estimates of the worldwide incidence of eighteen major cancers in 1985. *Int. J. Cancer*, **54**, 594–606
3. Pisani, P., Parkin, D.M. and Ferlay, J. (1993). Estimates of the worldwide mortality from eighteen major cancers in 1985. Implications for prevention and projections of future burden. *Int. J. Cancer*, **55**, 891–903
4. Newhouse, M.L., Pearson, R.M., Fullerton, J.M., Boesen, E.A. and Shannon, H.S. (1977). A case–control study of carcinoma of the ovary. *Br. J. Prev. Soc. Med.*, **31**, 148–53
5. Casagrande, J.T., Louie, E.W., Pike, M.C., Roy, S., Ross, R.K. and Henderson, B.E. (1979). 'Incessant ovulation' and ovarian cancer. *Lancet*, **2**, 170–3

6. Hildreth, N.G., Kelsey, J.L., LiVolsi, V.A., Fischer, D.B., Holford, T.R., Mostow, E.D., Schwartz, P.E. and White, C. (1981). An epidemiologic study of epithelial carcinoma of the ovary. *Am. J. Epidemiol.*, **114**, 398–405

7. Weiss, N.S., Lyon, J.L., Liff, J.M., Vollmer, W.M. and Daling, J.R. (1981). Incidence of ovarian cancer in relation to the use of oral contraceptives. *Int. J. Cancer*, **28**, 669–71

8. Cramer, D.W., Hutchinson, G.B., Welch, W.R., Scully, R.E. and Knapp, R.C. (1982). Factors affecting the association of oral contraceptives and ovarian cancer. *N. Engl. J. Med.*, **307**, 1047–51

9. Rosenberg, L., Shapiro, S., Slone, D., Kaufman, D.W., Helmrich, S.P., Miettinen, O.S., Stolley, P.D., Rosenshein, N.B., Schottenfield, D. and Engle, R.L. Jr. (1982). Epithelial ovarian cancer and combination oral contraceptives. *J. Am. Med. Assoc.*, **247**, 3210–12

10. Tzonou, A., Day, N.E., Trichopoulos, D., Walker, A., Saliaraki, M., Papapostolou, M. and Polychronopoulou, A. (1984). The epidemiology of ovarian cancer in Greece: a case–control study. *Eur. J. Cancer Clin. Oncol.*, **20**, 1045–52

11. La Vecchia, C., Decarli, A., Fasoli, M., Franceschi, S., Gentile, A., Negri, E., Parazzini, F. and Tognoni, G. (1986). Oral contraceptives and cancers of the breast and of the female genital tract: interim results from a case–control study. *Br. J. Cancer*, **54**, 311–17

12. Cancer and Steroid Hormone Study of the Centers for Disease Control and the National Institute of Child Health and Human Development (1987). The reduction in risk of ovarian cancer associated with oral contraceptive use. *N. Engl. J. Med.*, **316**, 650–5

13. Harlow, B.L., Weiss, N.S., Roth, G.J., Chu, J. and Daling, J.R. (1988). Case–control study of borderline ovarian tumors: reproductive history and exposure to exogenous female hormone. *Cancer Res.*, **48**, 5849–52

14. Wu, M.L., Whittemore, A.S., Paffenbarger, R.S. Jr, Sarles, D.L., Kampert, J.B., Grossner, S., Jung, D.L., Ballon, S., Hendrickson, M. and Mohle-Boetani, J. (1988). Personal and environmental characteristics related to epithelial ovarian cancer. I. Reproductive and menstrual events and oral contraceptive use. *Am. J. Epidemiol.*, **128**, 1216–27

15. Booth, M., Beral, V. and Smith, P. (1989). Risk factors for ovarian cancer: a case–control study. *Br. J. Cancer*, **60**, 592–8

16. Hartge, P., Schiffman, M.H., Hoover, R., McGowan, L., Lesher, L. and Norris, H.J. (1989). A case–control study of epithelial ovarian cancer. *Am. J. Obstet. Gynecol.*, **161**, 10–16

17. Shu, X.-O., Brinton, L.A., Gao, Y.T. and Yuan, J.M. (1989). Population-based case–control study of ovarian cancer in Shanghai. *Cancer Res.*, **49**, 3670–4

18. WHO Collaborative Study of Neoplasia and Steroid Contraceptives (1989). Epithelial ovarian cancer and combined oral contraceptives. *Int. J. Epidemiol.*, **18**, 538–45

19. Gwinn, M.L., Lee, N.C., Rhodes, P.H., Layde, P.M. and Rubin, G.L. (1990). Pregnancy, breast feeding, and oral contraceptives and the risk of epithelial ovarian cancer. *J. Clin. Epidemiol.*, **43**, 559–68

20. Harlow, B.L., Cramer, D.W., Geller, J., Willett, W.C., Bell, D.A. and Welch, W.R. (1991). The influence of lactose consumption on the association of oral contraceptive use and ovarian cancer risk. *Am. J. Epidemiol.*, **134**, 445–53

21. Parazzini, F., La Vecchia, C., Negri, E., Bocciolone, L., Fedele, L. and Franceschi, S. (1991). Oral contraceptive use and the risk of ovarian cancer: an Italian case–control study. *Eur. J. Cancer*, **27**, 594–8

22. Risch, H.A., Marrett, L.D. and Howe, G.R. (1994). Parity, contraception, infertility, and the risk of epithelial ovarian cancer. *Am. J. Epidemiol.*, **140**, 585–97

23. Rosenberg, L., Palmer, J.R., Zauber, A.G., Warshauer, M.E., Lewis, J.L. Jr, Strom, B.L., Harlap, S. and Shapiro, S. (1994). A case–control study of oral contraceptive use and invasive epithelial ovarian cancer. *Am. J. Epidemiol.*, **139**, 654–61

24. Ramcharan, S., Pellegrin, F.A., Ray, R. and Hsu, J.P. (1981). *A Prospective Study of the Side Effects of Oral Contraceptives. The Walnut Creek Contraceptive Study*, Vol. 3. NIH Publication No. 81-564 (Bethesda: National Institute of Health)

25. Willett, W.C., Bain, C., Hennekens, C.H., Rosner, B. and Speizer, F.E. (1981). Oral contraceptives and risk of ovarian cancer. *Cancer*, **48**, 1684–7

26. Beral, V., Hannaford, P. and Kay, C. (1988). Oral contraceptive use and malignancies of the genital tract. Results from The Royal College of General Practitioners' Oral Contraception Study. *Lancet*, **2**, 1331–5

27. Vessey, M.P. and Painter, R. (1995). Endometrial and ovarian cancer and oral contraceptives – findings in a large cohort study. *Br. J. Cancer*, **71**, 1340–2

28. La Vecchia, C., Franceschi, S., Bruzzi, P., Parazzini, F. and Boyle, P. (1990). The relationship between oral contraceptive use, cancer and vascular disease. *Drug Safety*, **5**, 436–46

29. Franceschi, S., Parazzini, F., Negri, E., Booth, M., La Vecchia, C., Beral, V., Tzonou, A. and Trichopoulos, D. (1991). Pooled analysis of 3 European case–control studies of epithelial ovarian cancer. III. Oral contraceptive use. *Int. J. Cancer*, **49**, 61–5

30. Whittemore, A.S., Harris, R., Itnyre, J. and the Collaborative Ovarian Cancer Group (1992). Characteristics relating to ovarian cancer risk:

collaborative analysis of 12 US case–control studies. II. Invasive epithelial ovarian cancers in white women. *Am. J. Epidemiol.*, **136**, 1184–203

31. Rosenblatt, K.A., Thomas, D.B., Noonan, E.A. and the WHO Collaborative Study of Neoplasia and Steroid Contraceptives (1992). High-dose and low-dose combined oral contraceptives: protection against epithelial ovarian cancer and the length of the protective effect. *Eur. J. Cancer*, **28A**, 1872–6

32. Harris, R., Whittemore, A.S., Itnyre, J. and the Collaborative Ovarian Cancer Group (1992). Characteristics relating to ovarian cancer risk: collaborative analysis of 12 US case–control studies. III. Epithelial tumors of low malignant potential in white women. *Am. J. Epidemiol.*, **136**, 1204–11

33. Horn-Ross, P.L., Whittemore, A.S., Harris, R., Itnyre, J., Casagrande, J.T., Cramer, D.W., Hartge, P., Kelsey, J.L., Lee, M., Lee, N.C., Lyon, J.L., Marshall, J.R., McGowan, L., Nasca, P.C., Paffenbarger, R.S. Jr, Rosenberg, L., Weiss, N.S. and Copley, G.D. (1992). Characteristics relating to ovarian cancer risk. Collaborative analysis of twelve US case–control studies. VI. Nonepithelial cancers among adults. *Epidemiology*, **3**, 490–5

34. Kaufman, D.W., Shapiro, S., Slone, D., Rosenberg, L., Miettinen, O.S., Stolley, P.D., Knapp, R.C., Leavitt, T. Jr, Watring, W.G., Rosenshein, N.B., Lewis, J.L. Jr, Schottenfeld, D. and Engle, R.L. Jr (1980). Decreased risk of endometrial cancer among oral-contraceptive users. *N. Engl. J. Med.*, **303**, 1045–7

35. Weiss, N.S. and Sayvetz, T.A. (1980). Incidence of endometrial cancer in relation to the use of oral contraceptives. *N. Engl. J. Med.*, **302**, 551–4

36. Hulka, B.S., Chambless, L.E., Kaufmann, D.G., Fowler, W.C. Jr and Greenberg, B.G. (1982). Protection against endometrial carcinoma by combination-product oral contraceptives. *J. Am. Med. Assoc.*, **247**, 475–7

37. Kelsey, J.L., LiVolsi, V.A., Holford, T.R., Fischer, D.B., Mostow, E.D., Schwartz, P.E., O'Connor, T. and White, C. (1982). A case–control study of cancer of the endometrium. *Am. J. Epidemiol.*, **116**, 333–42

38. Henderson, B.E., Casagrande, J.T., Pike, M.C., Mack, T., Rosario, I. and Duke, A. (1983). The epidemiology of endometrial cancer in young women. *Br. J. Cancer*, **47**, 749–56

39. CASH (Cancer and Steroid Hormone Study of the Centers for Disease Control and the National Institute of Child Health and Human Development) (1987). Combination oral contraceptive use and the risk of endometrial cancer. *J. Am. Med. Assoc.*, **257**, 796–800

40. WHO Collaborative Study of Neoplasia and Steroid Contraceptives (1988). Endometrial cancer and combined oral contraceptives. *Int. J. Epidemiol.*, **17**, 263–9

41. Koumantakis, Y., Tzonou, A., Koumantakis, E., Kaklamani, E., Aravantinos, D. and Trichopoulos, D. (1989). A case–control study of cancer of endometrium in Athens. *Int. J. Cancer*, **43**, 795–9

42. Levi, F., La Vecchia, C., Gulie, C., Negri, E., Monnier, V. and Franceschi, S. (1991). Oral contraceptives and the risk of endometrial cancer. *Cancer Causes Control*, **2**, 99–103

43. Shu, X-O., Brinton, L.A., Zheng, W., Gao, Y.T., Fan, J. and Fraumeni, J.F. Jr (1991). A population-based case–control study of endometrial cancer in Shanghai, China. *Int. J. Cancer*, **49**, 38–43

44. Jick, S.S., Walker, A.M. and Jick, H. (1993). Oral contraceptives and endometrial cancer. *Obstet. Gynecol.*, **82**, 931–5

45. Stanford, J.L., Brinton, L.A., Berman, M.L., Mortel, R., Twiggs, L.B., Barrett, R.J., Wilbanks, G.D. and Hoover, R.N. (1993). Oral contraceptives and endometrial cancer: do other risk factors modify the association? *Int. J. Cancer*, **54**, 243–8

46. Voight, L.F., Deng, Q. and Weiss, N.S. (1994). Recency, duration, and progestin content of oral contraceptives in relation to the incidence of endometrial cancer (Washington, USA). *Cancer Causes Control*, **5**, 227–33

47. Trapido, E.J. (1983). A prospective cohort study of oral contraceptives and cancer of the endometrium. *Int. J. Epidemiol.*, **12**, 297–300

48. Rosenblatt, K.A., Thomas, D.B. and The WHO Collaborative Study of Neoplasia and Steroid Contraceptives (1991). Hormonal content of combined oral contraceptives in relation to the reduced risk of endometrial carcinoma. *Int. J. Cancer*, **49**, 870–4

49. Schlesselman, J.J. (1995). Net effect of oral contraceptive use on the risk of cancer in women in the United States. *Obstet. Gynecol.*, **85**, 793–801

13

The association between oral contraceptive use and neoplasia of the cervix, vagina and vulva

K.L. Irwin

INTRODUCTION

The literature about the effect of oral contraceptives (OCs) on the risk of neoplasia of the uterine cervix, vagina and vulva is extensive and complex. This brief review focuses on studies of combined OCs published during this decade and complements previous reviews of earlier reports[1–4].

CERVICAL NEOPLASIA

Invasive cervical cancer is the second most common cancer among women world-wide and the most common cause of cancer among women in developing countries[5]. More than 80% of cervical neoplasia is of squamous cell origin. Preinvasive lesions of cervical dysplasia and carcinoma *in situ* (i.e. various grades of cervical intraepithelial neoplasia (CIN) or squamous intraepithelial neoplasia (SIL)) often precede the appearance of invasive cancer and therefore are considered early stages of a continuum of disease. Numerous risk factors for cervical neoplasia have been proposed (Table 1)[6]. Most experts believe that human papillomavirus (HPV) is necessary

145

Table 1 Reported risk factors for neoplasia of the cervix, vagina and vulva

Cervix
Human papillomavirus infection
Multiple sex partners
Sex partner with multiple sex partners
History of condyloma
Cervical dysplasia
Other viral genital infections (i.e. herpes simplex virus, human
  immunodeficiency virus)
Non-use of barrier contraceptives
? Oral contraceptive use
Nutritional deficiencies
Smoking

Vagina
HPV infection
Diethylstilbestrol exposure *in utero* (clear cell adenocarcinoma)
Chronic irritation (e.g. from pessaries)
Immunosuppressive therapy
Cervical neoplasia
Cervical radiation
Endometriosis
Previous hysterectomy for benign disease
Advanced age

Vulva
HPV infection
Chronic inflammatory disorders of the vulva
Compromised immunity
History of cervical neoplasia
Early age at menarche
Obesity
Diabetes
Smoking
Advanced age

for the development of most cervical neoplasia, possibly as an initiator of carcinogenesis[6]. However, other factors may be necessary for neoplasia to occur[6,7].

Despite extensive research on the association between OC use and cervical neoplasia, many experts remain uncertain if OC use increases risk. Many studies have suffered from one or more methodological limitation that might lead to spuriously increased or decreased risk estimates[1,2]. OC use may be associated with factors that influence the risk of cervical neoplasia, especially the sexual behavior of the women and their sex partners and the risk of exposure to HPV, and studies have inconsistently ascertained and controlled for these potentially confounding factors. OC users are more likely than non-users to have regular cervical smears because cytological screening is routinely offered as part of many family planning programs. More frequent screening of OC users would result in a relatively greater detection of preinvasive disease. Studies that have not adequately controlled for screening histories would find a spuriously increased risk of preinvasive disease among OC users and, if preinvasive disease were detected and treated earlier in OC users, a spuriously decreased risk of invasive disease. The use of inappropriate comparison groups has made some case–control and cohort studies difficult to interpret. For example, OC users may be overrepresented among hospitalized control patients as compared with population-based control patients. Studies comparing OC users with users of barrier methods (who are at reduced risk of cervical neoplasia) or with users of no contraceptive method (who may be at increased risk of neoplasia) may have yielded distorted risk estimates. Finally, until recently, most studies lacked data on HPV infection and thus could not assess the interaction of OCs and HPV.

These methodological concerns notwithstanding, several plausible mechanisms for a biological influence of OCs on cervical carcinogenesis have been proposed. Cervical cells are endowed with hormone receptors and undergo histological changes when OCs are used[2]. Steroids can promote development of cervical cancer in animals[2]. OCs may promote the carcinogenic effects of HPV by enhancing viral transcription or virus-induced cell transformation or by producing folate deficiency[2,8,9]. OCs may also heighten a woman's susceptibility to sexually transmitted infections by enlarging the area of cervical ectopy, changing cervical mucus, or altering immune response[2,10,11].

More than 50 case–control, cohort and cross-sectional studies have evaluated the association between OCs and invasive cancer, carcinoma *in situ*, or cervical dysplasia in the last two decades. Most studies have addressed the squamous cell type. The case–control and cohort studies published since 1990 have focused on combined OC users (Table 2)[12–31]. While some of these recent studies found no increased risk of invasive or *in situ* carcinoma associated with ever having used OCs, several studies have found that such use is associated with modestly increased risks: relative risk estimates have ranged from 1.3 to 2.2 in most well-controlled studies. Two recent studies of women with documented HPV infection found that the risk of invasive cancer was as much as six times greater among OC users than among non-users[13,14]. Another study of HPV-infected women suggests that risk of CIN III was twice as great among OC users than among non-users, although this difference was not statistically significant[15]. These findings are consistent with at least three earlier studies that found that the risk of neoplasia associated with OC use was higher among women with genital infections or multiple sex partners than among women without these characteristics[28,32,33]. These studies provide further evidence that OCs may promote carcinogenesis through interaction with HPV.

Several recent studies also support earlier findings that the risk of cervical neoplasia increases with longer duration of OC use and that increased risk is confined to women who have used OCs for 5 or more years, with risk estimated at nearly twice that of non-users in studies that controlled for the differences in sexual and cytological screening behaviors between OC users and non-users[20,22–26,28–30]. However, recent studies of the effects of age at first OC use remain conflicting: some indicate that women who first used the pill before age 18 are approximately twice as likely as those who never used it to develop invasive cancer[13,19], while other studies have observed no increased risk in this subgroup[17,18,22]. Thus, it remains uncertain if OC exposure at a critical period in the development of a woman's cervix influences the risk of neoplasia. Most studies that examined risk by recency of use found that the risk of high-grade intraepithelial neoplasia and *in situ* carcinoma was greater among current and recent users than among past users[18,22,30]. Enhanced cytological screening of OC users, i.e. detection bias, may explain this observation because CIN is usually diagnosed with routine cytology. However, late-stage carcinogenic effects of OCs cannot be ruled out.

Table 2 Recent studies of the relation between OC use and cervical cancer

First author	Disease type*	Number of cases	Adjusted relative risk estimate (95% CI)[†]
Squamous cell			
Becker[12]	CIN II/III	374	0.4 (0.2–0.9)
Bosch[13]	invasive	432	1.3 (0.9–2.0) (among all women)
		160	6.5 (1.3–31.4) (among HPV-infected women)[‡]
Brinton[16]	invasive	667	1.1 (0.8–1.5)
Brisson[17]	low-grade CIN	338	1.1 (0.6–1.9)
	high-grade CIN	546	1.4 (0.8–2.4)[‡]
Coker[18]	CIN II and III	103	0.7 (0.3–1.6)
Daling[19]	invasive	314	1.0 (0.6–1.6)[‡]
de Vet[20]	CIN I-III	257	2.3 (1.2–4.6)[‡]
Eluf-Neto[14]	invasive	197	1.3 (0.7–2.3)[‡]
		157	increased risk (among HPV-infected women)
Gram[21]	CIN I-III	401	1.5 (1.1–2.1)**
Jones[22]	*in situ*	293	1.8 (1.0–3.4)[‡]
Kjaer[23]	*in situ*	586	1.4 (0.9–2.1)[‡]
	invasive	59	1.3 (0.5–3.3)[‡]
Kohler[24]	CIN/invasive	309	3.5 ($p < 0.05$)[‡]
Mandelson[25]	invasive	140	2.2 (0.9–5.2)[‡]
Muñoz[15]	CIN III	249	1.3 (0.7–2.3)
Negrini[26]	high-grade SIL	19	2.7 (includes 1.0)[‡]
	low-grade SIL	208	0.9 (includes 1.0)[‡]
New Zealand Group[27]	dysplasia/carcinoma	318	no increased risk compared to IUD and MPA users**
Parazzini[28]	invasive	367	1.9 (1.0–3.1)[‡]
WHO[29]	invasive	998	1.3 (1.1–1.5)[‡]
Ye[30]	*in situ*	1110	1.3 (1.2–1.5)[‡]
Adenocarcinoma			
Brinton[16]	invasive	61	2.4 (1.3–4.6)
Daling[††]	*in situ*	54	2.0 (0.9–4.9)[‡]
Daling[††]	invasive	93	0.7 (0.4–1.2)
Ursin[31]	invasive	176	2.1 (1.1–3.8)[‡]

*CIN I, mild dysplasia; CIN II, moderate dysplasia; CIN III, severe dysplasia and carcinoma *in situ*; low-grade SIL, mild dysplasia; high-grade SIL, moderate and severe dysplasia and carcinoma *in situ*; [†]except where noted, all studies were of case–control design. Relative risk estimates adjusted for confounding factors are reported when available. Case number reflects number included in adjusted analyses when reported. 95% CI indicates 95% confidence interval; [‡]increased risk evident in long-term users only or risk increased with longer duration of use; **cohort study design; [††]unpublished data from ongoing study, J.R. Daling, personal communication, 1996

The effects of specific OC dosage and brands have not been studied in enough depth to draw meaningful conclusions at this time. At least two studies found increased risk of invasive and *in situ* carcinoma among women using OC formulations with high estrogen potency[32,33], although the effects of dose and duration of use were difficult to distinguish. However, as noted above, several studies have shown that users of lower-dose combined OCs used over the last two decades are also at modestly increased risk.

The effects of OC use on adenocarcinoma, which constitutes less than 20% of reported cervical cancer[6], have been less thoroughly studied. Several studies before 1990 concluded that the risk of adenocarcinoma associated with OC use was higher than the risk of squamous cell cancer[16,32], but other studies found no difference by histological type[1]. Studies published since 1990 also suggest an increased risk associated with OC use (Table 2)[16,24,31]. Preliminary data from the most recent US study of adenocarcinoma demonstrate that ever having used OCs is not associated with invasive adenocarcinoma. These data, however, suggest that women who use OCs for 5 or more years may have an increased risk of adenocarcinoma *in situ* (relative risk, RR 2.3, 95% confidence interval [CI]: 1.0–5.7) (J.R. Daling, personal communication, 1996). Some have proposed that the microglandular hyperplasia associated with OC use may be related to the development of adenocarcinoma[2].

VAGINAL NEOPLASIA

Vaginal cancer represents about 2% of gynecological malignancies. About 90% of tumors are of the squamous cell type[3]. Several risk factors for the squamous cell type, including HPV infection and prior cervical cancer, have been identified (Table 1)[3]. Only a few small studies have examined the effects of OC use because vaginal cancer remains extremely rare among women young enough to have used OCs during their reproductive years. To date, there is no evidence from published[34] or ongoing studies (J.R. Daling, personal communication, 1996) that ever-use or long-term use of OCs increases risk of *in situ* or invasive cancer.

Adenocarcinoma of the vagina, a rare histological type, has been linked with several risk factors, many of which are also associated with the squamous cell type[3]. *In utero* exposure to diethylstilbestrol is the only hormonal factor to be associated with incidence of vaginal adenocarcinoma[3]. There is no evidence that OCs affect the risk of this histological type.

VULVAR NEOPLASIA

Although invasive vulvar cancer is rare – constituting about 4% of genital tract malignancies – the incidence of high-grade vulvar intraepithelial neoplasia (VIN) in the United States has been increasing over the last two decades[35]. A clear progression from VIN to invasive disease is not well established because a considerable proportion of VIN may regress spontaneously[35]. About 80–90% of vulvar neoplasia is of the squamous cell type[35]. Various risk factors for the squamous type have been proposed (Table 1)[4]. Invasive disease may have multiple etiologies. Specifically, HPV appears to be associated with neoplasia in young women, especially those who smoke and have concurrent VIN. HPV does not seem to be associated with neoplasia among older women who do not smoke and lack concurrent VIN[35]. HPV has also been associated with some but not all histological types[4].

Few studies have addressed the effects of OC use on vulvar neoplasia because the disease is rare among women young enough to have used OCs. One study in 1984 found that women who had used OCs for 1–5 years were twice as likely as women who had never used OCs or had used them for less than a year to develop *in situ* carcinoma[36]. The risk was four times greater in women who had used OCs for 5 or more years. This study could not evaluate risk of invasive cancer because of the small number of case patients, but later studies that included larger numbers of women who used combined OCs have found no relation with *in situ* or invasive disease[37,38]. Preliminary data, however, from an ongoing case–control study of *in situ* carcinoma suggest a possibly increased risk among women who have used OCs for 5 or more years (RR 1.5, 95% CI 0.9–2.6) and who first used OCs before age 18 (RR 2.3, 95% CI 1.4–3.9) (J.R. Daling, personal communication, 1996).

SUMMARY OF RECENT LITERATURE

Like studies before 1990, recent studies of the association between OC use and cervical neoplasia are inconclusive because of methodological shortcomings and conflicting results. They provide, however, growing evidence that OC users, especially those who use OCs for 5 or more years, may be at a modestly increased risk of *in situ* and invasive carcinoma of the cervix of both the squamous cell and adenocarcinoma type. Recent research would support the conclusion of the 1992 WHO Scientific Group on Oral Contraceptives and Neoplasia that 'The extent to which this [increased risk] reflects a biological relationship is uncertain, particularly given the absence of reliable information on the role of possible infectious agents, such as HPV'[1]. Since 1992, evidence for HPV's role in cervical carcinogenesis has strengthened considerably, highlighting the need to address OC–HPV interactions in future studies. There is virtually no evidence that OC use increases risk of vaginal or vulvar neoplasia, although few studies have addressed these rare tumors. However, because vaginal and vulvar neoplasia are often associated with cervical neoplasia and HPV infection, an influence of OCs on primary tumors in these organs (possibly through interactions with HPV) cannot be ruled out without further study.

SCREENING AND PREVENTION OF NEOPLASIA OF THE LOWER GENITAL TRACT

Given these inconclusive data, how should clinicians approach screening for these malignancies among OC users? We are fortunate to have effective tools (i.e. cytology and colposcopy) for early detection of cervical cancer as well as reasonably sensitive methods for identifying women with genital HPV infection which increases a woman's risk for these malignancies. Periodic pelvic examination, that includes careful inspection of the entire perineum, vagina, cervix, and anus and cervical cytology are recommended for all sexually active women. Several groups have published recommendations regarding the frequency of cervical cytology[39]. While some recommendations have cautioned that women at high risk for cervical cancer may require screening at more frequent than standard intervals until they establish a pattern of normal smears, none has specifically defined OC users as being at high risk. (Chapter 14 discusses cervical cytology among OC users at length.) Available data do not support regular screening for vaginal or vulvar cancer (with either cytology or colposcopy) among current OC users because these malignancies are so rare in premenopausal women. However, the finding, that vaginal neoplasia is often diagnosed through abnormal cytology before symptoms arise, argues that periodic vaginal cytology in women with risk factors for this malignancy (especially those with anogenital warts, subclinical HPV infection, or cervical neoplasia) may be beneficial. Because vulvar neoplasia is often preceded by lesions or symptoms that a woman can readily detect, it is prudent to encourage women at high risk for this disease to periodically inspect their external genitalia (e.g. at the time of breast self-examination) and to report abnormalities to their clinician to allow for early biopsy of suspicious lesions. Finally, clinicians have an opportunity to prevent neoplasia of the cervix, vagina and vulva by counselling patients to avoid high-risk sexual behavior, to abstain from smoking, and to use barrier contraceptives that prevent exposure to sexually transmitted diseases.

REFERENCES

1. World Health Organization (1992). *Oral Contraceptives and Neoplasia: Report of a WHO Scientific Group*, WHO Technical Report Series 718, pp. 12–15. (Geneva: World Health Organization)
2. Brinton, L.A. (1991). Oral contraceptives and cervical neoplasia. *Contraception*, **43**, 581–95
3. Merino, M.J. (1991). Vaginal cancer: the role of infectious and environmental factors. *Am. J. Obstet. Gynecol.*, **165**, 1255–62
4. Crum, C.P. (1992). Carcinoma of the vulva: epidemiology and pathogenesis. *Obstet. Gynecol.*, **79**, 448–54
5. Tomatis, L. (ed.) (1990). *Cancer: Causes, Occurrence and Control.* (Lyon: International Agency for Research on Cancer), IARC Scientific Publications No. 100
6. Shiffman, M.H., Brinton, L.A., Devesa, S.S. and Fraumeni, J. (1996). Cervical cancer. In Schottenfeld, D. and Fraumeni, J. (eds.) *Cancer*

Epidemiology and Prevention, 2nd edn. (New York: Oxford University Press) In press

7. McDougall, J.K. (1994). Cofactors in the progression of HPV-associated tumors. In Giraldo, G., Salvatore, M., Chieco-Bianchi, L. and Beth-Giraldo, E. (eds.) *Advanced Technologies in Research, Diagnosis, and Treatment of AIDS in Oncology*, pp. 150–64. (Basel: Karger)

8. Mittal, R., Tsutsumi, K., Pater, A. and Pater, M.M. (1993). Human papillomavirus type 16 expression in cervical keratinocytes: role of progesterone and glucocorticoid hormones. *Obstet. Gynecol.*, **81**, 5–12

9. Pater, A., Bayatpour, M. and Pater, M.M. (1990). Oncogenic transformation by human papillomavirus type 16 deoxyribonucleic acid in the presence of progesterone or progestins from oral contraceptives. *Am. J. Obstet. Gynecol.*, **162**, 1099–103

10. Louv, W.C., Austin, H., Perlman, H. and Alexander, W.J. (1989). Oral contraceptive use and the risk of chlamydial and gonococcal infections. *Am. J. Obstet. Gynecol.*, **160**, 396–402

11. Franceschi, S., La Vecchia, C. and Talamini, R. (1986). Oral contraceptives and cervical neoplasia: pooled information from retrospective and prospective epidemiologic studies. *Tumori*, **72**, 21–30

12. Becker, T.M., Wheeler, C.M., McGouch, N.S., Stidley, C.A., Parmenter, C.A., Dorin, M.H. and Jordan, S.W. (1994). Contraceptive and reproductive risks for cervical dysplasia in southwestern Hispanic and non-Hispanic white women. *Int. J. Epidemiol.*, **23**, 913–22

13. Bosch, F.X., Muñoz, N., de Sanjose, S., Isarzugaza, I., Gili, M., Viladiu, P., Tormo, M.J., Moreo, P., Ascunce, N., Gonzalez, L.C., Tafur, L., Kaldor, J.M., Guerrero, E., Aristizabal, N., Santamaria, M., Alonso de Ruiz, P. and Shah, K. (1992). Risk factors for cervical cancer in Colombia and Spain. *Int. J. Cancer*, **52**, 750–8

14. Eluf-Neto, J., Booth, M., Muñoz, N., Bosch, F.X., Meijer, C.J.L.M. and Walboomers, J.M.M. (1994). Human papillomavirus and invasive cervical cancer in Brazil. *Br. J. Cancer*, **69**, 114–19

15. Muñoz, N., Bosch, F.X., de Sanjose, S., Vergara, A., del Moral, A., Muñoz, M.T., Tafur, L., Gili, M., Izarzugaza, I., Viladiu, P., Navarro, C., Alonso de Ruiz, P., Aristizabel, N., Santamaria, M., Orfila, J., Daniel, R.W., Guerroro, E. and Shah, K.V. (1993). Risk factors for cervical intraepithelial neoplasia grade III/carcinoma *in situ* in Spain and Columbia. *Cancer Epidemiol. Biomarkers Prevention*, **2**, 423–31

16. Brinton, L.A., Reeves, W.C., Brenes, M.M., Herrero, R., DeBritton, R.C., Gaitan, E., Tenorio, F., Garcia, M. and Rawls, W.E. (1990). Oral contraceptive use and risk of invasive cervical cancer. *Int. J. Epidemiol.*, **19**, 4–11

17. Brisson, J., Morin, C., Fortier, M., Roy, M., Bouchard, C., Leclerc, J., Christen, A., Guimont, C., Penault, F. and Meisels, A. (1994). Risk factors for cervical intraepithelial neoplasia: differences between low- and high-grade lesions. *Am. J. Epidemiol.*, **140**, 700–10

18. Coker, A.L., McCann, M.F., Hulka, B.S. and Walton, L.A. (1992). Oral contraceptive use and cervical intraepithelial neoplasia. *J. Clin. Epidemiol.*, **45**, 1111–18

19. Daling, J.R., Madeleine, M.M., McKnight, B., Carter, J.J., Ashley, R., Schwartz, S.M., Beckmann, A.M., Hagensee, M.E., Mandelson, M.T. and Galloway, D.A. (1996). The relationship of human papillomavirus-related cervical tumors to cigarette smoking, oral contraceptive use, and prior Herpes Simplex-2 infection (submitted)

20. de Vet, H.C., Knipschild, P.G. and Sturmans, F. (1993). The role of sexual factors in the aetiology of cervical dysplasia. *Int. J. Epidemiol.*, **22**, 798–803

21. Gram, I.T., Macaluso, M. and Stalsberg, H. (1992). Oral contraceptive use and the incidence of cervical intraepithelial neoplasia. *Am. J. Obstet. Gynecol.*, **167**, 40–4

22. Jones, C.J., Brinton, L.A., Hamman, R.F., Stolley, P.D., Lehman, H.F., Levine, R.S. and Mallin, K. (1990). Risk factors for *in situ* cervical cancer: results from a case–control study. *Cancer Res.*, **50**, 3657–62

23. Kjaer, S.K., Engholm, G., Dahl, C., Bock, J.E., Lynge, E. and Jensen, O.M. (1993). Case–control study of risk factors for cervical squamous-cell neoplasia in Denmark. III. Role of oral contraceptive use. *Cancer Causes and Control*, **4**, 513–19

24. Kohler, U. and Wuttke, P. (1994). Results of a case–control study of the current effect of various factors of cervical cancer risk. 2. Contraceptive behavior and the smoking factor. *Zentralbl. Gynakol.*, **116**, 405–9

25. Mandelson, M.T., Daling, J.R., White, E., Chu, J. and McKnight, B. (1990). Further evidence that duration and recency of oral contraceptive use are associated with invasive cervical cancer. *Am. J. Epidemiol.*, **132**, 77B (abstract)

26. Negrini, B.P., Schiffman, M.H., Kurman, R.J., Barnes, W., Lannom, L., Malley, K., Brinton, L.A., Delgado, G., Jones, S., Tchabo, J.G. and Lancaster, W.D. (1990). Oral contraceptive use, human papillomavirus infection, and risk of early cytologic abnormalities of the cervix. *Cancer Res.*, **50**, 4670–5

27. The New Zealand Contraception and Health Study Group (1994). Risk of cervical dysplasia in users of oral contraceptives, intrauterine devices or depot-medroxyprogesterone acetate. *Contraception*, **50**, 431–41

28. Parazzini, F., La Vecchia, C., Negri, E. and Maggi, R. (1990). Oral contraceptive use and invasive cervical cancer. *Int. J. Epidemiol.*, **19**, 259–63

29. WHO Collaborative Study of Neoplasia and Steroid Contraceptives (1993). Invasive squamous-cell cervical carcinoma and combined oral contraceptives: results from a multinational study. *Int. J. Cancer*, **55**, 228–36

30. Ye, A., Thomas, D.B. and Ray, R.M. (1995). Combined oral contraceptives and risk of cervical carcinoma *in situ*. WHO collaborative study of neoplasia and steroid contraceptives. *Int. J. Epidemiol.*, **24**, 19–26

31. Ursin, G., Peters, R.K., Henderson, B.E., d'Ablaing, G., Monroe, K.R. and Pike, M.C. (1994). Oral contraceptive use and adenocarcinoma of cervix. *Lancet*, **344**, 1390–4

32. Brinton, L.A., Huggins, G.R., Lehman, H.F., Jallin, K., Savitz, D.A., Trapido, E., Rosenthal, J. and Hoover, R. (1986). Long-term use of oral contraceptives and risk of invasive cervical cancer. *Int. J. Cancer*, **38**, 339–44

33. Brock, K.E., Berry, G., Brinton, L.A., Kerr, C., MacLennan, R., Mock, P.A. and Shearman, R.P. (1989). Sexual, reproductive, and contraceptive risk factors for carcinoma *in situ* of the uterine cervix in Sydney. *Med. J. Aust.*, **150**, 125–30

34. Brinton, L.A., Nasca, P.C., Mallin, K., Schairer, C., Rosenthal, J., Rothenberg, R., Yordan, E. and Richart, R.M. (1990). Case–control study of *in situ* and invasive carcinoma of the vagina. *Gynecol. Oncol.*, **38**, 49–56

35. Hacker, N.F. (1994). Vulvar cancer. In Berek, J.S. and Hacker, N.F. (eds.) *Practical Gynecologic Oncology*, pp. 403–40. (Baltimore: Williams and Wilkins)

36. Newcomb, P.A., Weiss, N.S. and Daling, J.R. (1984). Incidence of vulvar carcinoma in relation to menstrual, reproductive, and medical factors. *J. Natl. Cancer Inst.*, **73**, 391–6

37. Brinton, L.A., Nasca, P.C., Mallin, K., Baptiste, M.S., Wilbanks, G.D. and Richard, R.W. (1990). Case–control study of cancer of the vulva. *Obstet. Gynecol.*, **75**, 859–65

38. Sherman, K.J., Daling, J.R., McKnight, B. and Chu, J. (1994). Hormonal factors in vulvar cancer: a case–control study. *J. Reprod. Med.*, **39**, 857–61

39. US Preventive Services Task Force (1996). Screening for cervical cancer. In *Guide to Clinical Preventive Services*, 2nd edn., pp. 105–17. (Baltimore: Williams and Wilkins)

14

Cervical smears: when to start and how often to do

E. Buiatti

INTRODUCTION

The most appropriate age for starting Papanicolaou screening for cervical cancer, and the optimum time interval between tests have been widely debated during the last decade. The choice is not just a matter of maximizing the use of available resources. An appropriate (too early and/or intensive) screening program is likely to produce undesired or adverse effects, in addition to having a low cost–benefit ratio. In general, the age at starting and frequency of screening should be allowed to vary depending on the local availability of resources and organizational infrastructure, and on the characteristics of the population at risk. Thus, instead of defining specific starting ages and time intervals between tests, it may be better to produce criteria which may guide decision-making at the local level. A list of variables which need to be considered when establishing these screening characteristics is presented here, with special reference to pill users.

COMPLIANCE OF HIGH-RISK WOMEN

At present, users of combined oral contraceptives may be considered to be a group at moderately increased risk of developing

157

invasive cervical squamous cancer. For example, the relative risks among these women compared with the general population were estimated to be around 1.3 in a large international multicenter hospital-based case–control study, which included both high and medium–low risk areas[1]. Similarly, pill users have been shown to experience a moderately elevated risk of cervical dysplasia and carcinoma *in situ* compared to non-users[2,3]. Although significant, excess risk of cervical invasive carcinoma among pill users is much lower than geographical differences between high and low incidence areas, rate ratios between high and low incidence countries being approximately 12-fold (Brazil, Goiania: world standardized rate = 48.9 per 100 000 women; Israel, all Jews: world standardized rate = 4.2 per 100 000 women)[4].

High-risk populations and high-risk subgroups should represent a particular target group for a screening program. The participation by a large number of high-risk subjects should result in a significant impact on the incidence rates of invasive cancer and cause-specific mortality at a population level, as well as achieving a large positive test/total tests ratio and a gain in the cost–benefit ratio[5]. Indeed, the main factor limiting the impact of most cervical cancer screening programs is an over-representation of self-selected low-risk women and consequently the exclusion of high-risk individuals[6].

With respect to pill users, these observations suggest a need to increase in existing screening programs the participation of oral contraceptive users, especially those who have used these preparations for 4 or more years, and within the previous 8 years[3].

Not much information is available about the usual frequency of Papanicolaou smear screening in pill users compared to non-users. There is, however, a suggestion that pill users, unlike other high-risk subjects, already tend to be screened more often than the general population[3]. This observation is consistent with their frequent attendance at general and gynecological medical care facilities.

POLICY ON INTERVAL BETWEEN TESTS

Several studies have been published regarding the optimal interval between tests. Comparative results from two of these are presented in Figure 1 (reproduced from reference 7). The approaches underlying the two estimates differed. In the first[8], based on empirical estimates from screening and cancer registry data, screening-detected invasive cervical cancers were aggregated with clinically diagnosed cancers in order to calculate the 'relative protection' at progressively increasing intervals. In the second[7], which applied a statistical model to data from a cohort study for predicting the effect of different screening policies, and which assumed a given duration for the natural history of the disease, screening-detected cancers were excluded from the calculations, since by definition they could not be diagnosed in the interval between tests. This study assumed a fixed 4-year duration for the pre-clinical phase of invasive cancer, while varying the length of the pre-cancerous phases (dysplasia and carcinoma *in situ*), with a more rapid evolution in younger women. Thus, the estimated total duration for the natural history of the disease varied between 14 and 20 years. This estimate is consistent with those made by others[6].

Results according to the second approach are generally more optimistic. Furthermore, they predict a constant level of protection from invasive cancer for intervals of 1, 2, 3 and 4 years, because of the assumption that the phase of pre-clinical invasive cancer is fixed at 4 years. On the other hand, according to the first approach, there is a slight but continuous loss of protection as the interval increases, although the loss is steeper for intervals of 4 years or more. The highest cost–benefit ratio is obtained by a 3–4-year screening interval. Both approaches lead to the conclusion that a 3-year interval contributes to an excellent reduction in invasive cancer risk (preventing up to 90% of the cases), provided that the test has a reasonably good sensitivity[9]. According to the second approach, there is no reason to shorten the interval to less than 4 years, regardless of the available resources.

One reason for changing this strategy into one with shorter intervals might be the identification of subgroups in which the natural history of invasive cervical cancer is shortened (shorter 'sojourn time') compared to the cases deriving from the general population. Not much information is available about the effect of exposures with high cervical cancer risk on the natural history of the disease[10]. In fact, no data are available strongly supporting the hypothesis that

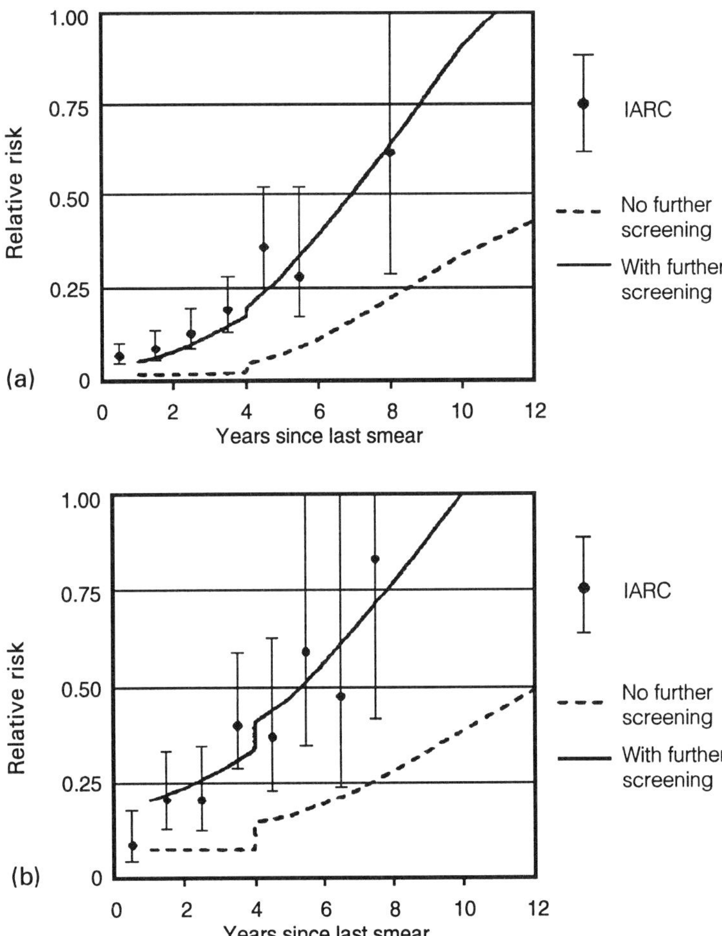

No further screening: only clinically diagnosed cancers, no further screening
With further screening: both clinically diagnosed cancers and invasive cancers
detected at further screening are taken into account
The IARC estimates in (a) and (b) are adapted from Table III and IV in the IARC study
paper, respectively

Figure 1 Comparison of estimated relative risks (mean and 95% confidence interval) of cervical cancer according to the IARC study, and model predictions for the best fitting estimates of the British Columbia data (– – – and ——) (a) For women aged 35–64 who had two or more negative smears; (b) for women < 35 years who had one negative smear. From reference 7 by permission of Oxford University Press

women in high-risk groups (such as those infected with highly carcinogenic human papillomavirus strains or, in the present case, pill users) who develop invasive cervical cancer have a shorter interval between dysplasia and clinically invasive carcinoma. Moreover, estimates of sojourn time in different birth cohorts show a high stability of the interval between dysplasia and invasive cancer, in spite of differences in incidence[6]. Apart from problems associated with the sensitivity of the test (see later), there is no theoretical basis for reducing the interval between tests in high-risk groups.

SENSITIVITY OF THE TEST AND ITS EFFECT ON THE INTERVAL STRATEGY

The sensitivity of the Papanicolaou test in identifying pre-cancerous lesions or invasive cancer depends on several factors including the proportion of unsatisfactory smears, the level of training of the program personnel, the time dedicated to assessing each smear, the use of quality assurance programs for the cytology laboratories and the strategy regarding ASCUS (atypical squamous cells of undetermined significance) cases[11]. Thus, the proportion of false-negative smears varies in the different conditions. A meta-analysis of Papanicolaou test accuracy, based on 62 studies, showed that the sensitivity of the test varied between 11 and 99%, while the specificity ranged from 14 to 97%[12]. Although some of the variation may be explained by differences in study quality and the level of verification bias[12], these results confirm the importance of planning and conducting screening programs with high standards of accuracy[5]. When the sensitivity of the test is low, rescreening after a short interval may be effective in identifying some of the false negatives from the previous test. In this situation, the policy of short intervals is not being made on the basis of the natural history of the disease, but as an inefficient way of avoiding missing too many cases. A follow-up study, conducted in New Zealand with a 1-year time interval between tests, found results for the incidence of pre-cancerous lesions which are consistent with this statement[2].

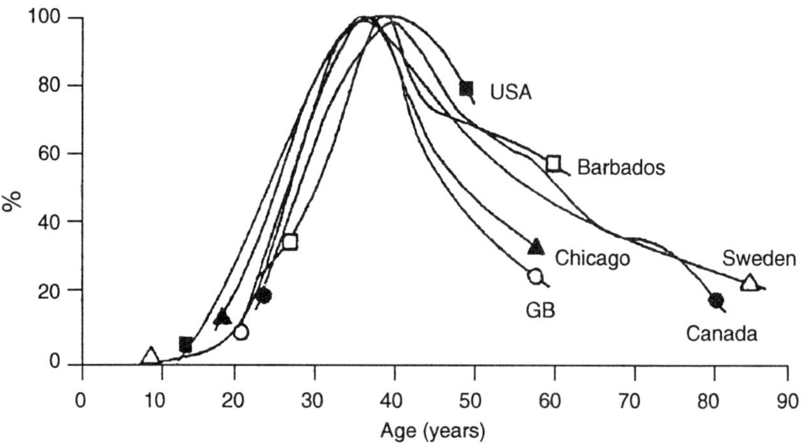

Figure 2 Age-specific prevalence rates of carcinoma *in situ* in six different geographical locations: Barbados (Barron, 1978), USA (Sadeghi *et al.*, 1988), Leeds/Wakefield, UK (Parkin *et al.*, 1981), British Columbia, Canada (Fiddler *et al.*, 1968), Chicago (Bibbo *et al.*, 1971) and Sweden (Gustafsson and Adami, 1990) as percentage of peak values. Smoothed by quadratic B splines. Reproduced from reference 6 by permission of John Wiley & Sons, Inc.

AGE AT STARTING THE SCREENING

Decisions about the age at which to start the screening are related to the age distribution of pre-cancerous lesions and invasive neoplasia. Measuring the incidence of pre-cancerous lesions, and their age distribution, is difficult because these lesions are asymptomatic and therefore their diagnosis depends on the level of screening activity. Several estimates, however, are available for different populations[6]. These show that the highest frequency of pre-cancerous lesions (from mild dysplasia to carcinoma *in situ*) occurs at 25–35 years of age (Figure 2), while invasive cancer is most frequent around age 45–50 (Figure 3)[6]. These results indicate that the first Papanicolaou test could reasonably be offered at 25 years of age, thus including the age groups at higher risk of the pre-cancerous lesions, which represent the main target of cervical cancer screening[5]. The curves presented in Figure 2, however, mostly refer to European populations

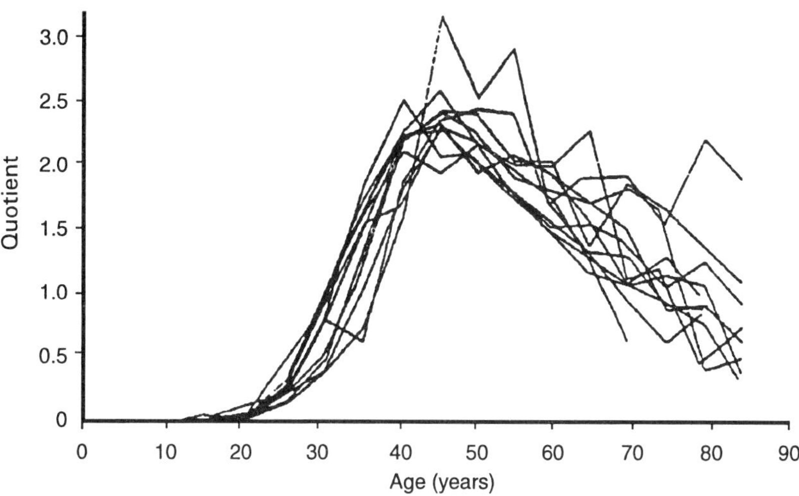

Figure 3 Weighted age-specific incidence of invasive cancer from 12 European countries (Denmark, former East Germany, England and Wales, Finland, Hungary, Norway, Poland, Romania, Scotland, Slovenia, Sweden, former West Germany). Curves with the largest irregularities contain only a few cases. To facilitate shape comparisons, quotients are computed by dividing age-specific incidence by cumulated age-specific incidence up to age 70. Reproduced from reference 6 by permission from John Wiley & Sons, Inc.

which excludes very high-risk areas. This could contribute some variability to the age distribution of the lesions. A case–control study based on two populations at different risk of cervical cancer (Colombia and Spain) suggested that the age when lesions developed could be related to the age at first intercourse[10]. The interval between first intercourse and disease was quite stable (around 30 years) and independent of the incidence of disease. Pill consumers could be characterized by an anticipated age for developing cervical lesions if this contraceptive method is associated with an anticipated age for first intercourse. No reliable data are available on this matter. If the hypothesis is confirmed, the proposed age at first test in pill users might need to be revised.

ADVERSE EFFECTS OF AN EXCESSIVE FREQUENCY OF SCREENING

Comparing the incidence and age distribution of the different precancerous lesions and of invasive carcinoma, it is clear that only a proportion of dysplasias transform themselves into carcinoma *in situ*, and, in turn, only some of these develop into invasive cancer. Perhaps 15% of lesions transform themselves into a more serious one at each step, while the remaining 85% heal spontaneously or remain unchanged. This proportion is independent of differences in disease incidence[6]. Unfortunately, no test is currently available which separates progressive lesions from those which tend to remain stable or to regress. These observations partially explain why cervical cancer screening programs result in overtreatment, this overtreatment being worse when screening is more frequent.

Another reason for overtreatment relates to the proportion of false positives made by the test. As with sensitivity, specificity can vary greatly in the different programs, inversely with respect to sensitivity[12]. In most programs, however, limitations in test sensitivity are a greater problem than limitations with test specificity.

Another important adverse effect of a program which screens too frequently is the exclusion of some women at risk, because the available resources are used in favor of a limited number of women who are excessively screened and overtreated. This problem is particularly serious in some undeveloped countries, where a small fraction of women is encouraged to have the test each year, whilst the majority of women, including those at highest risk, are not screened[9]. Even in developed countries, these considerations explain why a 3–4-year interval between screening is encouraged, with the aim of achieving good participation rates, high-quality standards and good management in all women, including pill users.

OTHER SCREENING STRATEGIES

Some other screening strategies in combination with, or instead of, one based on the Papanicolaou test are now under discussion. The aim is to overcome some of the problems related with the more traditional technique by:

(1)   Reducing the number of tests required during a woman's lifetime, thereby reducing some of the organizational problems associated with long-term participation in a screening program;

(2)   Reducing overtreatment by identifying the lesions which will tend to progress;

(3)   Reducing the population that needs to be invited, by concentrating on the very high-risk groups.

The first consideration is particularly relevant in high-risk countries with restricted resources, where it has been suggested that the testing be limited to once in a woman's lifetime, or once every 5–10 years, thereby using the available resources with a maximal cost–benefit ratio[9]. In fact, even Papanicolaou smears performed at 10-year intervals have been shown to prevent 65% of invasive cancers[13].

An interesting development in relation to the second and third points is the increasingly sophisticated, and cheaper, testing for type of human papillomavirus in infected persons. This may permit the differentiation between high- and very high-risk subjects, thereby enabling screening and therapeutic activities to be concentrated on the appropriate group. The prevalence of human papillomaviruses has been reported to be higher in invasive carcinomas from contraceptive users compared to non-users[14]. Although not confirmed by all studies[15], this finding has led to the hypothesis that contraceptives interact with viruses when determining cervical cancer risk. If confirmed, pill users who are human papillomavirus-positive may represent a group in which to concentrate special screening efforts.

REFERENCES

1. WHO Collaborative Study of Neoplasia and Steroid Contraceptives (1993). Invasive squamous-cell cervical carcinoma and combined oral contraceptives: results from a multinational study, *Int. J. Cancer*, **55**, 228–36

2. The New Zealand Contraception and Health Study Group (1995). An attempt to estimate the incidence of cervical dysplasia in a group of New Zealand women using contraception. *Epidemiology*, **6**, 121–6

3. Ye, Z., Thomas, D.B., Ray, R.M. and the WHO Collaborative Study of Neoplasia and Steroid Contraceptives (1995). Combined oral contraceptives and risk of cervical carcinoma *in situ*. *Int. J. Epidemiol.*, **24**, 19–26

4. Parkin, D.M., Muir, C.S., Whelan, S.L., Gao, Y-T., Ferlay, J. and Powell, J. (1992). *Cancer Incidence in Five Continents*, Vol. VI, IARC Sci. Publ. N. 120. (Lyon, France: IARC)

5. Coleman, D., Day, N., Douglas, G., Farmery, E., Lynge, E., Philip, J. and Segnan, N. (1993). European guidelines for quality assurance in cervical cancer screening. *Eur. J. Cancer*, **29A**, S1–37

6. Ponten, J., Adami, H.O., Bergstrom, R., Dillner, J., Friberg, L.G., Gustafsson, L., Miller, A.B., Parkin, D.M. and Trichopulos, D. (1995). Strategies for global control of cervical cancer. *Int. J. Cancer*, **60**, 1–26

7. Van Oortmarssen, G.J. and Habbema, J.D.F. (1995). Duration of preclinical cervical cancer and reduction in incidence of invasive cancer following negative Pap smears. *Int. J. Epidemiol.*, **24**, 300–7

8. IARC Working Group on Evaluation of Cervical Cancer Screening Programs (1986). Screening for squamous cervical cancer: duration of low risk after negative results of cervical cytology and its implication for screening policies. *Br. Med. J.*, **293**, 659–64

9. Richart, R.M. (1995). Screening. The next century. *Cancer Suppl.*, **76**, 1919–27

10. Moreno, V., Muñoz, N., Bosch, F.X., de Sanjose, S., Gonzales, L.C., Tafur, L., Gili, M., Izarzugaza, I., Navarro, C., Vergara, A., Viladiu, P., Ascunce, N. and Shah, K.V. (1995). Risk factors for progression of cervical intraepithelial neoplasm Grade III to invasive cancer. *Cancer Epidemiol. Biomarkers Prev.*, **4**, 459–67

11. Jones, III, H.W. (1995). Impact of the Bethesda system. *Cancer Suppl.*, **76**, 1914–18

12. Fahey, M.T., Irwig, L. and Macaskill, P. (1995). Meta-analysis of Pap test accuracy. *Am. J. Epidemiol.*, **141**, 680–9

13. World Health Organization (1986). Control of cancer of the cervix uteri. *Bull. WHO*, **64**, 607–18

14. Hildersheim, A., Reeves, W.C., Brinton, L.A., Lavery, C., Brenes, M., De La Guardia, M.E., Godoy, J. and Rawls, W.E. (1990). Association of oral-contraceptive use and human papillomaviruses in invasive cervical cancers. *Int. J. Cancer*, **45**, 860–4

15. Brinton, L.A., Reeves, W.C., Brenes, M.M., Herrero, R., DeBritton, R.C., Gaitan, E., Tenorio, F., Garcia, M. and Rawls, W.E. (1990). Oral contraceptive use and risk of invasive cervical cancer. *Int. J. Epidemiol.*, **19**, 4–11

15

Screening for ovarian cancer

J. Austoker

OVARIAN CANCER: THE CURRENT FACTS

Ovarian cancer is the fifth most common cancer in women, with 5750 new cases occurring in the UK in 1989[1]. Most (90%) cases occur in women over 45 years old. The overall prognosis is poor. In 1994, 4393 women died from ovarian cancer in the UK. It accounts for nearly 6% of all deaths from cancer in women and is the cause of more deaths in women than for all other gynecological malignancies combined.

Because of the lack of early symptoms, 65–75% of cases present at an advanced stage of disease. The overall 5-year relative survival rate is 28%, but the 5-year survival rate of stages III and IV combined is only 10%[2]. A 5-year survival rate greater than 90% may be achieved for the small minority of women with the disease confined to the ovary at diagnosis. The quality of initial surgery is an important prognostic factor and, recently, significant differences in survival have been reported between teaching and non-teaching hospitals[3].

PROSPECTS FOR SCREENING

The correlation between 5-year survival rates and stage at diagnosis has long suggested that early detection may improve prognosis. No randomized controlled studies of screening for ovarian cancer have yet been conducted (although three have just begun), so there is currently no evidence that early detection by screening reduces mortality from ovarian cancer. Some of the problems with screening for ovarian cancer are:

(1)   There is a lack of evidence that early detection reduces mortality;

(2)   There is lack of understanding how ovarian cancer develops;

(3)   No single test has both high enough sensitivity and high enough specificity to screen for early ovarian cancer, but a combination of tests looks promising;

(4)   Evidence is lacking on the balance of the benefit of screening to possible harm;

(5)   There is no conclusive evidence of the acceptability of currently available tests to the general population;

(6)   There is an inability at present to determine a high-risk population suitable for screening.

These problems underline the importance of conducting randomized trials of such screening.

SCREENING TESTS

During the past 10 years, large prospective studies have provided information about the use of the serum antigen marker CA 125, abdominal ultrasonography, transvaginal ultrasonography, and bimanual pelvic examinations in screening for ovarian cancer[4–7]. These studies have been uncontrolled and based on relatively small self-selected populations. Additional techniques, including other serum antigen markers, intraovarian color Doppler flow imaging, and radioimmunoscintography, are being evaluated for their ability to distinguish between early malignant and benign masses.

REQUIREMENTS FOR AN OVARIAN CANCER SCREENING TEST

The overall incidence of ovarian cancer in the general female population is low. This places limitations on the performance of prospective screening. In the UK, where the incidence for all ages is 1 in 5000, the use of a test with 100% sensitivity and 99% specificity for ovarian cancer in the general female population would result in one case of cancer being diagnosed for 5000 screened; 50 women would have a false-positive result[8]. As the likely consequence of an abnormal result on screening is surgery, the positive predictive value of an abnormal test must be high for the screening procedure to be acceptable. A positive predictive value of 10% would result in ten operations for each case of ovarian cancer detected. Since even a small fall in specificity would produce a large decrease in the positive predictive value, high specificity is an essential requirement for any screening test for ovarian cancer. The positive predictive value can be improved by targeting the screening tests at women at high risk, for example, those aged 45 and over. However, with an incidence in this age group of approximately 1 in 2500, a test with 100% sensitivity would require 99.6% specificity in order to have a positive predictive value of 10%. Ensuring a false-positive rate of less than 1% is thus critical, as women with positive results on screening will require laparotomy. The increased incidence of ovarian cancer among women with a family history of ovarian cancer reduces the level of specificity required to achieve an acceptable positive predictive value in this group. For the very few women with identified hereditary ovarian cancer syndromes, an even lower specificity would be acceptable.

SPECIFICITY AND SENSITIVITY OF SCREENING TESTS

The specificity of CA 125 or abdominal ultrasonography alone among postmenopausal women is about 97% and would result in more than 50 false-positive results for each case of ovarian cancer detected in this population[9]. Present evidence suggests that screening with CA 125 has a low sensitivity and may not be able to pick up cancer at a sufficiently early stage to improve prognosis. The sensitivity of serum CA 125 for identifying preclinical ovarian cancer is probably no greater than the 50% documented for clinically diagnosed stage I disease. Preliminary estimates suggest that the sensitivity of abdominal ultrasonography may be greater than that of CA 125, but the data are based on a small number of cases and incomplete follow-up. Transvaginal ultrasonography can achieve greater specificity and sensitivity than abdominal scanning[7]. It is also more comfortable because the bladder does not have to be full to achieve a good image. Specificity can be further improved by the use of color Doppler flow techniques as a secondary screening test. This helps to distinguish between benign and malignant ovarian masses, thus reducing the number of women who require surgical investigation having had a positive result on ultrasound screening.

The only strategy that has been shown prospectively to achieve a satisfactory positive predictive value on screening in the general population of postmenopausal women is the sequential combination of CA 125 with abdominal ultrasonography (positive predictive value 26.8%, specificity 99.9%). The lack of sensitivity of CA 125 in detecting early-stage disease is, however, a problem. Recent data suggest that the use of multiple markers in combination might improve sensitivity without the prohibitive decrease in specificity. Another study has shown that transvaginal ultrasonography, with color flow imaging as a secondary screening test, can effectively detect early ovarian cancer in women with a family history of ovarian cancer. The low false-positive rate achieved in this study (from 3.5% after ultrasonography alone to 0.9% after color Doppler flow imaging) has been confirmed in a pilot study of screening in the general population (Table 1).

BIMANUAL PELVIC EXAMINATION

Bimanual pelvic examination warrants special mention because it is currently performed routinely in clinical practice on asymptomatic women who attend for cervical screening. Bimanual pelvic examination has a low specificity (97.3%)[4] and sensitivity. When used alone, bimanual pelvic examination is not acceptable as a screening test for ovarian cancer because:

(1)   It has a low specificity;

(2)   It cannot distinguish between benign and malignant ovarian cysts;

Table 1 Screening parameters in published studies of asymptomatic women[10]

	Ultrasonography followed by color Doppler imaging		Tumor marker CA 125 followed by ultrasonography	
	Women with family history[7]	General population[11]	Women with family history[12]	General population[9]
Detection rate: sensitivity* (%)	100 (6/6)1		63 (5/8)	58 (11/19)
False-positive rate (%)	0.9	0.5	1.1	0.14
Prevalence of ovarian cancer	1 in 270	1 in 2500[†]	1 in 190	1 in 2500[†]
Odds of being affected, given a positive result	1:2.5	1:12[‡]	1:3	1:6

*With follow-up of 24 months; [†]estimate based on incidence of ovarian cancer in England and Wales among women aged 50–64 in 1987; [‡]based on detection rate in women with family history

(3) There is no convincing evidence that benign cysts have malignant potential;

(4) There is a high false-positive rate because of benign disease;

(5) It has low sensitivity.

Unpublished evidence suggests that the false-positive rate is high when examinations are performed by a gynecologist and may be even higher when performed by general practitioners and practice nurses (Ian Jacobs, personal communication). The false-positive rate is particularly high in premenopausal women. The precise sensitivity of pelvic examination is not known but seems to be very low. Moreover, pelvic examination does not seem to be effective in detecting early-stage disease. In two ultrasound studies in Sweden[13,14], four of the ten ovarian cancers detected by ultrasonography could not be detected by pelvic examination, and, in a further study, none of the four tumors detected by ultrasonography could be found by pelvic examination. In a study at King's College Hospital, London, only one of the five primary ovarian cancers could be detected by manual examination after ultrasonography[6]. The available evidence strongly suggests that bimanual pelvic examinations should not be performed in a routine screening procedure on asymptomatic women.

SCREENING WOMEN WITH A FAMILY HISTORY

In the absence of a documented reduction in mortality in a randomized controlled study, recommendations about ovarian cancer screening for high-risk women must be seen as contentious. Current opinion among many experts is that screening women with only one affected relative should be restricted to research protocols, but, for the few women from families with the hereditary ovarian cancer syndrome, the risk is sufficiently high to warrant annual ultrasound screening from the age of 25 or 5 years before the age at which cancer was detected in the youngest affected member of the family[8]. Because of the doubts about the efficacy of screening, prophylactic oophorectomy should be considered in the highest risk families once childbearing is completed. However, even bilateral oophorectomy does not guarantee complete protection against the development of cancer.

CONCLUSION

Currently, two screening procedures show promise: a combination of pre-screening with serum CA 125 and selective ultrasound examination (preferably using vaginal probes with color Doppler facility), and screening by transvaginal ultrasonography with color Doppler as a follow-up investigation. Three multicenter randomized trials have just commenced in the UK, USA and Europe.

Ultimately, both specificity and sensitivity may be improved by using a panel of complementary tumor markers as an initial screening test and transvaginal ultrasonography with color Doppler imaging as secondary tests. Recent advances in molecular genetics have raised the possibility that a high-risk population suitable for screening may be defined by genetic markers.

Until screening has been shown to reduce mortality from ovarian cancer in large randomized population-based trials, and the balance of potential benefit to costs, both to women and the health service, has been assessed, screening for ovarian cancer should not be offered routinely to asymptomatic women.

REFERENCES

1. Cancer Research Campaign (1995). *Scientific Yearbook* 1995–96
2. Cancer Research Campaign (1991). *Ovarian Cancer Factsheet 17*
3. Gillis, C.R., Hole, D., Still, R.M., Davis, J. and Kaye, S.B. (1991). Medical audit, cancer registration and survival in ovarian cancer. *Lancet*, **337**, 611–12
4. Jacobs, I., Stabile, I., Bridges, J. *et al.* (1988). Multimodal approach to screening for ovarian cancer. *Lancet*, **1**, 268–71
5. Jacobs, I., Prys Davies, A. and Oram, D. (1992). Role of CA 125 in screening for ovarian cancer. In Sharp, F. *et al.* (eds.) *Ovarian Cancer. Biology, Diagnosis and Management*, pp. 265–75. (London: Chapman and Hall Medical)
6. Campbell, S., Bhan, V., Royston, P. *et al.* (1989). Transabdominal ultrasound screening for early ovarian cancer. *Br. Med. J.*, **299**, 1363–7
7. Bourne, T.H., Campbell, S., Reynolds, K. *et al.* (1993). Screening for familial ovarian cancer with transvaginal ultrasonography and colour blood flow imaging. *Br. Med. J.*, **306**, 1025–9
8. Jacobs, I. (1994). Screening for epithelial ovarian cancer. *Lancet*, **343**, 337–8
9. Jacobs, I., Prys Davies, A., Bridges, J. *et al.* (1993). Prevalence of screening for ovarian cancer in postmenopausal women by CA125 measurement and ultrasonography. *Br. Med. J.*, **306**, 1030–4
10. Wald, N. (1994). *J. Med. Screening*, **1**, 135
11. Wald, N. and Parkes, C. (1993). Screening for ovarian cancer. *Br. Med. J.*, **306**, 1684
12. Bourne, T.H., Campbell, S., Reynolds, K.M. *et al.* (1996). The potential role of serum CA 125 in an ultrasound-based screening program for familial ovarian cancer. *Gynecol. Oncol.*, in press
13. Andolfe, E., Svalenius, F. and Astedt, B. (1986). Ultrasonography for early detection of ovarian carcinoma. *Br. J. Obstet. Gynaecol.*, **93**, 1286–9
14. Andolfe, E., Jorgensen, C. and Astedt, B. (1990). Ultrasound examination for detection of ovarian carcinoma in risk groups. *Br. J. Obstet. Gynaecol.*, **75**, 106–9

16

Relationship between oral contraceptives and pelvic inflammatory disease and associated sexually transmitted diseases

P. Wølner-Hanssen

Pelvic inflammatory disease is a general term used for infections of the endometrium, Fallopian tubes, and/or ovaries. Of specific interest is infection of the Fallopian tubes, acute salpingitis, because this condition is a common cause of infertility and tubal pregnancy. According to studies from different parts of Europe, *Chlamydia trachomatis* is the most common micro-organism associated with acute pelvic inflammatory disease and salpingitis in this part of the world[1-3]. A number of studies have shown that women with acute salpingitis are less likely to use oral contraceptives than controls without this condition[4-6]. On the other hand, several case–control, cross-sectional and cohort studies have shown that oral contraceptive users more often are culture positive for *C. trachomatis* or more often acquire the micro-organism than non-users[7,8]. Thus, we have a complex relationship between oral contraceptive use, chlamydial infection, and acute pelvic inflammatory disease.

Available data on the relationship between new low-dose oral contraceptives and chlamydia are limited. The most intriguing data were collected during the 1980s by a group of researchers who studied women who presented to Harborview Medical Center, the King County Sexually Transmitted Disease Clinic, or the Student Health Clinic in Seattle, USA. A number of papers have been, or are in the process of being, published from the data.

Analyses of 755 randomly selected women attending the sexually transmitted disease clinic, showed that *C. trachomatis* was cultured from the cervix, urethra, and/or rectum of 21% of oral contraceptive users, 15% of those using no contraceptives, and from 9% of users of other methods of birth control (odds ratio (OR) for oral contraceptive users versus other-method users, 2.7, $p < 0.001$) (unpublished data). Several demographic and behavioral variables were considered as potentially confounding the association between oral contraceptive use and positive *C. trachomatis* culture. However, even after adjustment for these confounders, oral contraceptive use remained significantly associated with *C. trachomatis* infection (adjusted OR for oral contraceptive users versus other-method users, 1.9, $p < 0.04$). The pills were categorized according to the type of progestogen that they contained. Four groups were large enough for meaningful analyses. The strongest associations between pill use and chlamydial infection were found among the 19 women using preparations containing levonorgestrel (42% of whom cultured positive), whether the comparison was with non-users (OR, 5.1; $p < 0.001$), users of no contraceptives (OR, 3.8; $p < 0.01$), or users of other methods of contraception (OR, 7.3; $p < 0.001$). The data were also stratified by the estrogen potency of the pills: low-dose pills contained 35 µg or less of ethinylestradiol ($n = 123$), medium-dose pills 50 µg ethinylestradiol or 80 µg mestranol ($n = 92$), and high-dose preparations 80 µg ethinylestradiol or 100 µg mestranol ($n = 21$). There was no clear dose relationship, the odds ratios for the association between oral contraceptive use and chlamydial infection being highest for low-dose and second highest for high-dose pills. Thus, the study showed that modern, low-dose pills are still associated with chlamydial infection.

Oral contraceptive use apparently has a protective effect against pelvic inflammatory disease. Not only is use of oral contraceptives negatively associated with pelvic inflammatory disease *per se*, but pill users who develop acute salpingitis appear to have laparoscopically milder tubal inflammation than non-users[5]. In addition, pill users with chlamydial pelvic inflammatory disease may develop less frequently perihepatitis and may have lower antibody titers against the micro-organism[9]. Following an episode of acute salpingitis, pill users less often experience tubal factor infertility than non-users[10].

In a recent study, based on the same Seattle population as mentioned previously, pelvic inflammatory disease patients and controls were stratified according to the presence of the infecting micro-organism[6]. Twenty-six women with chlamydial pelvic inflammatory disease were compared with 79 controls, who were also infected with *C. trachomatis* but who did not have pelvic inflammatory disease. Oral contraceptive use was significantly less common among cases than among controls (OR, 0.22; $p = 0.006$). When oral contraceptive users were compared with women not using any method of birth control, an even stronger negative association between pill use and pelvic inflammatory disease was found (OR, 0.17; $p = 0.002$). In multivariate analyses, adjustment was made for 11 potentially confounding variables, one at a time. The adjustments did not affect the magnitude of associations appreciably, irrespective of whether oral contraceptive users were compared with non-users (range of ORs, 0.2–0.3; range of p values, 0.005–0.066), or women not using any method of contraception (range of ORs, 0.16–0.24; range of p values, 0.004–0.063). In contrast, no association between pill use and pelvic inflammatory disease was found among women infected with *Neisseria gonorrhoeae*. In conclusion, the study corroborates older studies which suggest a protective effect of oral contraceptives against pelvic inflammatory disease, although this effect seems to be limited to women infected with *C. trachomatis*.

One might ask how it is possible that oral contraceptive users more frequently acquire chlamydial infection, yet once infected less often develop acute pelvic inflammatory disease. What initially seems like a paradox may not in fact be one. A number of studies have suggested that cervical ectopy enhances the susceptibility of the cervix to infection from *C. trachomatis*. Cervical ectopy regresses with age[11]. A recent study showed that oral contraceptive use might prolong the period when the ectocervix is covered with columnar epithelium, and thus prolong the period of increased susceptibility to *C. trachomatis*[11]. This might in part explain why oral contraceptive users are more often infected with this micro-organism.

It has been hypothesized that the cervical mucus of oral contraceptive users is impenetrable to micro-organisms as well as spermatozoa and thus constitutes a barrier against ascending genital infection. This hypothesis, however, is not supported by the finding that oral contraceptive use protects against chlamydial, but not gonococcal, pelvic inflammatory disease[6]. Moreover, there is increasing evidence that chlamydial salpingitis results not from a tissue-damaging effect of the micro-organism *per se*, but from a delayed type hypersensitivity response to specific *C. trachomatis* antigens, especially the 60 kDa heat-shock protein (hsp60)[12]. Hsp60 is the second most abundant protein in chlamydial whole cell lysates and is nearly identical to human hsp. Antibodies and cell-mediated immunity to natural and recombinant chlamydial hsp60 have been associated with pelvic inflammatory disease and its sequelae[12]. In experimental chlamydial infections in monkeys, challenge with chlamydial hsp60 caused a salpingeal delayed type hypersensitivity response in immunologically 'primed' animals but not control animals[13]. It has been hypothesized, therefore, that delayed type hypersensitivity responses to chlamydial hsp60 and the human counterpart in certain infected women result in tubal inflammation[12]. There is some evidence that cellular immunity might be depressed in oral contraceptive users. For example, oral contraceptive users may develop rheumatoid arthritis less often than non-users[14]. Thus, one might postulate that women using oral contraceptives who acquire a chlamydial infection have an inhibited or limited inflammatory response in the Fallopian tubes because of a reduced auto-immune response to human hsp. Much research is needed fully to understand the relationship between oral contraceptive use and pelvic inflammatory disease.

In conclusion, like the older oral contraceptives, modern low-dose pills appear to be associated with an increased risk of chlamydial infection. The protective effect of oral contraceptives against pelvic inflammatory disease seems to be limited to infection with *C. trachomatis*. Oral contraceptives should not, therefore, be prescribed as a protection against pelvic inflammatory disease. Decisions about whether pill users should be screened for *C. trachomatis* include economic considerations which depend on the prevalence of the infection in the target population.

REFERENCES

1. Gjønnæss, H., Dalaker, K., Ånestad, G., Mårdh, P.-A., Kvile, G. and Bergan, T. (1982). Pelvic inflammatory disease: etiological studies with emphasis on chlamydial infection. *Obstet. Gynecol.*, **59**, 550–5
2. Wølner-Hanssen, P., Svensson, L., Mårdh, P.-A. and Weström, L. (1985). Laparoscopic findings and contraceptive use in women with signs and symptoms suggestive of acute salpingitis. *Obstet. Gynecol.*, **66**, 233–8
3. Henry-Suchet, J., Catalan, F., Loffredo, V., Serfaty, D., Siboulet, A., Perol, Y., Sanson, M.J., Debache, C., Pigeau, F., Coppin, R., DeBrux, J. and Poynard, T. (1980). Microbiology of specimens obtained by laparoscopy from controls and from patients with pelvic inflammatory disease or infertility with tubal obstruction: *Chlamydia trachomatis* and *Ureaplasma urealyticum*. *Am. J. Obstet. Gynecol.*, **138**, 1022–5
4. Eschenbach, D.A., Harnisch, J.P. and Holmes, K.K. (1975). Pathogenesis of acute pelvic inflammatory disease: role of contraception and other risk factors. *Am. J. Obstet. Gynecol.*, **128**, 838–50
5. Svensson, L., Weström, L. and Mårdh, P.-A. (1984). Contraceptives and acute salpingitis. *J. Am. Med. Assoc.*, **251**, 2553–5
6. Wølner-Hanssen, P., Eschenbach, D.A., Paavonen, J., Kiviat, N., Stevens, C.E., Critchlow, C., DeRouen, T. and Holmes, K.K. (1990). Decreased risk of symptomatic chlamydial pelvic inflammatory disease associated with oral contraceptive use. *J. Am. Med. Assoc.*, **263**, 54–9
7. Svensson, L., Weström, L. and Mårdh, P.-A. (1981). *Chlamydia trachomatis* in women attending a gynecological outpatient clinic with lower genital tract infection. *Br. J. Vener. Dis.*, **57**, 259–62
8. Louv, W.C., Austin, H., Perlman, J. and Alexander, W.J. (1989). Oral contraceptive use and the risk of chlamydial and gonococcal infection. *Am. J. Obstet. Gynecol.*, **160**, 396–402
9. Wølner-Hanssen, P. (1986). Oral contraceptive use modified the manifestations of pelvic inflammatory disease. *Br. J. Obstet. Gynaecol.*, **93**, 619–24
10. Svensson, L., Mårdh, P.-A. and Weström, L. (1983). Infertility after acute salpingitis with special reference to *Chlamydia trachomatis*. *Fertil. Steril.*, **40**, 322–9
11. Critchlow, C. W., Wølner-Hanssen, P., Eschenbach, D.A., Kiviat, N.B., Koutsky, L.A., Stevens, C.E. and Holmes, K.K. (1995). Determinants of cervical ectopia and of cervicitis: age, oral contraception, specific cervical infection, smoking, and douching. *Am. J. Obstet. Gynecol.*, **173**, 534–43

12. Lehtinen, M. and Paavonen, J. (1995). Heat-shock proteins in the immunopathogenesis of chlamydial pelvic inflammatory disease. In Orfila, J., Byrne, G.L., Chernesky, M.A., Grayston, J.T., Jones, R.B., Ridgway, G.L., Saikku, P., Schachter, J., Stamm, W.E. and Stephens, R.S. (eds.) *Chlamydia Infections.* Proceedings of the Eighth International Symposium on Human Chlamydial Infections, pp. 599–610. (Cambridge: Cambridge University Press)

13. Patton, D.L., Sweeney, Y.T. and Kuo, C.C. (1994). Demonstration of delayed hypersensitivity in *Chlamydia trachomatis* salpingitis in monkeys: a pathogenic mechanism of tubal damage. *J. Infect. Dis.*, **169**, 680–3

14. Vandenbroucke, J.P., Valkenburg, H.A. and Boersma, J.W. (1982). Oral contraceptives and rheumatoid arthritis: further evidence for a preventive effect. *Lancet*, **2**, 839–42

17

Oral contraception and HIV

D.A. Hicks

INTRODUCTION

Unintended pregnancy and sexually transmitted disease (STD) represent the twin major risks of heterosexual sexual intercourse. Some women use oral contraception as a prophylactic against the former, and a barrier method to avoid the latter: the so-called 'double-Dutch' method. Most pill users, however, employ either no or intermittent prophylaxis against STD.

Among the various STDs, infection with the human immunodeficiency virus (HIV) is a major concern. Globally, most new infections from HIV result from heterosexual transmission and there are now more women with HIV than men.

Thus, with respect to women who only use oral contraception (OC), three questions arise:

(1) Does oral contraception increase or decrease the risk of transmission of HIV?

(2) What do we know about OC use in HIV-positive women?

(3) Can we use this information to help us rationalize our decisions about clinical and public health policy?

DOES ORAL CONTRACEPTION INCREASE OR DECREASE THE RISK OF TRANSMISSION OF HIV?

Theoretical considerations (Table 1)

The size of *cervical ectopy* is widely believed to be increased in users of combined oral contraceptives because of an estrogenic effect, although confirmatory data are limited[1]. Any association would probably be dose-dependent and presumably does not occur among users of progestogen-only pills.

If an ectopy were enlarged, then bleeding during coitus might follow, thereby increasing the probability of HIV transmission from an infected partner. Arguing against this mechanism are animal experiments which show that the presence of the cervix is not necessary for HIV transmission to occur.

Cervical infections leading to macro- or micro-ulceration of the genital tract epithelium could facilitate infection with HIV. STDs increase the pool of lymphocytes and macrophages in the genital tract, and these are the cells that the HIV prefers to infect. Concomitant or concurrent STDs, therefore, could increase infectivity in seropositive individuals and susceptibility in seronegative individuals.

Table 1 Postulated mechanisms for an increased or decreased risk of HIV transmission in association with OC use

Increased risk	Decreased risk
Increased cervical ectropion	thickened cervical mucus
Increased risk of other sexually transmitted diseases	reduced myometrial activity
	less cervical dilatation
	relative endometrial atrophy
Prolonged/chaotic menstrual bleeding	decreased menstrual bleeding
Immune effects	immune effects

Cervical infections with *Neisseria gonorrhoeae*[2] and *Chlamydia trachomatis*[2,3] have been associated with an increased risk of HIV 1 infection in prostitutes. Infection with both these agents has been found to be more frequent in women using oral contraception in a number of studies, although sexual behavior is likely to have confounded the results.

Hormonal influences produce physiological alterations amounting to *mechanical changes* which might be protective:

(1)   Changes in cervical mucus (preventing penetration by bacteria and semen);

(2)   Less dilatation of the cervix (limiting access to the endometrium);

(3)   Reduced myometrial activity (leading to less retrograde menses and reduced access to the pelvis for an infective agent);

(4)   Relative atrophy of the endometrium (less of a 'raw area' available for infection).

Menstrual bleeding leaves a raw endometrial area which could facilitate viral entry, and a pool of lymphocytes and macrophages which might be targeted by HIV. Any condition that increases the duration of menstrual bleeding or intermenstrual loss, such as poor cycle control in pill users or poor compliance, may theoretically contribute to an increased risk of acquiring HIV infection.

The great majority of pill users, however, have good cycle control with decreased menstrual loss, and may therefore enjoy a decreased risk from HIV infection.

Immunological changes in pill users have been documented, but there is no consensus as to whether any changes are clinically important[4,5].

Progesterone, certainly during pregnancy, appears to be weakly immunosuppressive and helps to prevent fetal rejection. Estrogen inhibits cell-mediated immune responses and facilitates the development of antibodies. Estrogen receptors are found on human T cells with the overall effect that both hormones produce a suppressive influence on the cellular rather than the humoral arm of the immune system.

Is this effect significant, though? In OC users, the observed 50% decrease in T-lymphocyte response to phytohemagglutinin may be responsible for the decreased incidence of rheumatoid arthritis[6] and several viral diseases (chickenpox, herpes simplex and rubella) have been shown to be associated with its use[7].

The female genital tract mucosa may well possess a privileged and different immune system to mucosa elsewhere[8]. Research into the effects of sex steroids upon it could provide a valuable insight into the transmission and prevention of HIV.

Clinical evidence

Two early and important studies performed on Nairobi prostitutes[9,10] revealed a positive association between OC use and HIV infection. The first found a significant association (OR = 1.8; 95% CI 1.1–2.9) ($p < 0.05$) between HIV seropositivity and current use of OCs. Of the HIV-positive women, 32% were current OC users versus 21% of HIV-negative women. This cross-sectional study was designed to look at the epidemiology of STDs and not *a priori* at the association between OC use and HIV seropositivity, but a step-wise logistic regression analysis confirmed the independent association. The results suggest that oral contraception may increase susceptibility to HIV, or may be a marker for other factors which increase the risk of acquisition.

This study has been criticized for its inherent design faults including selection and detection biases. Pill users with high-risk behavior were thought more likely to participate than non-users with high-risk behavior.

As a result of such criticisms, the authors looked prospectively at 196 HIV-seronegative female sex workers in Nairobi, enrolled by the incentive of free health care. Detection of HIV seroconversion was one of the study's objectives and the women were followed up for at least 12 months. Oral contraceptive use was associated with an increased risk of HIV infection (OR 3.1; 95% CI 1.1–8.6) ($p < 0.03$) although a large proportion of women were lost to follow-up (37%). Analysis of the data by other investigators yields different risk estimates, some of only borderline significance. Sampling bias could also have influenced this study's results.

Understandable concern was generated by these findings and a number of studies have been performed to look at this association. The available data have varied in quality, resulting in disparate conclusions.

Reviews of the current literature[11–13] conclude that differences in the populations studied, variations in duration of OC use and sometimes limited ability to control for confounding mean that no consistent association can be established. All suggest that studies need to be performed which include substantial numbers of more representative women who have used OCs for prolonged durations.

The World Health Organization and the International Planned Parenthood Federation have reviewed all the data and advise against changing oral contraception policy with respect to HIV.

WHAT DO WE KNOW ABOUT ORAL CONTRACEPTIVE USE IN HIV-POSITIVE WOMEN?

Less is known about the epidemiology, cause and consequences of HIV infection amongst women than in men. The effects from and upon different methods of contraception must be included in this ignorance.

The existing literature would suggest that the fertility rates of HIV-infected women do not differ significantly from matched uninfected women[14]. Most discussions in this context focus on prevention of viral dissemination from the woman rather than on preventing unwanted pregnancy. It should be noted, however, that HIV is not seen by seropositive women as a contraindication to pregnancy[15].

A summative depression in the immune system by the sex steroids acting in concert with immunosuppression from HIV itself could result in a shortened development time to AIDS. There is no information to support this speculation. Current knowledge, therefore, is insufficient to contraindicate OC use in women with HIV disease, provided no other contraindication to hormonal therapy is present. Disease transmission should be addressed separately but it should be remembered that adequate contraception by oral means might serve as a disincentive to the use of barrier techniques for some.

For the HIV-positive woman, drug interaction must also be considered. Many therapies are employed in this disease, not only to treat illnesses but also for prophylaxis.

OCs alter the metabolism of other drugs, notably through protein binding, inhibition of microsomal oxidation and demethylation, and enzyme induction in conjugation reactions. Consideration should be given to antibiotic therapy, particularly tetracyclines and rifampicin (reduced OC efficacy), tricyclic antidepressants (increased side-effects) and benzodiazepines.

Specific anti-HIV drugs such as zidovudine, zalcitabine and didanosine are not known to alter OC effectiveness (data on file, Glaxo-Wellcome, Roche and Bristol-Myers), but clinical information is scanty.

Current knowledge means that oral contraception is appropriate for HIV-positive women provided that no other contraindications exist. Prevention of transmission should be addressed separately and dealt with by barrier methods.

DECISIONS ON CLINICAL AND PUBLIC HEALTH POLICY

Can we use this information to help us rationalize our decisions about clinical and public health policy? There is no strong or consistent evidence that a policy of advising women to avoid or change from oral contraception will reduce the risk of the transmission of HIV to or from them. The use of barrier methods is much more likely to produce this desirable effect and the adaptation of behavior even more so.

The initiation of behavior change may well be best addressed when the woman seeks contraceptive advice. An adequate sexual history is therefore mandatory. Screening for HIV in women seeking such advice will depend upon local situations. The relatively high prevalence identified in some African studies will represent the screening of a totally different demographic and socioeconomic population from those found in European countries. The delivery of family planning provision is not uniform even across the individual countries of Europe.

At worst, if a correlation between OC use and HIV transmission were identified, at what level of risk would we take action? Even if OCs increased the underlying risk three- or four-fold, this increase may only be seen in users who frequently change their partner and/or who have a high background incidence of STD.

It would be tragic if women were influenced by an ill-informed media who sometimes seem keen only to emphasize certain harmful facts. This would cause women to abandon an excellent method of contraception with consequent profound implications in encountering either or both of the twin evils mentioned earlier.

REFERENCES

1. Critchlow, C.W., Wølner-Hanssen, P., Eschenbach, D.A., Kiviat, N.B., Kovitsky, L.A., Stevens, C.E. and Holmes, K.K. (1995). Determinants of cervical ectopia and of cervicitis: age, oral contraception, specific cervical infection, smoking and douching. *Am. J. Obstet. Gynecol.*, **173**, 534–43

2. Laga, M., Manoka, A., Kivuvu, M., Malele, B., Tuliza, M., Nzila, N., Goeman, J., Behets, F., Batter, V. and Alary, M. (1993). Non ulcerative sexually transmitted diseases as risk factors for HIV 1 transmission in women: results from a cohort study. *AIDS*, **7**, 95–102

3. Moss, G.B., Clemetson, D. and D'Costa, L. (1991). Association of cervical ectopy with heterosexual transmission of human immunodeficiency virus: results of a study of couples in Nairobi, Kenya. *J. Infect. Dis.*, **164**, 588–91

4. Baker, D.A. and Thomas, J. (1984). The effect of low dose oral contraceptives on the initial immune response to infection (1984). *Contraception*, **29**, 19–25

5. Fotherby, K. and Hamawi, W. (1984). Immunological aspects of contraceptive steroids. *J. Obstet. Gynaecol.*, **4** (Suppl. 1), 57–61

6. Spector, T.D., Roman, E. and Silman, A.J. (1990). The Pill, parity and rheumatoid arthritis. *Arthritis Rheum.*, **33**, 782–9

7. Royal College of General Practitioners (1974). *Oral Contraception and Health*. (London: Pitman Medical)

8. Forrest, B.D. (1991). Women, HIV and mucosal immunity. *Lancet*, **337**, 835–6

9. Simonsen, J.N., Plummer, F.A., Ngugi, E.N. *et al.* (1990). HIV infection among lower social economic strata prostitutes in Nairobi. *AIDS*, **4**, 139–44

10. Plummer, F.A., Simonsen, J.N., Cameron, D.W., Ndinya-Achola, J.O., Kreiss, J.K., Gakinga, M.N., Waiyaki, P., Cheong, M., Piot, P., Roland, A.R. and Ngugi, E.N. (1991). Co-factors in male to female transmission of Human Immunodeficiency Virus Type 1. *J. Infect. Dis.*, **163**, 233–9

11. Hicks, D.A. (1993). The oral contraceptive pill and HIV infection. *Br. J. Sex. Med.*, May, June, 32–5

12. Costello Daly, C., Helling-Giese, G.E., Mati, J.K. and Hunter, D.J. (1994). Contraceptive methods and the transmission of HIV: implications for family planning. *Genitourin. Med.*, **70**, 110–17

13. Taitel, H.F. and Kafrissen, M.E. (1995). A review of oral contraceptive use and risk of HIV transmission. *Br. J. Fam. Plann.*, **20**, 112–16

14. Selwyn, P.A., Carter, R.J., Schoenbaum, E.E., Robertson, V.J., Klein, R.S. and Rogers, M.I. (1989). Knowledge of HIV antibody status and decisions to continue or terminate pregnancy among intravenous drug users. *J. Am. Med. Assoc.*, **261**, 3567–71

15. Johnstone, F., Maccallum, L. and Riddell, R. (1990). Contraceptive use in HIV infected women. *Br. J. Fam. Plann.*, **16**, 106–8

18

Screening for sexually transmitted diseases in pill users

P.-A. Mårdh and S. Elshibly

It has been stated [see Chapter 16] that oral contraceptive (OC) use may increase the risk of acquiring sexually transmitted diseases (STD), such as gonorrhea and chlamydial infection. However, a number of confounding factors, such as sexual risk behavior (Table 1) and screening methodology, have to be considered before any statement of this nature can be taken for granted.

To be able to establish any possible risks or protective effect of OCs, it is essential to know the type of pill used, the agent by which the subject may have been infected, changes in vaginal flora and the prevalence of different STDs in the population studied, and the pattern of sexual risk taking in the study group[1]. Other confounding factors include age, parity, previous history of genital infection and partner-related factors (Table 2). If any risk of OCs is to be discussed, the relative risk of alternative contraception or non-use ought to be taken into consideration. It is notable that there has so far been no request from drug registration authorities to obtain any documentation of the influence of OCs on susceptibility and resistance to genital infections or changes in vaginal flora, or on the risks of developing genital complications and sequelae from their use.

Age may influence susceptibility to exogenous genital infectious agents and, therefore, may bias any evaluation of the possible risk of OCs, if not adjusted for. Evaluation of the risk of infertility as a consequence of STDs, having an ectopic pregnancy, or developing

Table 1 High-scoring factors for the risk of sexually transmitted diseases

Number of lifetime sexual partners

More than one partner in the previous month

More than one partner in the last 6 months

First intercourse within 1 week of meeting first lifetime partner

Non-use of contraceptive at first ever intercourse

Being drunk at first ever intercourse or at first intercourse with current partner

Partner being drunk at first ever intercourse or at first intercourse in current relationship

Table 2 Confounding factors that may influence the impact of contraceptives on the susceptibility and course of genital infections and their complications and sequelae

Type of contraceptive (oral contraceptive, condom, etc.)

Type and amount of hormone in pill

Age of user

Parity of user

Infecting organism

Earlier episode(s) of pelvic inflammatory disease

Changes in vaginal flora, bacterial vaginosis and other

Sexual behavior

Sexual technique(s) practised

Partner-related factors

chronic abdominal pain may thus all be age-correlated. This, among other factors, varies according to the immune status of the infected, i.e. the presence of immunocompetent cells in genital tract tissues which relates to previous exposure to microbes, not necessarily STD agents. Thus, women seem to develop a somewhat greater capacity to handle infectious agents in the lower genital tract with increasing age. The paucity of immunocompetent cells in young women in vaginal tissue sections stained by monoclonal antibodies is striking when compared to those seen in somewhat older women[2].

Recent work has suggested that high- as opposed to medium- and low-dose OCs are associated with greater risk of acquisition of human papilloma virus (HPV) types 16/18[3]. Whether this dose-related difference in susceptibility is seen with other STDs remains to be determined.

Our data (in contrast to those of Chapter 16, Ed.) do not indicate that chlamydial infections are more common in OC users than in non-users if adjustment is made for age and sexual risk behavior. On the other hand, OC use decreases the chance of *Chlamydia trachomatis* ascending to the upper genital tract[4]. This diminishes the risk of tubal damage. This important observation suggests that, in a woman with sexually risky behavior, OCs may well increase her risk of acquiring chlamydial cervicitis but, even if the infection ascends to the Fallopian tubes, she has a better chance of retaining her fertility than if she were not taking the pill. We found that almost all such women, as compared to 25–90% of non-OC users (depending on the number of earlier episodes of tubal infection) with laparoscopically confirmed pelvic inflammatory disease (PID), had retained their fertility when followed up one decade later[5]. The risk ratio for developing PID in OC users as compared to non-users is around 0.3[6]. OCs protect against ascent of chlamydial but not gonococcal infection[4].

The pill may not only influence the risk of developing chlamydial endometritis and salpingitis, but also reduce spread of infection to the abdominal cavity[7]. We found a difference in the prevalence of chlamydial perihepatitis between OC users and non-users: perihepatitis was found laparoscopically in 27% of Norwegian women with chlamydial salpingitis (none of whom were taking OCs), compared to 3% in Swedish women, the vast majority of whom were on the pill[8]. These latter women were also less likely to have periappendicitis, peritonitis and perisigmoiditis[7].

Further evaluation of the influence of OCs on PID should include consideration of changes in vaginal flora, by studying bacterial vaginosis. This condition occurs in 5–15% of all women of reproductive age, is also associated with PID[9], and is decreased by OC use. This fact may be taken into account when selecting contraceptive methods in women who later wish to conceive. Another reason to screen for bacterial vaginosis, apart from the obstetric complication of premature labor seen in women with this condition, may be the recently proposed increased risk of developing cervical cancer due to the presence of nitroamines produced by bacteria occurring in high number in women with bacterial vaginosis[9].

Both the mechanisms by which OC use seems to decrease the inflammatory reaction in Fallopian tubes, and by which *Chlamydia trachomatis* may establish chronicity and cause tubal damage via heat shock proteins[10], have been discussed previously (Chapter 16). This latter mechanism cannot be reversed by elimination of chlamydial organisms by antibiotic therapy. Therefore, as most infected individuals are symptomless, it is essential to develop comprehensive screening programs for *Chlamydia trachomatis* and *Neisseria gonorrhoeae* in both symptomatic and asymptomatic women, in order to treat positive cases and their partners, thereby hindering spread of the organisms to others.

Sweden seems to have been one of the very first countries to have introduced a nationwide diagnostic service for these infections, with use of chlamydial tissue cell cultures and high-quality gonococcal culture media. Some half a million samples are tested annually in Sweden (in a population of approximately 8.5 million). In 1987, the number of reported instances of genital/ocular chlamydial infections was 38 223, reducing to 14 275 by 1994. Gonorrhea has become very rare and has decreased from 2587 to 338 cases during the same period. Although a quicker and more pronounced reduction in the prevalence of genital chlamydial infection has been observed in Sweden than in most other European countries, annual reported cases still outnumber all the other reportable bacterial and parasitic infections together (e.g. *Salmonella, Campylobacter, Shigella, Neisseria gonorrhoeae, Neisseria meningitidis, Giardia lamblia*).

The trend in the reduction of reported chlamydial cases seems, however, to have halted last year in Sweden following the introduction of the more sensitive amplified DNA screening techniques of polymerase chain reaction (PCR) and ligase chain reaction (LCR). Nucleic acid-based tests, which can also detect gonorrhea, have opened up the chance to use non-invasive sampling for STD diagnosis, i.e. to test voided urine instead of urethral and cervical samples. This means one may avoid a gynecological examination, which has been a factor restricting the possibility of testing women for these infections. Thus any epidemiological evaluation should be considered in the light of this limitation. Increasing use of tests of voided urine allows more males and females to be tested in screening programs[11,12].

A wide variation in the percentage of chlamydia-positive samples, ranging from 4% to 10%, has been found across the different counties of Sweden. The explanation for this is not obvious, but it might be due in part to local differences in contact strategies being established between health-care units and the general population, as well as the ratio of symptomatic to asymptomatic cases being tested, and the percentage of never-before tested individuals. The male-to-female ratio among positive cases has traditionally been 1:3, but has recently reduced closer to parity, suggesting that more screening of men has started. Regional variation in partner notification patterns, and uptake of the newer tests, including non-invasive sampling methods, will also account for these changing differences.

Introduction of PCR and LCR screening has been essential because of the poor performance of the traditional enzyme immunoassay (EIA), as the prevalence of chlamydial infection has fallen. When the automated EIA test was introduced as an alternative to cell culture, the sensitivity generally decreased by 10–30% or even more. These methods have sensitivities ranging from only 50 to 85% when compared to PCR and LCR. The more widely used EIA test functions much more accurately in high rather than low prevalence settings, producing false-positive results. Thus the predictive value of a positive result in a low-prevalence (e.g. 2–4%) population may be only around 50%, which makes tossing a coin as good as an EIA test (and, of course, much cheaper). This means that the use of EIA may be accurate in symptomatic women attending an STD clinic, but completely unreliable in asymptomatic women attending a family planning unit where the prevalence may be low.

Pre-screening urine samples for polymorphs, using the leukocyte esterase test, before testing for *Chlamydia trachomatis* and *Neisseria gonorrhoeae* by (more expensive) microbiological methods has been performed in order to reduce costs by only having to test a subset (may be only 5–10%) of individuals. This selects a higher-prevalence sample subset only from a low-prevalence group, which may make EIA more satisfactory in this situation.

The amplified DNA-based techniques have the potential risk of delivering a false-positive result due to contamination at the clinic, or at the laboratory after amplification. However, with the most commonly used commercial kits (Roche – PCR, Abbott – LCR), this risk is more or less overcome by the introduction of closed devices for sampling and laboratory analysis, and by chemical sterilization of the amplified product. Discrepancies in sensitivity between different DNA-based tests might be due to how efficiently one has been able to deal with possible Taq-polymerase inhibitors[11] occurring in clinical samples. As more and more effective techniques have been developed, observations of products introduced on the market some time ago should not be compared to those more recently launched, as unfortunately has been reported.

In a recent study[13], we found that most European countries would save money from introducing chlamydial screening programs, with the following provisos:

(1)   The prevalence of infection in the population exceeds 6%;

(2)   A DNA test is used for detection; and

(3)   The single-dose antichlamydial drug, azithromycin, is used to treat positive cases.

In some European countries, the prevalence of chlamydial infection exceeds 6% in women attending family planning clinics without having any suspicion of being infected. Furthermore, even if the prevalence of gonorrhea is some 3–30 times lower than that of chlamydial infection in this type of setting, DNA testing the same samples for gonorrhea adds to the cost-effectiveness of screening. It is essential, however, that all screening activities for curable STDs should be accompanied by partner notification, and counselling of infected individuals about sexual risk behavior.

REFERENCES

1. Sikström, B., Hellberg, D., Nilsson, S., Brihmer, K. and Mårdh, P.-A. (1995). Smoking, alcohol, sexual behavior and drug use in women with cervical human papillomavirus infection. *Arch. Obstet. Gynecol.*, **256**, 131–7
2. Hill, J.A. and Anderson, D.J. (1996). Cellular defense mechanisms of the human cervico-vaginal compartment. *J. Reprod. Immunol.*, in press
3. Sikström, B., Hellberg, D., Nilsson, D. and Mårdh, P.-A. (1996). Cervical human papilloma virus infection: contraceptive and reproductive history. *Adv. Contracept.*, in press
4. Louv, C.M., Austin, H., Perlman, J. and Alexander, J.W. (1989). Oral contraceptive use and the risk of chlamydial and gonococcal infections. *Am. J. Obstet. Gynecol.*, **160**, 396–402
5. Svensson, L., Mårdh, P.-A. and Weström, L. (1983). Infertility after acute salpingitis with special reference to *Chlamydia trachomatis*. *Fertil. Steril.*, **40**, 322–9
6. Mårdh, P.-A., Paavonen, J., Weström, L. and Møller, B. (1996). Pelvic inflammatory diseases. In. Rein, M. (ed.) *Infectious Diseases Teaching Atlas*. (Philadelphia: Current Medicine)
7. Mårdh, P.-A., Paavonen, J. and Puolakkainen, M. (1989). *Chlamydia*. (New York: Plenum)
8. Gjønnaess, H., Dalaker, K., Ånestad, G., Mårdh, P.-A., Kvile, G. and Bergan, T. (1982). Pelvic inflammatory disease. Etiologic studies with emphasis on chlamydial infection. *Obstet. Gynecol.*, **59**, 551–5
9. Mårdh, P.-A., Eschenbach, D.A. and Martinez de Oliveira, J. (organizers) (1994). *Bacterial Vaginosis*. (Oxford: Oxford Clinical Communications)
10. Morrison, R.P. (1991). Chlamydial hsp 60 and the immunopathogenesis of chlamydial disease. *Semin. Immunol.*, **3**, 25–33
11. Domeika, M., Bassiri, M. and Mårdh, P.-A. (1994). Diagnosis of genital *Chlamydia trachomatis* infection in asymptomatic males by testing urine by PCR. *J. Clin. Microbiol.*, **32**, 2350–2
12. Bassiri, M., Hu, H.Y., Domeika, M., Burczak, J., Svensson, L.-O., Lee, H.H. and Mårdh, P.-A. (1995). Detection of *Chlamydia trachomatis* in urine specimens from women by ligase chain reaction. *J. Clin. Microbiol.*, **33**, 898–900
13. Genc, M. and Mårdh, P.-A. (1996). A cost effectiveness analysis of screening and treatment for *Chlamydia trachomatis* infection in asymptomatic women. *Ann. Intern. Med.*, **124**, 1–7

Section 4

Breast cancer and the pill

19

Breast cancer and oral contraceptives: the evidence so far

V. Beral and G. Reeves

INTRODUCTION

Breast cancer is the most common cancer among women worldwide. About one in 20 women is likely to develop breast cancer before the age of 75 and 600 000 new cancers are diagnosed each year[1]. More than 200 million women have used oral contraceptives and, if their use altered breast cancer risk even by a relatively small amount, large numbers of women would be affected, especially if there was a persistent effect many years after use ceased.

More than 60 epidemiological studies have investigated the relationship between breast cancer and use of oral contraceptives[2–65]. None of the studies has shown a substantial increase in breast cancer among all ever users of oral contraceptives, although some have reported an increased risk in one or more subgroups of women. It is impossible to tell from what has been published whether or not there are consistent findings across all studies. This is in part because results for various aspects of oral contraceptive use, such as duration of use or age at first use, have tended to be categorized in different ways from one study to another. Also there is a tendency for investigators to subdivide women into various subgroups, the divisions again tending to vary from one study to another, and extreme results in particular subgroups may well have arisen by chance in particular studies. Furthermore, various aspects of oral contraceptive use are highly correlated, for example women who have used oral contraceptives for long periods of time tend to have begun use comparatively long ago and to have ceased use comparatively recently. Women who have used the pill recently tend to be young. Thus, if a true relationship exists between breast cancer risk and a particular aspect of use, there will be indirect relationships with other aspects of use as well. These considerations need to be taken into account in any analysis, but most studies are too small to determine which relationships, if any, are direct and which are indirect.

THE COLLABORATIVE GROUP ON HORMONAL FACTORS IN BREAST CANCER

The Collaborative Group on Hormonal Factors in Breast Cancer was set up in 1992 to bring together, reanalyze and publish the worldwide epidemiological evidence on breast cancer risk in relation to hormonal contraceptive use, use of hormone replacement therapy and reproductive factors. The aim was to collect centrally data on individuals in each study and to analyze the data using similar definitions for each study of important aspects of oral contraceptive use, such as duration of use, age at first use, time since first use, time since last use, etc. The collaboration now includes about 90% of the epidemiological studies on the topic. Preliminary results have been discussed at meetings of collaborators in September 1993 and March 1995. Two reports have been prepared, one describing the main results for hormonal contraceptives and another giving details of the studies and women included in the collaboration, describing the methods, and presenting further results[66].

METHODS

Studies were identified from review articles, literature searches and by correspondence with colleagues. Special efforts were made to identify all studies that included relevant information, irrespective of whether results for oral contraceptives had been published. Principal investigators of studies that included at least 100 women with breast cancer were invited to participate in the collaboration. Data on individual women were sought on sociodemographic factors, on various aspects of the timing of oral contraceptive use and on factors that might conceivably confound any relationships observed. Data were checked centrally and a wide range of consistency checks was performed. Apparent inconsistencies and omissions were clarified with collaborators.

Data from different studies were examined separately and also combined, using a modification of the Mantel–Haenszel stratification technique[66]. All analyses were routinely stratified by study, single years of age, parity and the age a woman was when she first gave birth to a child and the age a woman was when her risk of conception ceased.

ANALYSIS STRATEGY

The main exposures examined relating to oral contraceptive use are duration of use, age at first use, time since first use and time since last use. Because these four indices of exposure are highly correlated, the approach to determining which relationships are direct and which are indirect has been, first, to examine the relationship with breast cancer separately for each of the four indices of exposure. Then that factor is held constant and the relationship with the other three factors is re-examined. After thus establishing the main relationships, their consistency is investigated across the different studies and study designs, for women of different ages and from different countries and ethnic groups, for women with and without a family history of breast cancer, for women of different heights, weights, etc.

Analyses are also performed of breast cancer risk in relation to type and dose of estrogen and progestogen and all analyses are repeated for tumors that were localized to the breast and had spread beyond it.

THE FUTURE

The results from this collaboration should be published later in 1996. The main findings should resolve many of the controversies that have plagued this field of research for more than a decade. However, most of the data relate to oral contraceptive use that began less than 25 years ago and to types of hormonal preparations that are no longer available, so there will continue to be the need for new studies of the relationship between breast cancer and oral contraceptive use.

REFERENCES

1. Parkin, D.M., Laara, E. and Muir, C.S. (1988). Estimates of the world-wide frequency of sixteen major cancers in 1980. *Int. J. Cancer*, **41**, 184–97
2. Ross, R.K., Paganini-Hill, A., Gerkins, V.R., Mack, T.M., Pfeffer, R., Arthur, M. and Henderson, B.E. (1980). A case–control study of menopausal estrogen therapy and breast cancer. *J. Am. Med. Assoc.*, **243**, 1635–9
3. Pike, M.C., Henderson, B.E., Krailo, M.D., Duke, A. and Roy, S. (1983). Breast cancer in young women and use of oral contraceptives: possible modifying effect of formulation and age at use. *Lancet*, **2**, 926–30
4. Vessey, M., Baron, J., Doll, R., McPherson, K. and Yeates, D. (1983). Oral contraceptives and breast cancer: final report of an epidemiologic study. *Br. J. Cancer*, **47**, 455–62
5. Hiatt, R.A., Bawol, R., Friedman, G.D. and Hoover, R. (1984). Exogenous estrogen and breast cancer after bilateral oophorectomy. *Cancer*, **54**, 139–44
6. Lê, M.G., Bachelot, A., Doyon, F., Kramar, A. and Hill, C. (1984). Oral contraceptive use and breast cancer or cervical cancer. Preliminary results of a French case–control study. In *Hormones and Sexual Factors in Human Cancer Aetiology*. (Amsterdam: Elsevier Scientific Publishers)
7. Talamini, R., La Vecchia, C., Franceschi, S., Colombo, F., Decarli, A., Grattoni, E., Grigoletto, E. and Tognoni, G. (1985). Reproductive and hormonal factors and breast cancer in a Northern Italian population. *Int. J. Epidemiol.*, **14**, 70–4

8. Hislop, T.G., Coldman, A.J., Elwood, J.M., Brauer, G. and Kan, L. (1986). Childhood and recent eating patterns and risk of breast cancer. *Cancer Detection and Prevention*, **9**, 47–58

9. Meirik, O., Lund, E., Adami, H.O., Bergstrom, R., Christoffersen, T. and Bergsjo, P. (1986). Oral contraceptive use and breast cancer in young women. A joint national case–control study in Sweden and Norway. *Lancet*, **2**, 650–4

10. Nomura, A.M.Y., Kolonel, L.N., Hirohata, T. and Lee, J. (1986). The association of replacement estrogens with breast cancer. *Int. J. Cancer*, **37**, 49–53

11. Alexander, F.E., Roberts, M.M. and Huggins, A. (1987). Risk factors for breast cancer with applications to selection for the prevalence screen. *J. Epidemiol. Comm. Hlth.*, **41**, 101–6

12. Lee, N.C., Rosero-Bixby, L., Oberle, M.W., Grimaldo, C., Whately, A.S. and Rovira, E.Z. (1987). A case–control study of breast cancer and hormonal contraception in Costa Rica. *J. Natl. Cancer Inst.*, **79**, 1247–54

13. McPherson, K., Vessey, M.P., Neil, A., Doll, R., Jones, L. and Roberts, M. (1987). Early oral contraceptive use and breast cancer: results of another case–control study. *Br. J. Cancer*, **56**, 653–60

14. Wang, D.Y., De Stavola, B.L., Bulbrook, R.D., Allen, D.S., Kwa, H.G., Verstraeten, A.A., Moore, J.W., Fentiman, I.S., Chaudary, M., Hayward, J.L. and Gravelle, I.H. (1987). The relationship between blood prolactin levels and risk of breast cancer in premenopausal women. *Eur. J. Clin. Oncol.*, **23**, 1541–8

15. Kay, C.R. and Hannaford, P.C. (1988). Breast cancer and the pill – a further report from the Royal College of General Practitioners' Oral Contraception Study. *Br. J. Cancer*, **58**, 675–80

16. Ravnihar, B., Primic Zakelj, M., Kosmelj, K. and Stare, J. (1988). A case–control study of breast cancer in relation to oral contraceptive use in Slovenia. *Neoplasma*, **35**, 109–21

17. Rohan, T.E. and McMichael, A.J. (1988). Oral contracpetive agents and breast cancer: a population-based case–control study. *Med. J. Aust.*, **149**, 520–6

18. Yuan, J.-M., Yu, M.C., Ross, R.K., Gao, Y.-T. and Henderson, B.E. (1988). Risk factors for breast cancer in Chinese women in Shanghai. *Cancer Res.*, **48**, 1949–53

19. Mills, P.K., Beeson, W.L., Phillips, R.L. and Fraser, G.E. (1989). Prospective study of exogenous hormone use and breast cancer in seventh-day adventists. *Cancer*, **64**, 591–7

20. Marubini, E., Decarli, A., Costa, A., Mazzoleni, C., Andreoli, C., Barbieri, A., Capitelli, E., Barlucci, M., Cavallo, F., Monferroni, N.,

Pastorino, U. and Salvini, S. (1988). The relationship of dietary intake and serum levels of retinol and beta-carotene with breast cancer. Results of a case–control study. *Cancer*, **61**, 173–80

21. Olsson, H., Moller, T.R. and Ranstam, J. (1989). Early oral contraceptive use and cancer among premenopausal women: final report from a study in southern Sweden. *J. Natl. Cancer Inst.*, **81**, 1000–4

22. Romieu, I., Willett, W., Colditz, G., Stampfer, M., Rosner, B., Hennekens, C.H. and Speizer, F.A. (1989). Prospective study of oral contraceptive use and the risk of breast cancer in women. *J. Natl. Cancer Inst.*, **81**, 1313–21

23. Siskind, V., Schofield, F., Rice, D. and Bain, C. (1989). Breast cancer and breast feeding: results from an Australian case–control study. *Am. J. Epidemiol.*, **130**, 229–36

24. Stanford, J.L., Brinton, L.A. and Hoover, R.N. (1989). Oral contraceptives and breast cancer: results from an expanded case–control study. *Br. J. Cancer*, **60**, 375–81

25. UK National Case–Control Study Group (1989). Oral contraceptive use and breast cancer risk in young women. *Lancet*, **1**, 973–82

26. Vessey, M.P., McPherson, K., Villard-Mackintosh, L. and Yeates, D. (1989). Oral contraceptives and breast cancer: latest findings in a large cohort study. *Br. J. Cancer*, **59**, 613–17

27. Bernstein, L., Pike, M.C., Krailo, M. and Henderson, B.E. (1990). Update of the Los Angeles study of oral contraceptives and breast cancer: 1981 and 1983. In Mann, R.D. (ed.) *Oral Contraceptives and Breast Cancer*, pp. 169–81. (Carnforth, UK: Parthenon Publishing)

28. Paul, C., Skegg, D.C.G. and Spears, G.F.S. (1990). Oral contraceptives and risk of breast cancer. *Int. J. Cancer*, **46**, 366–73

29. Schildkraut, J.M., Hulka, B.S. and Wilkinson, W.E. (1990). Oral contraceptives and breast cancer: a case–control study with hospital and community controls. *Obstet. Gynecol.*, **76**, 395–402

30. WHO Collaborative Study of Neoplasia and Steroid Contraceptives (1990). Breast cancer and combined oral contraceptives: results from a multinational study. *Br. J. Cancer*, **61**, 110–19

31. Clavel, F., Andrieu, N., Gairard, B., Bremond, A., Piana, L., Lansac, J., Breart, G., Rumeau-Rouquette, C., Flamant, R. and Renaud, R. (1991). Oral contraceptives and breast cancer: a French case–control study. *Int. J. Epidemiol.*, **20**, 32–8

32. Segala, C., Gerber, M. and Richardson, S. (1991). The pattern of risk factors for breast cancer in a Southern France population. Interest for a stratified analysis by age at diagnosis. *Br. J. Cancer*, **64**, 919–25

33. Weinstein, A.L., Mahoney, M.C., Nasca, P.C., Leske, M.C. and Varma, A.O. (1991). Breast cancer risk and oral contraceptive use: results from a large case–control study. *Epidemiology*, **2**, 353–8

34. Wingo, P.A., Lee, N.C., Ory, H.W., Beral, V., Peterson, H.B. and Rhodes, P. (1991). Age-specific differences in the relationship between oral contraceptive use and breast cancer. *Obstet. Gynecol.*, **78**, 161–70

35. Ewertz, M. (1992). Oral contraceptives and breast cancer risk in Denmark. *Eur. J. Cancer*, **28A**, 1176–81

36. Lee, H.P., Gourley, L, Duffy, S.W., Esteve, J., Lee, J. and Day, N.E. (1992). Risk factors for breast cancer by age and menopausal status: a case–control study in Singapore. *Cancer, Causes and Control*, **3**, 313–22

37. Miller, A.B., Baines, C.J., To, T. and Wall, C. (1992). Canadian National Breast Screening Study. I. Breast cancer detection and death rates among women aged 40–49 years. *Can. Med. Assoc. J.*, **147**, 1459–76

38. Rosenberg, L., Palmer, J.R., Clarke, E.A. and Shapiro, S. (1992). A case–control study of the risk of breast cancer in relation to oral contraceptive use. *Am. J. Epidemiol.*, **136**, 1437–44

39. Ursin, G., Aragaki, C.C., Paganini-Hill, A., Siemiatycki, J., Thompson, W.D. and Haile, R.W. (1992). Oral contraceptives and premenopausal bilateral breast cancer: a case–control study. *Epidemiology*, **3**, 414–19

40. Wang, Q.-S., Ross, R.K., Yu, M.C., Ning, J.-P., Henderson, B.E. and Kimm, H.T. (1992). A case–control study of breast cancer in Tianjin, China. *Cancer Epidemiology, Biomarkers and Prevention*, **1**, 435–9

41. Yang, C.P., Daling, J.R., Band, P.R., Gallagher, R.P., White, E. and Weiss, N.S. (1992). Non contraceptive hormone use and risk of breast cancer. *Cancer, Causes and Control*, **3**, 475–9

42. Calle, E.E., Martin, L.M., Thun, M.J., Miracle, H.L. and Heath, C.W. Jr (1993). Family history, age, and risk of fatal breast cancer. *Am. J. Epidemiol.*, **138**, 675–81

43. Ngelangel, C.A., Lacaya, L.B., Cordero, C. and Laudico, A.V. (1994). Risk factors for breast cancer among Filipino women. *Phil. J. Intern. Med.*, **32**, 231–6

44. Morabia, A., Szklo, M., Stewart, W., Schuman, L. and Thomas, D.B. (1993). Consistent lack of association between breast cancer and oral contraceptives using either hospital or neighbourhood controls. *Prevent. Med.*, **22**, 178–86

45. Tavani, A., Negri, E., Franceschi, S., Parazzini, F. and La Vecchia, C. (1993). Oral contraceptives and breast cancer in Northern Italy. Final report from a case–control study. *Br. J. Cancer*, **68**, 568–71

46. Schuurman, A.G., van den Brandt, P.A. and Goldbohm, R.A. (1995). Exogenous hormones and the risk of postmenopausal breast cancer.

Results from the Netherlands cohort study. *Cancer, Causes and Control,* **6**, 416–24

47. Newcomb, P.A., Storer, B.E., Longnecker, M.P., Mittendorf, R., Greenberg, E.R., Clapp, R.W., Burke, K.P., Willett, W.C. and MacMahon, B. (1994). Lactation and a reduced risk of premenopausal breast cancer. *N. Engl. J. Med.,* **330**, 81–7

48. Primic-Zakelj, M., Evstifeeva, T., Ravnihar, B. and Boyle, P. (1995). Breast cancer risk and oral contraceptive use in Slovenian women aged 25 to 54. *Int. J. Cancer,* **62**, 414–20

49. Rookus, M.A., van Leeuwen, F.E. for the Netherlands Oral Contraceptives and Breast Cancer Study Group (1994). Oral contraceptives and risk of breast cancer in women aged 20–54 years. *Lancet,* **344**, 844–51

50. White, E., Malone, K.E., Weiss, N.S. and Daling, J.R. (1994). Breast cancer among young US women in relation to oral contraceptive use. *J. Natl. Cancer Inst.,* **86**, 505–14

51. La Vecchia, C., Negri, E., Franceschi, S., Talamini, R., Amadori, D., Filiberti, R., Conti, E., Montella, M., Veronesi, A., Parazzini, F., Ferraroni, M. and Decarli, A. (1995). Oral contraceptives and breast cancer: a cooperative Italian study. *Int. J. Cancer,* **60**, 163–7

52. Rossing, M.A., Stanford, J.L., Weiss, N.S. and Habel, L.A. (1995). Oral contraceptive use and risk of breast cancer in middle-aged women. *Am. J. Epidemiol.,* in press

53. Brinton, L.A., Daling, J.R., Liff, J.M., Schoenberg, J.B., Malone, K.E., Stanford, J.L., Coates, R.J., Gammon, M.D., Hanson, L. and Hoover, R.N. (1995). Oral contraceptives and breast cancer risk among younger women. *J. Natl. Cancer Inst.,* **87**, 827–35

54. Paffenbarger, R.S., Fasal, E., Simmons, M.E. and Kampert, J.B. (1977). Cancer risk as related to use of oral contraceptives during fertile years. *Cancer,* **39**, 1887–91

55. Sartwell, P.E., Arthes, F.G. and Tonascia, J.A. (1977). Exogenous hormones, reproductive history and breast cancer. *J. Natl. Cancer Inst.,* **59**, 1589–92

56. Kelsey, J.L., Holford, T.R., White, C., Mayer, E.S., Kilty, S.E. and Acheson, R.M. (1978). Oral contraceptives and breast disease. An epidemiological study. *Am. J. Epidemiol.,* **107**, 236–44

57. Ravnihar, B., Seigel, D.G. and Lindtner, J. (1979). An epidemiologic study of breast cancer and benign breast neoplasias in relation to the oral contraceptive and estrogen use. *Europ. J. Cancer,* **15**, 395–405

58. Ramcharan, S., Pellegrin, F.A., Ray, R.M. and Hsu, J.-P. (1981). The Walnut Creek contraceptive drug study: a prospective study of the side effects of oral contraceptives. In *NIH Publication No. 81-564.*

Center for Population Research Monograph, volume III, pp. 43–69. (Bethesda: National Institutes for Health)

59. Janerich, D.T., Polednak, A.P., Glebartis, D.M. and Lawrence, C.E. (1983). Breast cancer and oral contraceptive use: a case–control study. *J. Chronic Dis.*, **36**, 639–46

60. Brownson, R.C., Blackwell, C.W., Pearson, D.K., Reynolds, R.D., Richens, J.W. and Papermaster, B.W. (1988). Risk of breast cancer in relation to cigarette smoking. *Arch. Intern. Med.*, **148**, 140–4

61. Jick, S.S., Walker, A.M., Stergachis, A. and Jick, H. (1989). Oral contraceptives and breast cancer. *Br. J. Cancer*, **59**, 618–21

62. Harris, R.E., Zang, E.A. and Wynder, E.L. (1990). Oral contraceptives and breast cancer risk: a case–control study. *Int. J. Epidemiol.*, **19**, 240–6

63. Wynder, E.L., MacCornack, F.A. and Stellman, S.D. (1978). The epidemiology of breast cancer in 785 United States caucasian women. *Cancer*, **41**, 2341–54

64. Harris, N.V., Weiss, N.S., Francis, A.M. and Polissar, L. (1982). Breast cancer in relation to patterns of oral contraceptive use. *Am. J. Epidemiol.*, **116**, 643–51

65. Rosenberg, L., Palmer, J.R., Rao, R.S., Zauber, A.G., Strom, B.L., Warshauer, M.E., Harlep, S. and Shapiro, S. (1996). Case–control study of oral contraceptive use and risk of breast cancer. *Am. J. Epidemiol.*, **143**, 25–37

66. Collaborative Group on Hormonal Factors in Breast Cancer (1996). Breast cancer and hormonal contraceptives: further results. *Contraception*, in press

20

Screening for breast cancer in young women

H. Cuckle

INTRODUCTION

In 1988, on the recommendation of a committee chaired by Sir Patrick Forrest[1], the Department of Health established a routine National Health Service breast screening program in the UK. All women registered with a general practitioner are invited for a mammogram at age 50 and routinely recalled every 3 years until age 64; quality control and monitoring ensure a high standard of performance[2]. The efficacy of this approach rests on the results of several studies of women screened at age 50 years or older, including randomized trials which avoid potentially strong statistical biases. Whilst comparable data in young women are available from 11 published studies (see Table 1), none of them included sufficient numbers of deaths reliably to estimate the mortality effect.

HEALTH INSURANCE PLAN STUDY

Carried out in New York in the 1960s, women aged 40–64 years old in the screening arm were offered a series of four screens by clinical examination and mammography at annual intervals. Approximately 15 000 women in each arm were aged 40–49 years at entry, and, although there was a 25% reduction in breast cancer mortality in the

Table 1 Mammographic screening in young women: effect on mortality in 11 studies

Study	Age group (years)	Screening interval (years)	Relative risk*	95% Confidence interval
Randomized trials				
Health Insurance Plan[3]	40–49	1	0.75	0.52–1.10
Two-counties[4,5]	40–49	2	0.92	0.52–1.60
Malmö[6]	45–54	1½–2	1.29	0.74–2.25
Stockholm[7]	40–49	2	1.09	0.40–3.00
Swedish overview[8†]	40–49	1½–2	0.87	0.63–1.20
Edinburgh[9]	45–49	2	0.98	0.45–2.11
Canada[10]	40–49	1	1.36	0.84–2.20
Geographical control				
Trial of Early Detection of Breast Cancer[11‡]	45–49	2	0.74	0.54–1.01
Case–control studies				
Breast Cancer Detection Demonstration Project[12]	35–49	1	0.89	0.75–1.03
Nijmegen[13]	35–49	2	1.25	0.36–4.30
Florence[14]	40–49	2–3	0.83	0.37–1.85

*Estimated change in breast cancer mortality given screening offered: for the case–control studies it is given as screening accepted; †includes data from the Two-counties, Malmö and Stockholm trials together with a trial in Gothenberg; ‡includes the screening arm of the Edinburgh trial

screening arm, this did not achieve statistical significance. A recent re-analysis restricted to breast cancer cases did show ignificance[15], but this is potentially biased.

The Health Insurance Plan Study results in young women are difficult to interpret. First, the lack of statistical significance does not count against a true effect. With the relatively small numbers included, there is a 50% chance that a true reduction as great as 30% would be missed. Second, some of the reduced mortality in women aged 45–49 at entry is attributable to the cancer being detected by screening when the women were over 50 years old. However, there was also a 36% mortality reduction in the 40–44-year age group which cannot be accounted for in this way.

SWEDISH TWO-COUNTIES STUDY

This was carried out at a time when there had been technical improvements in the quality of mammography. Screening by single-view mammography was offered to women aged 40–74 years with a routine recall period of nearly 3 years for older women and 2 years for the approximately 20 000 women aged 40–49 years. Whilst only a small mortality reduction was observed compared with 15 000 young controls, statistical power was even lower than for the Health Insurance Plan Study: follow-up was shorter and the breast cancer mortality in the control arm was considerably lower.

MALMÖ, STOCKHOLM AND THE SWEDISH OVERVIEW

Two other Swedish trials initially reported even less promising results among young women. In Malmö, the study was for those aged 45–69 years old but approximately 8000 were aged 45–54 in each of the screening and control arms. However, mortality was in fact higher in the screening arm. In Stockholm, of the overall population aged 40–64 years, approximately 14 000 and 7000 in the screening and control arms, respectively, were aged 40–49 years and no mortality reduction was seen. Recently, all the results from Swedish studies have been brought up to date and combined with an unpublished randomized trial in Gothenberg. Each of them now has a similar mortality reduction overall which amounts to 13%, on average, at age 40–49.

EDINBURGH STUDY

Women aged 45–64 years were randomized according to their general practitioner and there appears to have been a chance allocation to the screening arm of those who were at increased risk of breast cancer. After 7 years follow-up, there was little mortality reduction in those aged 45–49 (approximately 6000 in each arm). With a longer follow-up, the mortality reduction has increased but, as with the

Health Insurance Plan Study, some of this may be due to screening after age 50.

CANADIAN STUDY

With approximately 25 000 women aged 40–49 years in each arm, this is the only published trial specifically designed to have sufficient power to detect a mortality benefit in younger age groups. Beginning in 1988, all participants had a clinical examination at entry; those in the screening arm also had a mammogram at entry with both clinical examination and mammography annually thereafter for 5 years. There was a large excess breast cancer mortality in the screening arm, but this has been largely attributed to the chance occurrence of a high number of advanced tumors in this arm at entry. Also the trial has been criticized for poor-quality mammography, particularly in its early years.

NON-RANDOMIZED STUDIES

The UK Trial of Early Detection of Breast Cancer included women aged 45–64 years and compared the mortality from breast cancer in two screening centers with that in four centers in which no screening had taken place[16]. One of the screening centers is Edinburgh and this forms the screening arm of the randomized trial. Screening by mammography and physical examination was biannual with a physical examination only in the intervening years. After 10 years of follow-up, the mortality reduction in young women almost reached statistical significance.

The US Breast Cancer Detection Demonstration Project was not population-based. Instead, open access to mammography and physical examination was provided for five annual screens in 29 centers. The effect on mortality has been derived by comparing the observed number of deaths in attenders with that expected from the SEER (Surveillance, Epidemiology and End Results) program, a research-orientated registry of cases followed up for mortality. Overall (age 35–74 years), the observed mortality was less than expected and, although the effect was smaller in younger women, it almost reached statistical significance because of the size of the study (over 200 deaths in young women).

The two other studies in Nijmegen and Florence compared mortality in attenders with that in those who did not attend. Overall, mortality was reduced by about one-half in both centers but part of this large difference was caused by the 'healthy screenee' effect, whereby those accepting the offer of screening have reduced mortality *a priori*. The same effect may also be distorting the results in the younger women.

NEW VENTURES

In setting up the NHS Breast Screening Program, the Forrest Committee recommended that research be an integral part of its activity, and the age at which screening should start was highlighted as a priority area. Consequently, the UK Co-ordinating Committee for Cancer Research launched a large randomized trial of mammography starting at age 40–41. To date, 21 National Health Service Breast Screening Program centers are taking part. Eligible women are identified from Family Health Service Authority lists and randomized to a study arm (65 000) or control (130 000). Mammography is offered annually and a 10-year follow-up period is anticipated. A similar European trial is also being planned and it is hoped that the results can eventually be combined with the above UK trial.

CONCLUSION

Taken together, the 11 published studies do not argue strongly either in favor or against a mortality reduction in young women. A clearer conclusion may eventually emerge from them with longer follow-up. Since prognosis is more favorable than in older women, very long follow-up may be needed before a mortality benefit emerges, as it did in the Health Insurance Plan Study after 18 years. However, some of the studies (e.g. Two-counties) have begun to offer screening to those reaching age 50 years, thereby shortening the average length of unbiased follow-up.

The best hope for this important issue to be clarified will depend on the outcome of the UK Coordinating Committee for Cancer Research and European trials. Until these are completed, there are no scientific grounds for the routine screening of young women. This conclusion applies equally to those at increased risk of breast cancer as to young women in general.

REFERENCES

1. Forrest, A.P.M. (1986). *Breast Cancer Screening: Report to the Health Ministers of England, Wales, Scotland, and Northern Ireland.* (London: Her Majesty's Stationery Office)
2. Chamberlain, J., Moss, S.M., Kirkpatrick, A.E., Michell, M. and Johns, L. (1993). National Health Service breast screening programme results for 1991–2. *Br. Med. J.,* **307**, 353–6
3. Shapiro, S., Venet, W., Strax, P. and Venet, L. (1988). Periodic screening for breast cancer. In *The Health Insurance Plan Project and its Sequelae, 1963–86.* (Baltimore & London: Johns Hopkins University Press)
4. Tabar, L., Fagerberg, C.J.G., Gad, A. *et al.* (1985). Reduction in mortality from breast cancer after mass screening with mammography. *Lancet,* **1**, 829–32
5. Tabar, L., Fagerberg, G., Duffy, S.W., Day, N.E., Gad, A. and Grontoft, O. (1992). Update of the Swedish Two-Counties Program of Mammographic Screening for Breast Cancer. *Radiol. Clin. N. Am.,* **30**, 187–210
6. Andersson, I., Aspegren, K., Janzon, L. *et al.* (1988). Mammographic screening and mortality from breast cancer: the Malmö mammographic screening trial. *Br. Med. J.,* **297**, 943–94
7. Frisell, J., Eklund, G., Hellström, L. *et al.* (1991). Randomized study of mammography screening – preliminary report on mortality in the Stockholm trial. *Breast Cancer Res. Treatment,* **18**, 49–56
8. Nyström, L., Rutqvist, L.E., Wall, S., Lindgren, A. *et al.* (1993). Breast cancer screening with mammography: overview of Swedish randomised trials. *Lancet,* **341**, 973–8
9. Roberts, M.M., Alexander, F.E., Anderson, T.J. *et al.* (1990). Edinburgh trial of screening for breast cancer: mortality at seven years. *Lancet,* **335**, 241–6

10. Miller, A.B., Baines, C.J., To, T. and Wall, C. (1992). Canadian National Breast Screening Study. 1. Breast cancer detection and death rates among women aged 40 to 49 years. *Can. Med. Assoc. J.*, **147**, 1459–88

11. UK Trial of Early Detection of Breast Cancer Group (1993). Breast cancer mortality after 10 years in the UK trial of early detection of breast cancer. *Breast*, **2**, 13–20

12. Morrison, A.S., Brisson, J. and Khalid, N. (1988). Breast cancer incidence and mortality in the Breast Cancer Detection Demonstration Project. *J. Natl. Cancer Inst.*, **80**, 1540–7

13. Peeters, P.H.M., Verbeek, A.L., Hendriks, J.H. and Bon, M.J. (1989). Screening for breast cancer in Nijmegen. Report of 6 screening rounds, 1976–1986. *Int. J. Cancer*, **43**, 226–30

14. Palli, D., Rosselli Del Turco, M.R., Buiatti, E., Carli, S., Ciatto, S., Toscani, L. and Maltoni, G. (1986). A case–control study of the efficacy of a non-randomized breast cancer screening program in Florence (Italy). *Int. J. Cancer*, **38**, 501–4

15. Chu, K.C., Smart, C.R. and Tarone, R.E. (1988). Analysis of breast cancer mortality and stage distribution by age for the Health Insurance Plan clinical trial. *J. Natl. Cancer Inst.*, **14**, 1125–32

16. UK Trial of Early Detection of Breast Cancer Group (1988). First results on mortality reduction in the UK Trial of Early Detection of Breast Cancer. *Lancet*, **2**, 411–16

21

Screening for breast cancer in young women using breast self-examination

A.K. Hackshaw

INTRODUCTION

Breast self-examination is a procedure for detecting breast cancer which has been promoted for many years by public health services as a safe and relatively simple method. It is a technique whereby women are taught to examine their breasts on a regular basis. Routine mammographic screening has been shown significantly to reduce mortality in women aged over 50 years[1]. Since mammographic screening has not yet been shown to reduce mortality in women under 50 years, it might be argued that there is a case for using breast self-examination in younger women, and also in populations where mammography is not available. It could also be proposed that young women prescribed oral contraceptives should be taught breast self-examination if it is shown that they increase the risk of breast cancer. Young women are more likely to practice breast self-examination than older women, but there is no firm evidence that it will save lives.

Table 1 The proportion of female students aged 17–30 years who practice breast self-examination (1988–91)

Country	Percentage of women who practice breast self-examination*
Austria	45
Belgium	25
Denmark	31
Finland	66
France	29
Germany (East)	57
Germany (West)	56
Greece	17
Hungary	34
Iceland	20
Ireland	24
Italy	18
Netherlands	35
Norway	31
Poland	32
Portugal	33
Spain	17
Sweden	23
Switzerland	39
UK	31
USA	(8)[†]
All	33

*More than once a year; [†]this is comparable to the 8% of women who practice breast self-examination at least ten times a year in all the other countries (excluding USA) listed above
Source: Wardle *et al.* (1995)[2]

BREAST SELF-EXAMINATION PRACTICE AND INCIDENCE OF BREAST CANCER IN YOUNG WOMEN

Table 1 shows the percentage of female students aged 17–30 years in 20 European countries and the USA who practice breast self-examination. Although most of these countries recommend breast self-examination, only one-third of these women, on average, practice it on a regular basis. This figure is likely to be less in the general population. Practice of breast self-examination varied between countries and was particularly low in countries such as Italy and Spain. The yearly incidence of breast cancer in young women is relatively low – about 2–3 per 100 000 women aged 15–30 years[3,4]. In the UK it is about 3 per 100 000 women aged 15–29 years (47 per 100 000 in women aged 15–49 years). The number of annual deaths from breast cancer in young women is also low, for example, in the UK there are only about six deaths per million women aged 15–29 years[5] (14 per 100 000 in women aged 15–49 years). For comparison, in women aged 50–69 years, the incidence is 227 per 100 000 and the mortality is 102 per 100 000[5].

EVIDENCE ON THE EFFECTIVENESS OF BREAST SELF-EXAMINATION

Although this article relates to younger women, few studies have given results by age and therefore overall results are shown.

Detection of breast cancer

Most of the studies have been retrospective and were based on women diagnosed with breast cancer. Many looked at the use of breast self-examination and not necessarily cancers actually detected during breast self-examination. Table 2 shows those studies in which cancers were actually detected by breast self-examination. Overall, 23% of cancers were identified during breast self-examination – all the others were detected by the woman by accident or a physician examination. The one study which gave results by age[12] showed that only 14% (8/59) [95% CI, 5–22%] of women aged under 35 years with cancer were detected by breast self-examination. In women aged 35–44 years, the figure was 9% (21/230) [95% CI, 5–13%]. Table 2 also shows the proportion of stage I (or less) cancers identified in women who detected their cancer during breast self-examination. There is a suggestion that breast self-examination is associated with detecting less advanced cancer. There are, however, the problems of biases in these studies (lead-time bias, length-biased sampling and selection bias) when comparing cancers in

Table 2 The percentage of women with breast cancer detected by breast self-examination (BSE) in retrospective studies and the percentage with stage I and localized tumors

Study	Percentage of cancers detected by BSE	Stage I or less			In situ and local		
		BSE[†]	No BSE	Difference	BSE[†]	No BSE	Difference
Greenwald et al., 1978[6]	19 (55/284)	22 (12/55) 38 (20/53)	18 (37/210) 30 (62/204)	4* 8**	—	—	—
Smith et al., 1980[7]	49 (108/220)	—	—	—	59 (63/107)	60 (67/111)	−1
Feldman et al., 1981[8]	30 (302/996)	—	—	—	—	—	—
Huguley et al., 1981[9]	21 (431/2083)	27 (118/431)	26 (428/1652)	1*	—	—	—
Gould-Martin et al., 1982[10]	22 (60/274)	—	—	—	52 (31/60)	63 (135/214)	−11
Hislop et al., 1984[11]	23 (93/404)	—	—	—	—	—	—
Owen et al., 1985[12]	9 (189/2063)	—	—	—	58 (109/189)	54 (1006/1874)	4
Smith and Burns, 1985[13]	51 (185/360)	—	—	—	59 (110/185)	54 (94/175)	5
Devitt, 1989[14]	15 (54/367)	—	—	—	—	—	—
Kuroishi et al., 1992[15]	—	37 (132/355)	29 (383/1327)	8**	—	—	—
Farwell et al., 1993[16]	17 (363/2164)	—	—	—	—	—	—
Senie et al., 1994[17]	58 (421/729)	—	—	—	—	—	—
All	23 (2261/9944)	27 (130/486) 37 (152/408)	25 (465/1862) 29 (445/1531)	2* 8**	58 (313/541)	55 (1302/2374)	3

[†]Cancers detected by BSE; *pathological stage; **clinical stage

breast self-examination groups and non-breast self-examination groups and so no firm conclusion can be made from these studies.

There have been published results from two non-randomized trials of breast self-examination (the UK Trial of early detection of breast cancer[18] and the Mama study[19]) and one randomized controlled trial in Russia[20] (still in progress). The results are in Table 3. There have been no published results from another randomized controlled trial in China. Although the non-randomized studies showed a higher proportion of cancers in the breast self-examination group, the randomized trial showed no difference at all after 5 years. Benign biopsy rates were higher in breast self-examination groups. The UK trial[18] found a higher malignant : benign ratio for the younger group of women (45–49 years) when compared to all women (45–64 years), suggesting a higher recall rate in younger women who practice breast self-examination.

Survival and mortality

Five retrospective studies[15,21–25] have shown a higher survival rate in women who use breast self-examination (not necessarily with cancers detected during breast self-examination). These studies looked at women with breast cancer and observed what proportion of these were still alive after 5 years. In women of all ages there was, on average, a 10% higher survival rate. One study[15], however, compared women with cancer detected during breast self-examination to those detected by chance and, although there was a significant difference in survival at 5 years, there was no significant difference at 10 years. The only study to look at survival by age[21,22] showed a difference in survival rate of about 12% in women aged 22–49 years who used breast self-examination compared to those who did not. These studies are, however, as mentioned before, subject to various biases and no firm conclusion can be made. The increased survival could be accounted for by lead time and length biases.

The two non-randomized trials[18,19] showed conflicting results (Table 3). The UK trial showed no effect on mortality (relative risk 1.01). The Mama study showed a 25% reduction in mortality. In women aged 20–40 years there was a significant reduction of 35%

Table 3 Trials of breast self-examination (BSE)

Study	Age range (years)	Cancer prevalence per 1000 women*		Benign biopsies per 1000 women		Malignant : benign ratio		Percentage change in mortality (95% CI)
		BSE	Non-BSE	BSE	Non-BSE	BSE	Non-BSE	
Non-randomized trials								
UK[18]	45–64	13.3	12.1	9.1	6.1	1:0.7	1:0.5	+1 (–14, +17)
	45–49	12.1	10.8	15.3	12.0	1:1.3	1:1.1	—
Finland[19]	20–80	19% more cancers in the BSE group than expected						–25 (–39, –8)
	20–40	54% more cancers in the BSE group than expected						–35 (–79, +53)
Randomized controlled trial								
Russia[20]	40–64	3.2	3.2	7.8	4.6	1:2.4	1:1.4	—
	40–49	2.4	2.5	—	—	—	—	—

*The number of diagnosed breast cancers per 1000 women

and in women aged 40–49 years the reduction was 31% (rate ratio 0.69, 95% CI 0.42–1.08). Results on mortality from the trials in Russia and China will not be available for several years.

There is, at present, no satisfactory evidence to show that breast self-examination saves lives at any age. Even if the two trials in Russia and China show an effect, the least benefit is likely to be in young women in whom the incidence and mortality rates are relatively low compared to those in older women.

CONCLUSION

Table 4 shows the advantages and disadvantages of a mass routine screening policy using breast self-examination. Screening young women using breast self-examination would not be worthwhile. Young women have relatively little to gain from breast self-examination, and, even if it is shown to reduce mortality, the number of unaffected women having surgical biopsies (false-positives) is likely to be large in relation to the gain. This is in agreement with previous views[26,27]. In women who practice breast self-examination, most cancers are not found during the examination. Young women are as likely to detect a cancer themselves in daily activities such as washing and dressing as with a formal monthly self-examination. If, in

Table 4 The advantages and disadvantages of a mass screening policy using breast self-examination in young women

Advantages	*Disadvantages*
Technique is relatively simple and safe	low incidence
More likely to detect the cancer than no checking of the breasts	low mortality
Probably identifies less advanced cancers	no proven reduction in mortality high number of unnecessary biopsies increased anxiety in false-positives most cancers are missed high cost of teaching effective self-examination to all young women

the future, it is shown that oral contraceptives increase the risk of breast cancer, the actual incidence and mortality in young women will still be low. Young women should not be taught breast self-examination because they are prescribed oral contraceptives. Women, however, should be encouraged to seek medical advice if they discover an abnormality. This is known as 'breast awareness'[28], but is a part of good general health self-care where a woman should notice an abnormality in *any* part of her body which should then be investigated by a doctor. Consultations discussing 'breast awareness' can be used as a vehicle for educating women about breast cancer and encourage women to attend for a mammographic examination later in life when the risk of breast cancer increases dramatically and screening (using mammography) is effective.

ACKNOWLEDGEMENT

I thank Malcolm Law, Nicholas Wald and Judith Ibison for their helpful comments.

REFERENCES

1. Wald, N.J., Chamberlain, J. and Hackshaw, A. (1993). Report of the European Society for Mastology Breast Cancer Screening Evaluation Committee (1993). *Breast*, **2**, 209–16
2. Wardle, J., Steptoe, A., Smith, H., Groll-Knapp, E., Koller, M., Smith, D. and Brodziak, A. (1995). Breast self-examination: attitudes and practices among young women in Europe. *Eur. J. Cancer Prev.*, **4**, 61–8
3. *Cancer Incidence in Five Continents* (1982). IARC Scientific Publications, Volume IV, number 42
4. Cancer Research Campaign Factsheet 6.1 (1991)
5. Office of Population, Censuses and Surveys (1986). OPCS Mortality Statistics: Cause. Series DH2, number 13
6. Greenwald, P., Nasca, P.C., Lawrence, C.E., Horton, J., McGarrah, R.P., Gabriele, T. and Carlton, K. (1978). Estimated effect of breast self-examination and routine physician examinations on breast-cancer mortality. *N. Engl. J. Med.*, **229**, 271–3

7. Smith, E.M., Francis, A.M. and Polissar, L. (1980). The effect of breast self-exam practices and physician examinations on extent of disease at diagnosis. *Prev. Med.*, **9**, 409–17

8. Feldman, J.G., Carter, A.C., Nicastri, A.D. and Hosat, S.T. (1981). Breast self-examination, relationship to stage of breast cancer at diagnosis. *Cancer*, **47**, 2740–5

9. Huguley, C.M. and Brown, R.L. (1981). The value of breast self-examination. *Cancer*, **47**, 989–95

10. Gould-Martin, K., Paganini-Hill, A., Casagrande, C., Mack, T. and Ross, R.K. (1982). Behavioral and biological determinants of surgical stage of breast cancer. *Prev. Med.*, **11**, 429–40

11. Hislop, T.G., Coldman, A.J. and Skippen, D.H. (1984). Breast self-examination: importance of technique in early diagnosis. *Can. Med. Assoc. J.*, **131**, 1349–52

12. Owen, W.L., Hoge, A.F., Asal, N.R., Anderson, P.S., Owen, A.S. and Cucchiara, A.J. (1985). Self-examination of the breast: use and effectiveness. *Southern Med. J.*, **78**, 1170–3

13. Smith, E.M. and Burns, T.L. (1985). The effects of breast self-examination in a population-based cancer registry. *Cancer*, **55**, 432–7

14. Devitt, J.E. (1989). False alarms of breast cancer, *Lancet*, **2**, 1257–8

15. Kuroishi, T., Tominaga, S., Ota, J., Horino, T., Taguchi, T. *et al.* (1992). The effect of breast self-examination on early detection and survival. *Jpn. J. Cancer Res.*, **83**, 344–50

16. Farwell, M.F., Foster, R.S. and Costanza, M.C. (1993). Breast cancer and earlier detection efforts. Realized and unrealized impact on stage. *Arch. Surg.*, **128**, 510–14

17. Senie, R.T., Lesser, M., Kinne, D.W. and Rosen, P.P. (1994). Method of tumor detection influences disease-free survival of women with breast carcinoma. *Cancer*, **73**, 1666–72

18. Ellman, R., Moss, S.M., Coleman, D. and Chamberlain, J. (1993). Breast self-examination programmes in the trial of early detection of breast cancer: ten year findings. *Br. J. Cancer*, **68**, 208–12

19. Gastrin, G., Miller, A.B., To, T., Aronson, K.J., Wall, C., Hakama, M., Louhivuori, K. and Pukkala, E. (1994). Incidence and mortality from breast cancer in the Mama Program for breast screening in Finland, 1973–1986. *Cancer*, **73**, 2168–74

20. Semiglazov, V.F., Moiseyenko, V.M., Bavli, J.L., Migmanova, N.S. *et al.* (1992). The role of breast self-examination in early breast cancer detection (results of the 5-years USSR/WHO randomized study in Leningrad). *Eur. J. Epidemiol.*, **8**, 409–502

21. Costanza, M.C. and Foster, R.S. (1984). Relationship between breast self-examination and death from breast cancer by age groups. *Cancer Detec. Prev.*, **7**, 103–8
22. Foster, R.S. and Costanza, M.C. (1984). Breast self-examination practices and breast cancer survival. *Cancer*, **53**, 999–1005
23. Huguley, C.M., Brown, R.L., Greenberg, R.S. and Clark, W.S. (1988). Breast self-examination and survival from breast cancer. *Cancer*, **62**, 1389–96
24. Bonett, A., Dorsch, M., Roder, D. and Esterman, A. (1990). Infiltrating ductal carcinoma of the breast in South Australia. Implications of trends in tumour diameter, nodal status and case-survival rates for cancer control. *Med. J. Aust.*, **152**, 19–23
25. Le Geyte, M., Mant, D., Vessey, M.P., Jones, L. and Yudkin, P. (1992). Breast self examination and survival from breast cancer. *Br. J. Cancer*, **66**, 917–18
26. Frank, J.W. and Mai, V. (1985). Breast self-examination in young women: more harm than good? *Lancet*, **2**, 655–7
27. Morrison, A.S. (1991). Is self-examination effective in screening for breast cancer? *J. Natl. Cancer Inst.*, **83**, 226–7
28. Austoker, J. (1994). Cancer prevention in primary care. Screening and self examination for breast cancer. *Br. Med. J.*, **309**, 168–74

Section 5

Other aspects of pill prescribing

22

Problems of postpartum pill use

D.R. Bromham

INTRODUCTION

The postpartum period offers a recently delivered woman the opportunity of discussing and planning future contraception at a time when informed professional advice is more likely to be available and when the chance of conception is seen as being relatively remote, allowing a less pressurized decision. Conversely, it has been argued that the remoteness of the chance of conception demands that contraception with a method having any inherent dangers or increased risk for the mother or, indeed the infant, be avoided by not commencing use until really needed[1].

Estimates of the interval between delivery and return of female fertility vary but it has been suggested[2] that in non-breastfeeding women 40% will have menstruated within 6 weeks. Although as many as 50% of these menstruations may follow anovulatory cycles, it seems that 15% of non-breastfeeders have ovulated by 6 weeks. Ovulation as early as 25 days after delivery may occur[2]. For breastfeeding women, the pattern is very different. The contraceptive effects of lactational amenorrhea are outside the scope of this review, but it is relevant to remark that the effectiveness of this natural method is dependent on the completeness of breastfeeding[3]. Where infant feeding practices follow a mixed pattern, fertility may rapidly return and one review suggests that as many as 5% of breastfeeders may ovulate within 6 weeks of delivery[2].

229

To result in conception there must also be a resumption of sexual intercourse. Here there is considerable presumption that, for esthetic, religious and psychological reasons, intercourse does not resume until several weeks after delivery[4]. Although this reflects Biblical references to a 'period of uncleanliness' (Leviticus XII) there are very little data to indicate the rate at which sexual activity recommences. However, it seems reasonable to suppose that, in women who breastfeed, return of sexual activity is more likely to precede ovulation which in any event is unpredictable. Lactation is therefore inappropriately considered as a contraindication to other contraceptive methods, particularly where mixed infant feeding practices are likely. The balance between need and risk is particularly evident when considering the use of the combined oral contraceptive pill in the postpartum period. Conventional guidelines on usage of the pill by postpartum women reflect three potential effects that have been acknowledged and debated for many years.

ADDITIONAL RISK OF VENOUS THROMBOEMBOLISM POSTPARTUM

Although recognized for some 25 years[5] as an estrogen-related risk for pill users, venous thromboembolism has not been studied directly in association with postpartum usage of this method of contraception. Perceptions that the puerperium was a contraindication to pill usage because of this risk owe as much to recognized major venous thromboembolism risks where high doses of estrogen had been used, prior to the advent of alternative methods, to suppress lactation[6]. However, it has been pointed out[1] that alteration in clotting mechanisms present during, and persisting for a short time after, pregnancy resemble those seen in hematological studies of pill users. Although these pill-induced changes are less marked with low-estrogen dose pills[7] there remains the possibility of synergism with the hematological changes of pregnancy. These usually return to normal within 4 weeks of delivery, in most cases much earlier[8]. Some factors associated with an increased risk of venous thromboembolism that may be present at delivery would be regarded as temporary contraindications to pill usage, e.g. Cesarean section, prolonged labor with or without dehydration, prolonged immobility, but are short-term situations. Others may take longer to resolve, e.g. severe varicose veins. In this context, it should be recognized that the World Health Organisation data[9] show that among European women a history of hypertension in pregnancy is associated with a significant increase for venous thromboembolism in pill users. Although some prothrombotic states have been postulated as associated with hypertension in pregnancy, the more practical constraint after a hypertensive pregnancy is the need to confirm a return to a normotensive state before commencing the pill, persistent significant hypertension being a contraindication.

There appears to be little evidence that continuation of lactation has any influence on cardiovascular risks with the pill, and breastfeeding requires consideration for reasons independent of this.

EFFECT ON LACTATION

Again, the practice of using high doses of estrogen to suppress lactation has colored our perceptions of pill usage by lactating women. One study[10] using high-dose pills started on the 5th day postpartum failed to confirm that pill use suppressed lactation; similar continuations of breastfeeding were observed over a 6-week period in pill users and controls. The numbers were, however, very small. Although this sort of experience led some observers to deny any adverse effect of the combined pill on breastfeeding, larger multinational studies have been less encouraging. Use of the pill in the first few weeks postpartum is associated with a reduction in milk volume of up to 40%[11,12]. Although the effect on volume and duration of breastfeeding is less marked with low-dose pills, it is still apparent[11–13]. Others have identified a negative effect on milk composition and infant growth[14,15]. However, there is significant variation in the methodologies used in these studies and difficulties with interpretation[16]. The American Academy of Pediatrics has concluded that the evidence for an effect on milk composition is inconclusive and that suppression of lactation is of less importance if the pill is not commenced in the immediate postpartum period[17]. The Academy subsequently defined the combined pill as a drug compatible with breastfeeding[18]. Although adverse nutritional effects of pill usage during lactation may be relatively unimportant in developed societies, they would be of more major concern in the developing world.

STEROID SECRETION IN BREAST MILK

Although detectable amounts of contraceptive steroids may be found in breast milk[13], they are very low and do not exceed the amounts that would be found in the event of an ovulation occurring in a breastfeeding woman. There is little evidence to support the concept that this may cause major problems for the infant ingesting them. Although effects such as breast enlargement have been postulated, reporting is largely anecdotal[19,20]. Nonetheless, the remote possibility that such problems might occur has contributed to recommendations that the combined pill is not started in breastfeeders until 6 weeks postpartum, that being a stage at which infant organ systems may be less vulnerable and at which enzyme systems to metabolize these steroids are believed to be established[21].

CONCLUSIONS

'An absence of evidence is not evidence of absence'

From the foregoing it seems that international guidelines[22] regarding the commencement of oral contraception in the postpartum period, while not based entirely on intuitive assumptions or extrapolation from other situations, do have some circumstantial evidence to support them. For any woman it is important to consider the existence of any contraindication to pill use including persisting changes associated with the pregnancy and delivery. If these are not present, then the suggestion that pill usage could commence 3 weeks after delivery seems an appropriate compromise – giving protection against the first ovulation *and* avoiding synergism with residual prothrombotic factors in the vast majority (but not all!) of cases. The bulk of research data suggests some adverse effect on lactation.

However, with low-dose pills commenced after lactation is established, this is probably minor. None the less, it seems appropriate with a lactating patient to regard the combined pill as a secondary choice compared to alternatives such as progestogen-only methods. If the additional contraceptive security of the combined pill is required, it is probably best to commence this at about 6 weeks postpartum. This is again a compromise – minimizing both the risks of conception and of lactation suppression without totally avoiding either.

In addition to clarification of the impact on lactation and infant nutrition, we must look to further research to elucidate the link between hypertension in pregnancy and venous thromboembolism in pill users which as yet remains a significant conundrum.

REFERENCES

1. WHO Task Force on Oral Contraceptives (1987). Contraception during the postpartum period and during lactation: the effects on women's health. *Int. J. Gynaecol. Obstet.*, **25** (Suppl.), 13–26
2. Vorherr, H. (1973). Contraception after abortion and post partum. *Am. J. Obstet. Gynecol.*, **117**, 1002–25
3. Saarikoski, S. (1993). Contraception during lactation. *Ann. Med.*, **25**, 181–4
4. Sharman, A. (1968). Oral contraception after delivery. *Nursing Mirror*, 1 March, 28–9
5. Farmer, R.D.T. and Preston, T.D. (1995). The risk of venous thromboembolism associated with low dose oral contraceptives. *J. Obstet. Gynaecol.*, **15**, 195–200
6. Daniel, D.G., Campbell, H. and Turnbull, A.C. (1967). Puerperal thromboembolism and suppression of lactation. *Lancet*, **2**, 287
7. Bonnar, J. (1991). Changes in coagulation and fibrinolysis with low dose oral contraceptives. *Adv. Contracept.*, **7** (Suppl. 3), 285–91
8. Forbes, C.D. and Greer, I.A. (1992). Physiology of haemostasis and the effect of pregnancy. In Greer, I.A., Turpie, A.G.G. and Forbes, C.D. (eds.) *Haemostasis and Thrombosis in Obstetrics and Gynaecology*, pp. 1–25. (London and New York: Chapman & Hall Medical)
9. WHO Collaborative Study of Cardiovascular Disease and Steroid Hormone Contraception. (1995). Venous thromboembolic disease and

combined oral contraceptives: results of international multicentre case-control study. *Lancet*, **346**, 1575–82

10. Gambrell, R.D. (1970). Immediate postpartum oral contraception. *Obstet. Gynecol.*, **36**, 101–6

11. Borglin, N. and Sandholm, L. (1971). Effect of oral contraceptives on lactation. *Fertil. Steril.*, **22**, 39–41

12. Croxatto, H.B., Diaz, S., Peralta, O., Juez, G., Herreros, C., Casado, M.E., Salvatierra, A.M., Miranda, P. and Duran, E. (1983). Fertility regulation in nursing women. IV. Long-term influence of a low-dose combined oral contraceptive initiated at day 30 postpartum upon lactation and infant growth. *Contraception*, **27**, 13–25

13. Nillson, S., Meilbin, T., Hofvander, Y., Sundelin, C., Valentin, J. and Nygren, K.G. (1986). Long-term follow-up of children breastfed by mothers using oral contraceptives. *Contraception*, **34**, 443–57

14. World Health Organisation. (1988). Effects of hormonal contraceptives on breast milk composition and infant growth. *Stud. Fam. Plann.*, **6**, 361–9

15. Hull, V.J. (1981). The effects of hormonal contraception on lactation: current findings, methodological considerations, future priorities. *Stud. Fam. Plann.*, **12**, 134–155

16. Sweezy, S.R. (1992). Contraception for the postpartum woman. *NAACOG's Clinical Issues*, **2**, 209–25

17. American Academy of Pediatrics Committee on Drugs. (1981). Breastfeeding and contraception. *Pediatrics*, **68**, 138–40

18. American Academy of Pediatrics Committee on Drugs. (1989). Transfer of drugs and other chemicals into human milk. *Pediatrics*, **84**, 924–36

19. Harforche, J.K. (1977). Appearance of contraceptive steroids in human milk: effects on the child. *J. Biosoc. Sci.*, **4** (Suppl.), 165–79

20. Johansson, E. and Odlind, V. (1987). Passage of exogenous hormones into breast milk: possible effect. *Int. J. Gynaecol. Obstet.*, **25**, 111–14

21. Diaz, S. and Croxatto, H.B. (1993). Contraception in lactating women. *Curr. Opin. Obstet. Gynecol.*, **5**, 815–22

22. Blumenthal, P.D. and McIntosh, N. (1995). *Pocket Guide for Family Planning Service Providers*, pp. 46–7. (Baltimore: JHPIEGO Corporation)

23

Problems associated with pill use during adolescence

M. Oliveira da Silva

INTRODUCTION

Adolescents who wish to use oral contraception have several particular medical and compliance problems. Among the medical considerations are concerns that young women may use the pill before their bodies have fully developed. In addition, most adolescents are unlikely to be in a long-term stable relationship. Doctors must therefore take into account their special need for protection against sexually transmitted diseases.

In adolescents, are there any additional contraindications to modern oral contraception which require the special screening of young women? Two main medical concerns have been raised. The first relates to the possibility that the use of the pill by a young adolescent before her reproductive hypothalamic–pituitary–ovarian axis has fully matured will permanently damage it[1]. The second is related to the possibly negative effect that estrogens might have on an individual's height[2].

INITIATION OF CONTRACEPTION

The fundamental question regarding the maturity of the endocrinological axis is whether a teenager can take the pill before she has

235

started to menstruate regularly. Certainly, several authors have recommended that young women should wait until they are menstruating regularly. There is, however, conflicting opinion about when this event can be considered to have occurred.

Louise Tyrer, one of the first authors to write about this issue, recommended in 1975 that a teenager should not start the pill until she had had 1 or 2 years of regular menstruation. By this recommendation, gynecologists tried to avoid postpill amenorrhea and possible subsequent infertility in adolescents who wanted to take the pill. Some gynecologists, however, thought that this delay was much too long and, instead, suggested that 'once a woman has three consecutive, spontaneous, ovulatory menstrual cycles, oral contraceptives will not alter hypothalamic–pituitary–ovarian function'[2].

Irrespective of the stated minimum number of ovulatory cycles required to start oral contraception, irregular menstruation after menarche was accepted as a *relative contraindication* to pill use during the 1980s[3].

Five years ago, when the hormonal content of the pill was already much lower than those used 20 or 30 years ago, Tyrer, at the time the Vice-President for Medical Affairs of the American Planned Parenthood Federation, stated 'It is advisable that clinicians assure that onset of regular ovulation and menses has occurred prior to initiation of oral contraceptives for teenagers'[4].

Not all authors support this point of view. Indeed, the current trend of opinion is clearly to the contrary, as illustrated by the opinion of Goldzieher and Speroff. Goldzieher states that 'There is no basis for the notion that the adolescent hypothalamic–pituitary axis is adversely affected, temporarily or permanently, by oral contraceptive use'[5]. Leon Speroff has also written 'There is no evidence that early use of oral contraception has… any adverse effects on the reproductive tract'[6].

Evidence from data collected for over 30 years with different oral contraceptives (OCs) (most of which were of high dosage and no longer in existence) does not indicate a deleterious effect of the pill on either the endocrine axis or the fertility of women who take the pill at (or since) the start of their adolescence.

EFFECTS ON BONE GROWTH

The other important biological issue is whether the pill affects bone growth. Although an interesting hypothesis, there is a paucity of consistent and scientific data to support it. Nevertheless, it created a myth and unsubstantiated fear amongst gynecologists and general practitioners. As a result, clinical practice was, and still is, affected by it.

Goldzieher states that 'The idea that OCs stunt a girl's growth is hypothetical but not unreasonable, since high doses of estrogens have been used successfully to halt the growth of girls threatening to become excessively tall'[5]. The hypothesis arose because an effect of estrogen is to fuse the distal epiphyses of the long bones. However, the concern that a premature fusion of the distal epiphyses would result in a decrease in an individual's potential height was rejected by others who state that 'Once menarche has occurred, the final height cannot be altered by the administration of exogenous estrogen'[2].

Recently, the American College of Obstetricians and Gynecologists has officially endorsed this position[7]. 'Oral contraceptives in currently available low dosages do not cause premature closure of the epiphyses or inhibit skeletal growth. By the time menarche occurs, endogenous estrogen production has already initiated epiphyseal closure, and this process cannot be altered by small doses of exogenous steroids.'

Moreover, 'there are no data in normal-height girls to show that $30–35$-μg estrogen OCs or phasic preparations adversely affect ultimate height. In any event, a pregnancy (wanted or unwanted) is more likely to end the statural growth than OC therapy'[5]. Indeed, the hormonal milieu of an adolescent pregnancy can be more adverse than taking an OC. It is noteworthy that ethinylestradiol, the only estrogen present in currently available OCs, is a synthetic estrogen ten times more potent than natural estradiol. During pregnancy, there is a hyperestrogenic state in which, near term, the amount of estriol is 1000 times higher than that existing in non-pregnant women; estradiol and estrone levels are about 100 times higher.

The hypothetical effect of this hyperestrogenic state on the skeletal growth of young pregnant teenagers generated a profuse, speculative and conflicting literature during the 1970s and the 1980s. Notwithstanding the very obvious ethical and scientific difficulties in clarifying such a question, the most recent data do not support the hypothesis that ongoing maternal growth is affected by a pregnancy during adolescence[8]. There is now probably a consensus that OCs do not damage skeletal growth.

CHOICE OF PREPARATION

If there are no particular medical or biological problems associated with a young woman taking OCs, which pill should she take? Ideally, the prescribed pill should be of the lowest possible potency (do not confuse hormone potency with dosage) while maintaining the highest efficacy and tolerance. In adolescents, perhaps more than in any other group of women, these three objectives are not always compatible. For instance, the 20-µg pill sometimes appears to be the ideal preparation for adolescents, due to its reduced estrogen side-effects, but efficacy and tolerance can be compromised particularly when missed pills occur and/or spotting increases (a frequent problem in this age group). Although phasic pills were developed in an attempt to reduce the hormonal content of OCs, there are no data to suggest that young adolescents should use them rather than monophasic formulations, or vice-versa.

As in many other practical aspects of oral contraception, the empirical individualized approach is still the golden rule. If an adolescent has persisting side-effects with a monophasic pill, it is best to change her either to a different monophasic preparation (with different estrogen dosage and/or a different progestogen), or to a phasic pill. In adolescents who have polycystic ovarian syndrome – that is excess androgen production, its cosmetic manifestations (acne, hirsutism or seborrhea), irregular menses or oligomenorrhea – combined oral contraceptives containing cyproterone acetate will be the first choice. When mutual monogamy is not practiced, oral contraception should be used with a barrier method, and perhaps also a spermicide, in order to provide maximum protection against pregnancy and sexually transmitted diseases.

COMPLIANCE

Problems of compliance among adolescents are well recognized. Whatever the reasons for this poor compliance, obvious and universally accepted answers do not exist, since cultural and social situation strongly affect fruitful interventions. Compliance can be related with legal, economic and ethical aspects. Good compliance is associated with broader educational goals and a low incidence of side-effects. Unfortunately, factors associated with public education are beyond the strict intervention of doctors, although health personnel working with adolescents should never avoid assuming their educational role.

The consultation should occur at a convenient time after a short waiting time. Ideally, adolescents should be seen in a clinic which is separate from that used by adult women. Health personnel have to be able to build trust, a basic requirement of a successful interaction[6]. The consultation should not be restricted just to contraception, but should include family life, school or job behavior. Clinicians must be non-judgmental and able to identify adolescents' fears. The use of the package should be demonstrated. The beneficial and non-contraceptive effects of oral contraceptives should be emphasized, namely the reduction of dysmenorrhea and of pelvic inflammatory disease. A desk between the patient and the doctor should be avoided. The elimination of the pelvic examination during the first consultation has been defended and is quite acceptable: delaying this examination may increase access and compliance[6].

Fears and concerns should be identified in advance, and particular attention should be given to fear of weight gain. Adolescents should be told that low-dose OCs do not cause weight gain[9].

Although most authors believe that the 28-day package can improve compliance, I believe that its success mainly depends on its use among adult women, which is presently not the situation in the majority of European countries.

REFERENCES

1. Tyrer, L.B. and Granzig, W.A. (1975). Contraceptives for the teenager: things to know before prescribing. *Consultant*, **15**, 170–9
2. Brenner, P.F. (1983). Contraception. In Quilligan, E.J. (ed.) *Current Therapy in Obstetrics and Gynecology*, Vol. 2, p. 228. (Philadelphia: W.B. Saunders)
3. Greydanus, D.E. (1985). Contraception. In Lavery, J.O. and Sanfilippo, J.S. (eds.) *Pediatric and Adolescent Obstetrics and Gynecology*, p. 243. (New York: Springer-Verlag)
4. Tyrer, L. (1991). Teenagers and OCs. In Dickey, R.P. (ed.) *Managing Contraceptive Pill Patients*, 6th edn., pp. 54–155. (Durant: Emis)
5. Goldzieher, J. (1989). Oral contraceptive use in adolescence. In Goldzieher, J. (ed.) *Hormonal contraception: Pills, Injections and Implants*, pp. 102–3. (Dallas: Emis)
6. Speroff, L. and Darney, P. (1992). Clinical guidelines for contraception at different ages. In Speroff, L. and Darney, P. (eds.) *A Clinical Guide for Contraception*, p. 248. (Baltimore: Williams and Wilkins)
7. American College of Obstetricians and Gynecologists. (1992). Safety of oral contraceptives for teenagers. *J. Adol. Health Care*, **13**, 333–6
8. Stevens-Simon, C. and McAnarney, E.R. (1993). Skeletal maturity and growth of adolescent mothers: relationship to pregnancy outcome. *J. Adol. Health Care*, **13**, 428–32
9. Carpenter, S. and Neinstein, L.S. (1986). Weight gain in adolescent and young adult oral contraceptive users. *J. Adol. Health Care*, **7**, 342–8

24

Combined oral contraception and the perimenopausal woman

M. Short

'Age cannot wither her nor custom fade her infinite variety.'
Shakespeare

INTRODUCTION

Women continue to have a sexual life long after their desire to bear children but our knowledge of the safety, side-effects and effectiveness of different contraceptive methods during the last decade of reproductive life has not been a primary interest of researchers in fertility control. Slow and unpredictable physiological changes occur in this age group yet adequate studies of the requirements of these women have not been done. None the less, there is perhaps not a more compliant group than perimenopausal women, for they are well aware of the inherent problems of pregnancy at this age, both for themselves and for the fetus.

THE NEED FOR CONTRACEPTION

There is a high degree of fetal loss in older women, partly because the frequency of trisomy abnormalities increases with age. Clinically recognized spontaneous abortion occurs in only 12% of women

241

younger than 20 years but the incidence more than doubles in women over 40 years. The overall miscarriage risk (recognized and unrecognized) in women over 40 years is thought to be 75%[1] and more than two-thirds (70%) of these are due to chromosomal abnormalities[2]. A quarter of pregnancies in this age group go to term (in theory at least); the potential for a congenital abnormality, such as Down syndrome, is very high. Chromosomal abnormalities are not the only problem though; in a study from the Rotunda Hospital[3], Milner and colleagues found a significant increase in the risk of gestational diabetes, antepartum hemorrhage, fetal distress, prematurity, low birth weight and perinatal mortality among older mothers.

Increasing age also affects testicular function, with consequences both for the individual man and his progeny. From around the age of 30, the number and quality of spermatozoa begin to decline. Diminishing endocrine function occurs about 10 years later. Paternal aging, therefore, may be responsible for chromosomal abnormalities. It may also be the source of dominant and recessive mutations which manifest themselves in the descendents[4].

With statistics like this, contraception for both men and women in their forties is an important public health issue. This article assesses the risks and benefits of combined oral contraception in this age group, and considers some of the available alternatives.

OTHER CONTRACEPTIVES CURRENTLY AVAILABLE

Progestogen-only preparations must be included among the alternatives to combined oral contraception. Although the progestogen-only pills become more efficacious with age, there are the attendant problems of poor cycle control with irregular bleeding or amenorrhea[5]. Irregular menstruation at this time of life may create much tension and anxiety particularly when pregnancy is associated with an increased risk of fetal abnormality. Amenorrhea may also be a problem; counselling may reassure the woman that she is not pregnant, but anxiety about osteoporosis after 5 years of amenorrhea may remain. The same considerations apply to other progestogen-based contraceptives such as Depoprovera and Norplant. In addition to this problem is the local one of the progestogenic thickening of cervical mucus, making intercourse more difficult than it need be. The effects of long-term use of progestogens on a lipid profile and bone mass also have yet to be fully evaluated. On the other hand, progestogen-only pills have a much less suppressive effect on gonadotropins. Raised levels of follicle stimulating hormone (FSH) on two separate occasions in a woman using progestogen-only pills usually indicate ovarian failure[6]. There is no interference, therefore, with the biochemical diagnosis of the menopause.

Intrauterine contraceptive devices are another contraceptive option especially with the new progestogen-releasing devices. Intrauterine devices, however, are not without their problems, particularly with regard to their insertion and subsequent sequelae like spotting and cramps. They may, however, be a good way to administer progestogens during the perimenopause with the minimum of side-effects.

Barrier methods, particularly condoms, are often suggested as a method of contraception for perimenopausal couples. When couples have been used to more esthetically pleasing methods of contraception though, condoms and diaphragms can be both difficult to use and off-putting. Indeed, perimenopausal users of diaphragms often experience difficulty with insertion due to increased vaginal dryness, and concomitant cystitis. Given these problems, what are the benefits of using a combined oral contraceptive in perimenopausal women?

ADVANTAGES OF COMBINED ORAL CONTRACEPTION

Apart from the primary advantage of effective contraception in a very compliant population, another major advantage would be cycle control. Lighter periods may result in fewer hospital admissions for dilatation and curettage procedures, and perhaps fewer hysterectomies[7]. It is reasonable to assume that combined oral contraceptives protect against hot flushes. They may also protect against osteoporosis[8,9]. Other benefits of oral contraceptives, such as protection against ovarian cysts, endometriosis, endometrial and ovarian cancer occur in women older than 40 years as well as younger users.

Ovarian cysts

In virtually all studies, the incidence of ovarian cysts among pill users has been found to be reduced. Functional cysts are caused by abnormalities of ovulation. Since ovulation is more erratic among older women, this benefit of oral contraception may be important in this age group[5].

Ovarian cancer

Ovarian cancer is an important disease particularly in terms of mortality in women[10]. The literature consistently shows substantial reductions in the risk of all types of epithelial ovarian cancers among oral contraceptive users[11]. On average, the risk of ovarian cancer is reduced by 30% in ever users and by 50% or more in those exposed for 5 years or more. This effect seems to persist for 10 or more years after oral contraceptives are discontinued. The possible public health implications of these findings are significant as a substantial number of lives could be saved among women taking combined oral contraceptive preparations.

Endometrial cancer

The association between oral contraceptive use and endometrial carcinoma in women under the age of 60 years has been reviewed by Schlesselman[12]. Fifteen case–control studies provide consistent evidence of a protective effect which increases with duration of use. Four years of use leads to a 51% reduction in risk, while 12 years duration results in a 70% reduction in risk. Moreover, these protective effects do not appear to diminish for many years after stopping the pill.

Benign breast disease

Cystic disease of the breast occurs most frequently during the period of involution, i.e. in the 40–50-year age group. It has been estimated that some 50% of premenopausal women suffer from cystic disease of the breast[13]. A meta-analysis of available data showed an overall protective effect of combined oral contraceptive preparations on benign cystic disease.

DISADVANTAGES OF COMBINED ORAL CONTRACEPTIVES

The main concern of most researchers appears to be the possibility of an enhanced risk of cardiovascular disease with age (be it venous or arterial). Until the most recent pill controversy, it was felt that the use of oral contraceptives by non-smoking healthy women over the age of 40 did not confer any appreciable risk of cardiovascular disease[14].

While several epidemiological studies have investigated the problem of increased cardiovascular disease among oral contraceptive users much of the work relates to young healthy women. Most studies have recruited women younger than 35 years, where effectiveness is often paramount[15].

Myocardial infarction, thrombotic stroke and venous thrombosis are rare in young women, although the risk rises exponentially with increasing age. The prevalance of many associated risk factors also increases with age. Factors such as hypertension, family history, cigarette smoking, previous thrombotic episode and migraine[16] should all be taken into account when considering whether to prescribe the combined oral contraceptive pill in this age group – this is none other than good medical practice. Premenopausal women are often treated with high doses of progestogens to achieve cycle control and for the management of menorrhagia. The possible cardiovascular effects of such treatment have not been evaluated, but data gathered from mainly postmenopausal hormonal therapy suggest that progestogens may have an unfavorable effect on plasma lipids, especially the androgenic variety[7]. It might, therefore, be possible that the risk from taking the contraceptive pill is no greater than the risk from long-term use of high doses of progestogens.

Breast cancer

The controversy over oral contraception and breast cancer has not yet been resolved. While there is no evidence to suggest an increased risk of breast cancer among older users of oral contraceptives, any elevation could be important given the high incidence of breast cancer in many countries. In a review of breast cancer and contraception, Dexeus points out that, although the risk of breast cancer may be raised in young nulliparous women who have used oral contraceptives for a long duration, most of the available data relate to the use of older high-dose pills by older women[17]. Neither La Vecchia nor Harlap found consistent evidence of an association with oral contraception in women diagnosed after the age of 40–45[18,19]. The controversy concerns younger women, where studies have found positive relationships, including an association with a young age at starting oral contraception.

MENOPAUSAL DIAGNOSIS

It is known that 9% of women over the age of 45 years with a history of 6 months amenorrhea will resume menstruation and that ovulation can occur right up to the menopause in spite of hormone profiles suggesting a postmenopausal status. In 1988, Metcalf and colleagues[20] suggested that, as long as menstruation remains regular, women over the age of 40 years continue to ovulate in 98% of cycles. Kaufert[21] in interviews with perimenopausal women over a 3-year period provided evidence that there is no steady progress from a pre- to postmenopausal state. Indeed, women appeared to oscillate between the peri- and premenopausal states. Hence postmenopausal biochemical parameters were no guarantee of a postmenopausal state. The most sensitive marker for declining ovarian function in women with regular cycles is an elevated FSH level in the follicular phase. Lenton and colleagues[22] found that FSH levels rise dramatically from about 40 years of age, so that, by the age of 46–47 years the concentrations had almost doubled with a further increase in the 48–49-year age group. On the other hand, mean concentrations of luteinizing hormone (LH) remained static until the age of 48–49 whereupon they doubled. The estrogen-containing oral contraceptive prevents ovulation by the suppression of gonadotropin secretion and will mask the symptoms of ovarian failure as the progestogen component will ensure regular monthly withdrawal bleeds irrespective of menopausal status. In premenopausal women, LH and FSH levels are suppressed by at least 50% and may be undetectable by current assays. In postmenopausal women an 80% suppression of FSH has been reported for women given 50 µg of ethinylestradiol. The question of how to define the menopause therefore arises in women who become amenorrheic when stopping the pill. FSH levels are still valuable provided sufficient time has elapsed since stopping the pill to allow the recovery of endogenous gonadotropin production. There are data to show that gonadotropin levels return to normal within 1 week of stopping. Since a woman is unlikely to present for 6–8 weeks after stopping the pill, the FSH levels should no longer be affected.

Clearly, use of oral contraception masks the menopause and determining the correct time for transition from contraception to hormone replacement therapy (HRT) may be difficult. Since standard HRT is not a contraceptive, two approaches can be adopted to ensure adequate contraceptive cover. The first is to advise continuation of contraception up to the age of 55 years even if the woman is taking HRT. Alternatively, two measurements of FSH levels, 4–8 weeks apart, may be taken while the woman is off all hormonal preparations. Raised levels together with amenorrhea may be taken to indicate significant loss of ovarian function. Current recommendations then state that women aged more than 50 should use contraception for 1 year following 1 year of amenorrhea, while younger women use contraception for 2 years[6]. Very little is mentioned in the literature regarding oral contraception at this transition time, although the Food and Drug Administration in America has no upper limit on the use of oral contraception.

It is estimated that approximately 9% of women take HRT and fewer take it for any significant length of time, most stopping after 3 months. Perhaps we should be advocating the use of combined oral contraceptive preparations in perimenopausal women, not only for their contraceptive effects but for the very real beneficial side-effects that continue to occur in this age group.

CONCLUSION

Combined oral contraceptives have important benefits, regardless of age. We must weigh up, however, the benefits of an effective contraceptive which alleviates menopausal symptoms and perhaps protects against osteoporosis, against the possible cardiovascular risks in women over the age of 45 years. The risks of pregnancy, delivery or abortion in this age group should not be underestimated. Contrary to popular belief, women over a certain age do have intercourse. Although older women do not necessarily become pregnant easily, they still need effective contraception, for the sake of their health if not their sanity.

REFERENCES

1. Kruitwagen, R.F.P.M., Poels, L.G., Willemsen, W.N.P., Jap, P.H.K., Thomas, C.M.G. and Rolland, R. (1991). Endometrial epithelial cells in peritoneal fluid during the early follicular phase. *Fertil. Steril.*, **55**, 297
2. Jenkins, S., Olive, D.L. and Haney, A.F. (1986). Endometriosis: pathogenic implications of the anatomic distribution. *Obstet. Gynecol.*, **67**, 335
3. Milner, M., Barry-Kinsella C., Unwin, A. and Harrison, R.F. (1992). The impact of maternal aging on pregnancy and its outcome. *Int. J. Gynaecol. Obstet.*, **38**, 281–6
4. Auroux, M. (1995). *Fertility and Sterility: A Current Overview*, pp. 321–2. (Carnforth, UK: Parthenon Publishing)
5. Guillebaud, J. (1993). *Contraception: Your Questions Answered*, 2nd edn., pp. 228–34. (London: Churchill Livingstone)
6. Whitehead M.I. and Godfree, V. (1992). *Hormone Replacement Therapy: Your Questions Answered*, pp. 217–18. (Edinburgh: Churchill Livingstone)
7. Nesheim, B.I. (1994). Contraception towards the menopause. *Lakemedelsverket, Sweden*, **2**, 177–83
8. Corson, S. L. (1993). Oral contraceptives for the prevention of osteoporosis. *J. Reprod. Med.*, **38** (Suppl. 12), 1015–20
9. Volpe, A., Silfieri, M., Genazzani, A.D. and Genazzani, A.R. (1993). Contraception in older women. *Contraception*, **47**, 29–39
10. Stanford, J.L. (1991). Oral contraceptives and neoplasia of the ovary. *Contraception*, **43**, 543–56

11. Hanai, A. (1990). Trends and differentials in ovarian cancer incidence, mortality and survival experience. *Ampis*, **98** (Suppl. 12), 1–20

12. Schlesselman, J.E. (1991). Oral contraception and neoplasia of the uterine corpus. *Contraception*, **43**, 557–80

13. De Oliveira, C.F. (1995). Oral contraceptives and benign breast disease. *Fertil. Control Rev. Medicom*, **4**, 19–22

14. Luukainen, T. (1992). Contraception after 35. *Acta Obstet. Gynaecol. Scand.*, **71**, 169–74

15. Archer, D.F. (1992). Reversible contraception for women over 35 years of age. *Curr. Opin. Obstet. Gynaecol.*, **4**, 891–6

16. Lidegaard, O. (1995). Oral contraceptives and smoking, migraine, hypertension, diabetes and previous thrombosis; a risk assessment. *Fertil. Control Rev. Medicom*, **4**, 14–15

17. Dexeus, S. (1995). *Contraception and Breast Cancer*. Proceedings of the 3rd Congress of the ESC, Entopia, Athens, pp. 105–9

18. La Vecchia, C. (1992). Oral contraceptives and breast cancer. *Breast*, **2**, 76–81

19. Harlap, S. (1991). Oral contraceptives and breast cancer: cause and effect? *J. Reprod. Med.*, **36**, 374–95

20. Metcalf, M.G., Donald, R.A. and Livesey, J.H. (1982). Pituitary ovarian function before, during and after the menopause; a longitudinal study. *Clin. Endocrinol.*, **17**, 489–94

21. Kaufert, P.A., Gilbert, P. and Tate, R. (1987). Defining menopausal status: the impact of longitudinal data. *Maturitas*, **9**, 217–36

22. Lenton, E.A., Sexton, L., Lee, S. and Cooke, I.D. (1988). Progressive changes in LH and FSH and LH:FSH ratio in women throughout reproductive life. *Maturitas*, **10**, 35–43

25

The appropriateness of urinalysis as a routine screening test before oral contraceptive prescription

M. Thorogood and S. Langham

INTRODUCTION

A recent survey of delegates attending a meeting of the European Society of Contraception revealed an almost unanimous consensus on the importance of measuring blood pressure in women using oral contraceptives[1]. The same survey also found that as many as 40% of the delegates reported that they would routinely test the urine of women before prescribing combined oral contraceptives, most testing for the presence of both glucose and protein. Nearly 11% of delegates would measure blood glucose (Table 1). Oral contraceptives are widely used and any screening test routinely undertaken in users will represent a significant demand on health service resources. Moreover, the requirement to provide a specimen of urine or a blood sample may act as a barrier to seeking contraception in some women[2].

Although advice from the UK Department of Health is that the urine of women using oral contraceptives should be checked regularly[3], there are reasons to question the cost-effectiveness of such a procedure. In this paper, we review the evidence for the value of routine urine testing, and provide some estimates of the cost of this

251

Table 1 Reported usual practice regarding testing amongst 121 delegates at the European Society of Contraception Conference 1994 (percentages)

	Tests			
Usual practice	*Urinary glucose*	*Urinary protein*	*Measure blood pressure*	*Blood glucose*
Do in all or almost all women	19.0%	18.2%	95.1%	10.7%
Do as part of general health care, but may postpone until later	21.6%	19.8%	0.8%	9.1%

procedure. We also compare these cost estimates with those for measuring blood pressure in oral contraceptive users, a screening procedure which is performed by almost all prescribers.

ROUTINE SCREENING TESTS AND DETECTION OF PREVIOUSLY UNDIAGNOSED DISEASE

A screening test can only be of value if there is the possibility of improving the health of individuals by an earlier diagnosis of the condition, and if there is a sufficient prevalence of undiagnosed cases of the condition in the community. Evidence from screening studies can be used to estimate this prevalence.

With the development of the cheap, convenient, and accurate blood glucose monitoring kits, research-based screening programs which use dipstick urinalysis to identify undiagnosed cases of diabetes have disappeared. For this reason, data on the likely yield of such programs come from studies carried out in the 1960s. We have identified three studies which provided sufficient data on age and sex to indicate the likely prevalence of undiagnosed diabetes in young women[4-6], and the results are summarized in Table 2. Screening was given to 6379 women (assuming that the younger age group in the Newcastle upon Tyne study had a similar proportion of

Table 2 Results of three studies of diabetes in the community: prevalence of glycosuria and undiagnosed diabetes in women under 40 years

Location and sample	Age group (years)	Number of patients	% with glycosuria	% with previously undiagnosed diabetes
Newcastle upon Tyne	10–19	284*	—	0.0
One general practice,	20–29	284*	—	0.0
random 20% of practice list	30–39	323*	—	0.0
Essex	10–19	431	0.9	0.0
Halstead community,	20–29	302	2.0	0.0
97% of resident population	30–39	392	0.8	0.0
Bedford	10–19	—	—	—
Bedford community,	20–29	2007	2.8	0.1
67% of resident population (aged >20)	30–39	2801	2.2	0.4

* Total number of male and female patients tested

women as the overall sample, 50.1%). Fourteen women with undiagnosed diabetes were found (all in one study). From these studies, then, the likely prevalence of undiagnosed diabetes lies between 0.2% and 0.3%, with a 'false-positive' prevalence (of glycosuria not found to indicate diabetes) of between 1.2% and 1.9%. With improvements in medical surveillance and increased public awareness of the symptoms of diabetes, it is likely that the proportion of undetected diabetes would now be lower.

The assumption of a lower proportion of undiagnosed diabetics is confirmed by more recent evidence of the prevalence of undiagnosed diabetes which comes from the results of the 1993 Health Survey for England and Wales[7,8]. Glycosolated hemoglobin was measured in a random sample of 2931 women aged under 45 years old, and 13 (0.4%) of them had a level above 5.2% (a level taken to signify diabetes). Only one of these 13 women had not been previously diagnosed as a diabetic (Table 3), giving an estimated prevalence of undiagnosed diabetes of 0.03%.

Table 3 Health survey for England 1993: glycosolated hemoglobin level in women

Age group (years)	Number (%) with level >5.2%	Number diagnosed as diabetic	Number of women
16–24	1 (0.15)	1	633
25–34	6 (0.52)	6	1143
35–44	6 (0.52)	5	1155

So far, we have assumed that users of oral contraceptives are distributed evenly in the age range 16–44 years. In 1993, however, 68% of pill users were younger than 30 years[9]. If 68% of the routine urinalysis undertaken in oral contraceptive users is carried out in women aged under 30, then the estimated proportion of undiagnosed diabetics is even smaller. From the figures in Table 2, it would appear that the prevalence of undiagnosed diabetes detected on urinalysis might be as low as 0.1% in these younger women compared with 0.4% in the smaller older age group, giving an overall prevalence in potential oral contraceptive users of around 0.2%, with a further 2% of women requiring fasting blood glucose tests before a diagnosis of diabetes was excluded. The figures given in Table 3, however, are more recent and suggest that less than 0.03% of screened women will be detected as having undiagnosed diabetes.

There are very few data on the proportion of young women in whom undiagnosed renal disease might be found as a result of a urine test. In 1964 a group of researchers in Middlesex carried out urinalysis screening on 2052 women *of all ages*. Only 15 (0.7%) were found to have significant albuminuria and no new chronic disease was found[10].

In the 1993 Health Survey[11], blood pressure was measured by an automatic machine on a sample of over 3000 women aged 16–44 years (Tables 4 and 5). Three percent of the sample had hypertension (defined in Table 5), and two-thirds of them (2% of the population) were not receiving any hypotensive treatment, implying that the hypertension was either unknown or was being inadequately controlled.

Table 4 Health survey for England 1993: blood pressure readings in women (%)

Blood pressure reading (mmHg)	*Age group* (years)		
	16–24 (n = 889)	*25–34* (n = 1352)	*35–44* (n = 1185)
Diastolic < 85	98	93	88
Diastolic 85–94	2	6	9
Diastolic 95+	0	1	3

Table 5 Health Survey for England 1993: blood pressure grouping in the age group 16–44 years (n = 3511)

Blood pressure grouping	*%*
(1) Normotensive untreated Systolic less than 160 mmHg and diastolic less than 95 mmHg and not currently taking drugs prescribed for high blood pressure	97
(2) Normotensive treated Blood pressure levels as above (1) but taking drugs prescribed for high blood pressure	1
(3) Hypertensive treated Systolic greater than 159 mmHg and/or diastolic greater than 94 mmHg currently taking drugs prescribed for high blood pressure	0
(4) Hypertensive untreated Blood pressure levels as above (3) and not currently taking drugs prescribed for high blood pressure	2

There is no evidence that early detection and treatment of asymptomatic diabetes or asymptomatic infections of the renal tract prevent the onset of disease[12]. In contrast, the detection, management and treatment of asymptomatic hypertension can prevent the occurrence of both stroke and heart disease in later life[13].

USE OF ORAL CONTRACEPTIVES BY WOMEN WITH DIABETES OR IMPAIRED GLUCOSE TOLERANCE

It may be that clinicians want to screen all women for diabetes in order to avoid prescribing the pill to those with diabetes. Use of the pill may slightly increase insulin requirements in diabetic women, and some authors recommend that such women should use combined oral contraceptives for the shortest time possible, and should preferably use progestogen-only preparations[14]. A non-randomized trial in Copenhagen, however, has provided some evidence that use of oral contraceptives does not adversely affect the cardiovascular risk profile of otherwise healthy women with diabetes[15], although there is general agreement that diabetic women with pre-existing cardiovascular disease should be counselled strongly against using oral contraceptives[16]. Young undiagnosed diabetics, however, are extremely unlikely to have concomitant vascular problems. There is consistent evidence that use of oral contraceptives does not increase the incidence of overt diabetes in women not already known to have the condition[17–19].

USE OF ORAL CONTRACEPTIVES BY WOMEN WITH RENAL DISEASE

We have not found any evidence that use of oral contraceptives will adversely affect the outcome of any renal disease.

USE OF ORAL CONTRACEPTIVES BY WOMEN WITH ELEVATED BLOOD PRESSURE

A well-established adverse effect of oral contraceptives is a small elevation in blood pressure. It has been estimated that this is in the region of 5 mmHg of systolic pressure and around 2 mmHg of diastolic pressure[20], even with modern low-dose preparations. Moreover, the oral contraceptive pill continues to be associated with an increased risk of venous thromboembolism, myocardial infarction, and cerebrovascular accident. Subjects with even mildly elevated blood pressure are already at increased risk of stroke[21] and coronary heart disease[22] and to elevate that risk further by using the pill is unwise. Guillebaud[14] recommends that a diastolic blood pressure of 95 mmHg or more should be regarded as an *absolute* contraindication to use of oral contraceptives, while a diastolic blood pressure between 85 and 95 mmHg should be regarded as a relative contraindication, to be assessed along with the presence of other risks and the importance of avoiding pregnancy. One percent of women aged 16–44 in the 1993 Health Survey for England had a diastolic blood pressure of 95 mmHg or above, and a further 6% had a diastolic blood pressure between 85 and 94 mmHg (Table 4).

COST ESTIMATES OF CARRYING OUT THESE SCREENING TESTS

The technical procedures involved in carrying out screening tests can be costed, and in this section we describe some of those costs. There are other costs which are much more difficult to evaluate but which may be equally important. We cannot, for example, determine how many women are deterred from seeking contraceptive advice because they expect to be asked to provide a urine sample.

The cost of a urinalysis test varies, depending on whether the dipsticks are designed to test single or multiple constituents. On average, the test costs about £0.95 per patient (Table 6) but this estimate excludes certain important costs which will be incurred once a screening program is undertaken. These include:

(1)   Quality assurance procedures;

(2)   Follow-up tests to confirm the diagnosis (for example fasting blood tests, followed by glucose tolerance tests for those with equivocal results);

(3)   Treatment of the disease if the diagnosis is confirmed;

(4)   Unnecessary anxiety in those patients with positive screening tests, but in whom the diagnosis is not confirmed.

Table 6 Costs incurred in urinalysis screening program for diabetes

Item	Estimated cost (£)
Cost of a urine analysis test conducted by a nurse	
One Clinistix*	0.05
Specimen jar[†]	0.50
2 min of nurse time (Grade G)	0.40
Total procedure costs	0.95
Cost of follow-up fasting blood test to confirm diagnosis, conducted by a nurse	
Autolet[†] and Glucometer*	0.10
Glucostix*	0.27
Lancet for Autolet	0.01
5 min of nurse time (Grade G)	1.00
Total procedure costs	1.38

*Source: British National Formulary 1993 inflated by 5.6% to 1994 prices; [†]NHS Supplies catalogue November 1994

Note: these costs are based on the assumption that the equipment is used for 400 tests over 4 years

Most of these costs are impossible to estimate without extensive collection of further data, although the cost of a follow-up fasting blood test to confirm the diagnosis is likely to be around £1.38 (Table 6). Thus, screening 3000 oral contraceptive users would cost about £2850 for urinalysis, a further £83 for fasting blood samples in the 60 (2%) with suspicious results, and an additional cost for glucose tolerance tests on those with equivocal results (cost not estimated), and would probably detect *no more than* one case of undiagnosed diabetes.

The cost of measuring a blood pressure level with a sphygmomanometer is little more than the cost of the medical personnel's time (approximately £1.00 for 5 min of G-grade nurse time). Some further costs would be incurred in confirming or excluding the presence of hypertension in those women with a single elevated blood pressure. These women would typically be seen at least twice more for blood pressure measurements and may also have a 24 h blood pressure monitoring procedure. There is clear evidence that the cost of early treatment of patients with hypertension using antihypertensive drugs is more than offset by savings in other areas of health

Table 7 Cost-effectiveness of various health-care interventions (1990 prices) (Teeling Smith, 1992)[23]

Intervention	*Cost/quality-adjusted life year*
Cholesterol testing and diet only (all adults 40–69 years)	£200
General practitioner advice to stop smoking	£270
Neurosurgical intervention for subarachnoid hemorrhage	£490
Antihypertensive therapy to prevent stroke (aged 45–64 years)	£940
Pacemaker implantation	£1 100
Hip replacement	£1 180
Cholesterol testing and treatment (all adults aged 40–69 years)	£1 480
Coronary artery bypass graft (left main disease, severe angina)	£2 090
Breast cancer screening	£5 780
Home hemodialysis	£17 260
Coronary artery bypass graft (one-vessel disease, moderate angina)	£18 830
Hospital hemodialysis	£21 970
Neurosurgical intervention for malignant intracranial tumors	£107 780

care, for example hospitalization as a result of stroke later in life[23]. Teeling Smith has compiled a list of estimated cost per quality-adjusted life year of various health-care interventions, including the treatment of hypertension, which shows that drug treatment for patients aged 45–64 years with hypertension is cost-effective relative to other health-care interventions (Table 7)[24].

CONCLUSIONS

Screening young asymptomatic women by urinalysis for the presence of diabetes or renal disease is unlikely to reveal more than one new case of diabetes in 3000 women screened at a cost of around

£3000. Early, presymptomatic, diagnosis of diabetes does not prevent the onset of the disease, although awareness of the presence of the disease should increase the alertness and caution of the physician prescribing oral contraceptives. Moreover, the requirement to provide a urine sample may act as a barrier to seeking contraception in some women. Testing the urine of women seeking a prescription for oral contraceptives cannot be justified.

By contrast, measurement of blood pressure is a simple, non-intrusive procedure and treatment of hypertension with drug therapy has been shown to be cost-effective. Approximately one woman in 14 in the age range 16–44 years is likely to have a diastolic blood pressure of a level which is considered at least a relative contraindication to use of oral contraceptives and one in 100 will have a diastolic pressure above 95 mmHg, at which point oral contraceptives should not be prescribed.

ACKNOWLEDGEMENTS

We are grateful to the ESRC Data Archive for providing data from the Health Survey for England, and to B. Naidoo for data analysis. We are also grateful to Drs P. McCartney, A. McPherson and P. Hannaford who read and commented on an earlier version of this paper.

REFERENCES

1. Owen-Smith, V., Hannaford, P. and Webb, A. (1996). What do family planning providers do before prescribing combined oral contraceptives? *Br. J. Fam. Plann.*, in press
2. Shelton, J.D., Angle, M.A. and Jobstein, R.A. (1992). Medical barriers to access to family planning. *Lancet*, **340**, 1334–5
3. Standing Medical Advisory Committee. (1990). *Handbook of Contraceptive Practice*. (London: Department of Health)
4. Rehead, I.H. (1960). Incidence of glycosuria and diabetes mellitus in a general practice. *Br. Med. J.*, **1**, 695–9
5. Butterfield, W.J.H. (1964). Summary of results of the Bedford diabetes survey. *Proc. R. Soc. Med.*, **57**, 196–200

6. Harkness, J. (1962). Prevalence of glycosuria and diabetes mellitus. *Br. Med. J.*, **2**, 1503–7

7. Bennett, N., Dodd, T., Flattley, J., Freeth, S. and Bollong, K. (1995). *Health Survey for England 1993*. (London: HMSO)

8. Analysis of data set from *Health Survey for England 1993*. Data provided by the ESRC Data Archive, University of Essex

9. Foster, K., Jackson, B., Thomas, M., Hunter, P. and Bennett, P. (1993). *General Household Survey Series*. GSH 24. (London: HMSO)

10. Baddeley, H., Baddeley, H. and Sell, F.K. (1964). Mass urinalysis in general practice. *Lancet*, **1**, 925–6

11. Bennett, N., Dodd, T., Flattley, J., Freeth, S. and Bolling, K. (1993). *Health Survey for England*. (London: HMSO)

12. Mant, D. and Fowler, G. (1990). Urine analysis for glucose and protein: are the requirements of the new contract sensible? *Br. Med. J.*, **300**, 1053–5

13. Collins, R., Peto, R., MacMahon, S., Hebert, P., Fiebach, N.H., Eberlein, K.A., Godwin, J., Qizilbash, N., Taylor, J.O. and Hennekens, C.H. (1990). Blood pressure, stroke, and coronary heart disease. Part 2, short-term reductions in blood pressure: overview of randomised drug trials in their epidemiological contact. *Lancet*, **335**, 827–38

14. Guillebaud, J. (1991). Combined oral contraceptive pills. In Louden, N. and Baird, D.T. (eds.) *Handbook of Family Planning*, p. 63. (Edinburgh: Churchill Livingstone)

15. Petersen, K.R., Skouby, S.O., Sidelmann, J., Mølsted-Pedersen, L. and Jespersen, J. (1994). Effects of contraceptive steroids on cardiovascular risk factors in women with insulin-dependent diabetes mellitus. *Am. J. Obstet. Gynecol.*, **171**, 400–5

16. Mestman, J.H. and Schmidt-Sarosi, C. (1993). Diabetes mellitus and fertility control: Contraception management issues. *Am. J. Obstet. Gynecol.*, **168**, 12–20

17. Hannaford, P.C. and Kay, C.R. (1989). Oral contraceptives and diabetes mellitus. *Br. Med. J.*, **299**, 1315–6

18. Grice, D., Villard-Mackintosh, L., Yeates, D. and Vessey, M. (1991). Oral contraceptives and diabetes mellitus. *Br. J. Fam. Plann.*, **17**, 39–40

19. Rimm, E.R., Manson, J.E., Stampfer, M.J., Colditz, G.A., Willett, W.C., Rosner, B., Hennekens, C.H. and Speizer, F.E. (1992). Oral contraceptive use and risk of type 2 (non-insulin dependent) diabetes mellitus in a large prospective study of women. *Diabetologia*, **35**, 967–72

20. Prentice, R.L. (1988). On the ability of blood pressure effects to explain the relation between oral contraceptives and cardiovascular disease. *Am. J. Epidemiol.*, **127**, 213–9

21. Prospective Studies Collaboration (1995). Cholesterol, diastolic blood pressure, and stroke: 13 000 strokes in 450 000 people in 45 prospective cohorts. *Lancet*, **346**, 1647–53
22. MacMahon, S., Peto, R., Cutler, J., Collins, R., Solie, P., Neaton, J., Abbott, R., Godwin, J., Dyer, A. and Stamler, J. (1990). Blood pressure, stroke, and coronary heart disease. Part 1, prolonged differences in blood pressure: prospective observational studies corrected for the regression dilution bias. *Lancet*, **335**, 765–74
23. Teeling Smith, G. (1990). The economics of hypertension and stroke. *Am. Heart J.*, **119**, 725–8
24. Teeling Smith, G. (1992). Health economics in hypertension control. *J. Hypertens. Control*, **2**, 2–4

26

Do currently available combined oral contraceptives cause weight gain and other minor side-effects?

A.M.C. Webb

There is a huge literature about combined oral contraceptives (COCs) and most major studies have concentrated on the effects on mortality and major morbidity. This is both understandable and expected but there is a large number of so called minor side-effects which are usually mentioned in passing in these studies but which loom large in the concerns of women, especially young ones, expressed prior to and during pill taking[1]. These are also responsible for up to 20% of discontinuations[2]. The list is long and includes headaches, weight gain, irregular bleeding, breast tenderness, increase in breast size, changes in libido, depression, mood changes and acne.

What evidence is there that the pill causes or is even associated with any of the above? Surprisingly little. Some conditions, like acne, can be seen to improve on less androgenic pills[3] although differences between brands are less obvious even when comparing cyproterone acetate with a third-generation progestogen. There is no doubt that, overall, COCs regulate and lighten cycles and that the incidence of irregular bleeding is present in small percentages only, especially after the first three cycles. What is not quantified is how much of this bleeding is due to irregular pill-taking and no studies were found where those with irregular bleeding have been screened for chlamydia. In practice, when irregular bleeding occurs, the numbers that are not easily explained by irregular taking or infection are very small indeed. Breast tenderness is often glossed over and not easy to quantify. As to increase in breast size, no studies appear to have looked at this, despite a considerable number of women reporting an increase and a few complaining quite markedly.

A small number of studies have looked at psychological symptoms but a recent one showed that, however careful the design, quite different results can be obtained in different groups[4]. Looking at well-being and sexuality in a double-blind, placebo-controlled trial, no effect was noted in the Philippines, whereas COCs adversely affected sexuality in Edinburgh with nearly half also reporting reduced sexual interest. There is some difference in how COCs affect women in different countries but it is probably linked to their expectations. Most studies look at one brand of COCs alone or at most compare one brand with another. Very few look at COC use in comparison to no hormones or a placebo. However, as long ago as 1971, Goldzieher and colleagues[5] showed that headache, nervousness, depression, weight gain, nausea and vomiting occurred in women not taking hormones, and that the true incidence of drug-related complaints was likely to be much lower than that suggested by uncontrolled investigations. Double-blind studies can also show up other problems. In one study where all volunteers had to read the package insert for progesterone used for treatment of amenorrhea, 62% of placebo patients reported progesterone-type side-effects[6].

One of the most commonly mentioned side-effects, and certainly one that is firmly associated with COCs in the mind of many women, is weight increase. There are large, mainly phase III and IV, studies looking at the acceptability of modern pills. Looking at those that studied more than 500 women, they all state that the overall effect on weight was insignificant[7–12] and, where mentioned, only between less than 1.0 and 4% withdrew because of weight gain. Only one study looked at the women who gained weight and those who lost weight separately and noted that 70% of women had no change in weight at 2 years, 18% had increased by more than 2 kg and 12% had a loss of more than 2 kg[13]. Weight changes through life are common and some weight gain in the late teenage years is part of normal development, which was demonstrated by the fact that the majority of those gaining more than 2 kg were under 20 years old.

No real comment can be made about the cause of any of the weight changes unless COC users are compared with another group not using COCs. There is one small but detailed study looking at not only weight, but also body composition and fat distribution in young women[14]. All taking part were 16–21 years old, and 49 started using COCs with 31 acting as controls. Diet and activity were similar in both groups. It was found that in both groups many women gained and lost over 0.5 kg and in those that gained, the accumulation was of body fat, not water.

Overall, the effect of COCs on weight is at most small, and possibly non-existent, but there is no proof either way to determine if there is a small subgroup of particularly susceptible women. It is unlikely that there is, in view of the small numbers of women dropping out of studies due to weight gain, although there is a theoretical pathway for sex hormones triggering appetite via noradrenaline-regulated brain functions[15].

Gross obesity is associated with a variety of health problems, but most of the weight changes of which women taking COCs complain do not fall under this category and are far more influenced by fashion which imposes an ideal which is, if anything, too thin and has other associated health problems. Women who are grossly obese may be better off not using COCs as they are associated with an increased risk of thromboembolism to which, as a group, they may already be vulnerable. No one needs a set of scales to detect the women in whom this is a concern. Weighing the obese as a baseline towards helping them reduce weight with dietary and other advice is legitimate, but it should be very clear that this measurement is nothing to do with the COCs. In borderline cases, weighing can spot small changes which may clarify a decision on whether or not to continue COC use, but again it must be very clear that the reason for weighing is the management of obesity.

What about the majority of women who are not worried about their weight or where their concern is to do with fashion? Should they be weighed at any stage and, if so, how often? The arguments in favor include that it is easy, cheap, non-invasive and only takes a minute. Having a baseline weight can help to counteract claims from the woman that she feels fatter, and, in women prone to obesity, it may act as an early warning system to institute dietary advice at an early stage.

Nearly all women on the pill are fit and healthy. They do not come to see us because they are ill. They come because they wish to avoid a normal physiological consequence of the most essential human behavior, sex. By training, most doctors, apart from those with a psychotherapeutic background, are used to carrying out procedures and associate this with good practice. If a client comes and only a conversation takes place, many may feel, at some level, that they have not performed adequately. When women come for follow-up, if we do not even weigh them, they may well ask why they have to see a doctor. 'Why should I pay if you are not going to do anything, not even weigh me?' Maybe, therefore, some of us weigh out of habit, out of something to do and write down. Boxes ticked may reassure us of a job well done.

Looking at the arguments for weighing in detail, it is easy up to a point. How accurate are our scales? Most which I have tried can vary by one or two kilograms simply by gentle rocking of the platform. If more accurate balanced scales are used, this takes more time. How much clothing is worn at the time of weighing? What is worn can vary significantly between the seasons and, certainly in Britain, much of the fashion footwear that young women use is heavy and takes 5 or 10 minutes to unlace and lace up again. Once again, either clothing is mostly removed using up time or the measurement becomes very inaccurate and probably irrelevant. Is it cheap? Most clinics will have a set of scales but they do need maintenance and replacement and, if funds are limited, a set of scales is considerably less important than ensuring that the consultation room is private or that there are facilities for sterilization of instruments.

The argument for recording weight as a defense for the future tends to imply that doctors feel insecure about their ability to communicate with their client without ammunition to defend themselves. It also implies a certain distrust or patronizing attitude towards the client. The stance on early warning for obesity can be defended, but should then be used in all women who have a serious weight problem regardless of contraceptive method as the problem is not COCs but weight, and their overeating tendency will apply whatever they use.

Will weighing or not weighing make prescription of the pill any safer? Except in the very obese, COC safety related to weight is not an issue whereas acceptability is affected far more, so the question should be – does weighing women increase or decrease the acceptability? In view of the very strong social pressures associated with excess weight, asking a woman to be regularly weighed in front of someone in a position of authority will only emphasize concerns about weight in those who are already unreasonably pressured by society's fashion requirements. Some will view it as an invasion of their privacy, especially if they are asked partially or almost entirely to take off their clothes.

At the first visit, women often express concerns about weight gain related to COC use. Strong reassurance that there is no established link should be given, not only to those who express this concern but to all, and this should be reflected in the literature that is handed out. If, at the same time as giving reassurance, weight is measured a mixed message is given which will at some level be taken on. A few may verbalize it but for the majority it will be subliminal. The pill does not make you put on weight but let us check just in case! This implies we perhaps do not believe our own reassurance. It could be argued that a baseline weight may be taken just like an obstetric history or cytology history. They would not affect whether the pill is prescribed or not but are part of a general health baseline that might affect future management. If this is the case, this should be explicitly mentioned and firmly disassociated from COC prescription.

At follow-up visits for COC prescription, routine weight measurements need not be made. It wastes useful communication time and implies we believe there could be a problem. If scales are available and the woman expresses a concern about her weight, this needs to be addressed, but again reassurance given that any fluctuation is extremely unlikely to be pill-related. If the weight gain is great enough to cause medical concern, this needs to be addressed as an issue in itself. The direct cause of weight gain in the otherwise healthy is always related to excessive eating and the only way to address it is by reducing calorific intake, although the means to achieve this may vary. We must resist colluding with clients who may firmly blame the pill and deny eating more.

Future research may wish to concentrate, not on mean weight changes, but on the small group that gain or lose more than 2 kg and study them in greater detail. It would be surprising if any difference is found, but at least there would be proof which could be widely publicized and slowly, hopefully, affect general knowledge about COCs and increase acceptability.

In summary, there is little proof that the combined oral contraceptive is associated with, let alone causal of, many symptoms which women link to it. It is essential that those who prescribe the pill do not explicitly or implicitly by their actions reinforce these links which lead to reduced satisfaction with the combined oral contraceptive and subsequent unnecessary reduction in contraceptive choice.

REFERENCES

1. Emans, S.I., Grace, E., Woods, E.R., Smith, D.E., Klein, K. and Merola, J. (1987). Adolescents' compliance with the use of oral contraceptives. *J. Am. Med. Assoc.*, **257**, 3377–81
2. Pratt, W.F. and Bachrach, C.A. (1987). What do women use when they stop using the pill? *Fam. Plann. Perspect.*, **19**, 257–66
3. Dhieben, Th.O.M., Vromans, L., Theeuwes, A. and Coelingh-Bennink, H.J.T. (1994). The effects of CTR-24, a biphasic oral contraceptive combination compared to Diane-35 in women with acne. *Contraception*, **50**, 373–82
4. Graham, C.A., Ramos, R., Bancroft, J., Maglaya, C. and Farley, T.M.M. (1995). The effects of steroidal contraceptives on the well-being and sexuality of women: A double-blind, placebo controlled, two centre study of combined and progestogen-only methods. *Contraception*, **52**, 363–9
5. Goldzieher, J.W., Moses, L.E., Averkin, E., Scheel, C. and Taber, B.Z. (1971). A placebo controlled double-blind crossover investigation of the side effects attributed to oral contraceptives. *Fertil. Steril.*, **22**, 609–23
6. Shangold, M.M., Tomai, T.P., Cook, J.D., Jacobs, S.L., Zinaman, M.J., Chin, S.Y. and Simon, J.A. (1991). Factors associated with withdrawal bleeding after administration of oral micronised progesterone in women with secondary amenorrhoea. *Fertil. Steril.*, **56**, 1040–6

7. Fotherby, K. (1995). Twelve years of clinical experience with an oral contraceptive containing 30 mcg ethinyloestradiol and 150 mcg desogestrel. *Contraception*, **51**, 3–12

8. Akerlund, M., Røde, A. and Westergaard, J. (1993). Comparative profiles of reliability, cycle control and side effects of two oral contraceptive formulations containing 150 mcg desogestrel and either 30 mcg or 20 mcg ethinyloestradiol. *Br. J. Obstet. Gynaecol.*, **100**, 832–8

9. Walling, M. (1992). A multicentre efficacy and safety study of an oral contraceptive containing 150 mcg desogestrel and 30 mcg ethinylestradiol. *Contraception*, **46**, 313–26

10. Runnebaum, B., Grunwald, K. and Rabe, T. (1992). The efficacy and tolerability of norgestimate/ethinylestradiol (250 micrograms of norgestimate/35 micrograms of ethinylestradiol): results of an open, multicentre study of 59 701 women. *Am. J. Obstet. Gynecol.*, **166**, 1963–8

11. Düsterberg, B. and Brill, K. (1990). Clinical experiences with a low dose oral contraceptive containing gestodene. *Adv. Contracept.*, **6**, 37–50

12. Lammers, P. and Op, Ten Berg. M. (1991). Phase III clinical trial with a new oral contraceptive containing 150 mcg desogestrel and 20 mcg ethinylestradiol. *Acta Obstet. Gynecol. Scand.*, **70**, 497–500

13. Rekers, H. (1988). Multicentre trial of a monophasic oral contraceptive containing ethinylestradiol and desogestrel. *Acta Obstet. Gynecol. Scand.*, **67**, 171–4

14. Reubinoff, B.E., Grubstein, A., Meirow, D., Berry, E., Schenker, J.G. and Brzezinski, A. (1995). Effects of low-dose estrogen oral contraceptives on weight, body composition and fat distribution in young women. *Fertil. Steril.*, **63**, 516–21

15. Moller, S.E., Maach-Moller, B., Olesen, M., Madsen, B., Madsen, P. and Fjalland, B. (1995). Tyrosine metabolism in users of oral contraceptives. *Life-Sci.*, **56**, 687–95

Section 6

Increased availability of combined oral contraceptives

27

Can the pill be given to women with particular needs? Epilepsy and drug interactions

D.J. Back

It is estimated that epilepsy occurs in approximately 1% of the population[1]. Although frequently manifesting itself early in life, epilepsy persists in the woman into and beyond childbearing years. There are good reasons for wishing to maintain adequate contraceptive control in this patient population. An unintended pregnancy in a woman taking antiepileptic drugs raises concerns of possible complications of seizures during pregnancy, such as maternal injury, fetal injury and neonatal distress. There is also the worry of possible birth defects for the baby since some antiepileptic drugs have teratogenic potential[1].

In most countries there is now a choice of nearly 20 antiepileptic drugs. Thus physicians need to be well informed on how to choose between treatments. Very often choices are based on familiarity with particular drugs and keeping costs down. Antiepileptic drug treatment is highly successful in the majority of patients developing seizures for the first time, with complete control in approximately 70% of such patients[2]. Antiepileptic monotherapy is the rule in initial treatment, and, in the event of treatment failure, drugs tend to be exchanged rather than added. Even so, 10–15% of patients are better controlled with combination therapy. In making therapeutic decisions, the physician has to consider:

Table 1 Major antiepileptic drugs and reported interactions with oral contraceptive steroids

Drugs reported to interact	Drugs for which there is no evidence of interactions
Phenobarbitone	ethosuximide
Phenytoin	diazepam
Primidone	clonazepam
Carbamazepine	valproic acid (sodium valproate)
Oxcarbazepine	clobazam
	vigabatrin
	lamotrigine
	gabapentin

(1) The efficacy spectrum;

(2) Tolerability;

(3) Ease of use;

(4) Cost;

(5) Interaction potential.

The latter point is extremely important since the long-term nature of epilepsy treatment means that the possibility of an antiepileptic drug interaction is high.

Historically, a number of antiepileptic drugs have been implicated as causing breakthrough bleeding or failure of contraception in women taking oral contraceptives[3–10] (Table 1). Phenytoin has been the most commonly reported interacting anticonvulsant. Between 1973 and 1984, 43 cases of contraceptive failure in women taking anticonvulsants during oral contraceptive use were reported to the United Kingdom Committee on Safety of Medicines (CSM)[11]. Some women were using more than one drug. Phenytoin accounted for 25 cases and phenobarbitone for 20 cases with smaller numbers for other anticonvulsants. The CSM monitors adverse drug reactions by means of a reporting system. However, it is estimated that less than 10% of adverse reactions are actually reported to the CSM[12], the

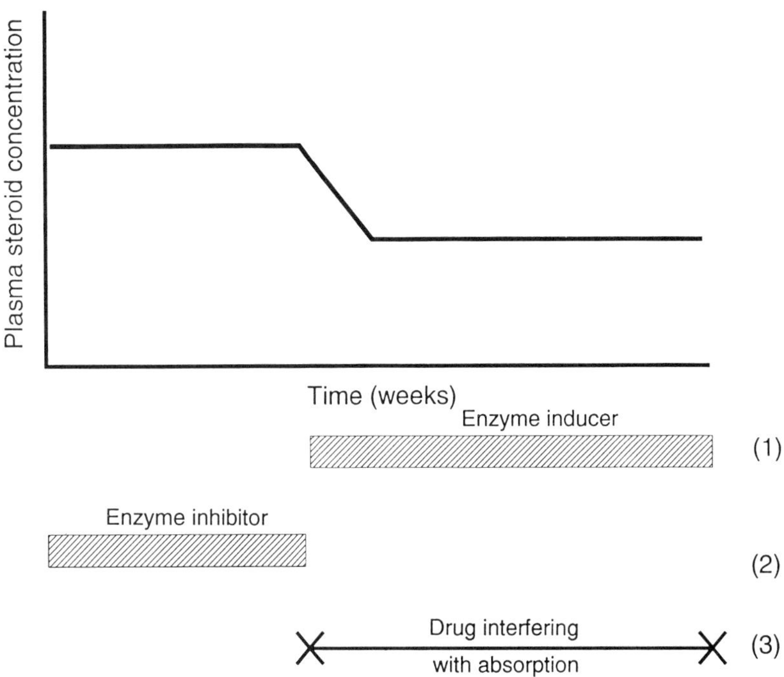

Figure 1 Steady-state plasma oral contraceptive steroid concentrations will decline on: (1) the addition of enzyme inducer; (2) the withdrawal of enzyme inhibitor, and (3) interference with absorption

main reasons being that the reaction was too trivial or already well known, or there was uncertainty of a causal relationship. If the same degree of under-reporting applies to the oral contraceptive–drug interactions, then the 43 pregnancies noted during the 11-year study period are a poor estimate of what actually occurred.

The drugs listed in Table 1 as interfering with oral contraceptive efficacy are all enzyme-inducing drugs and consequently increase the clearance of the pill. Although the clinical pharmacokinetic data of the interactions are sparse, they are nevertheless convincing and leave little room for doubting that many women will have reduced steroid concentrations on conventional dosage regimens (Figure 1). Pharmacokinetic data from two studies[13,14] involving single-dose administration of an oral contraceptive (50 µg ethinylestradiol, EE_2 and 250 µg levonorgestrel, LNG) to women before, and 8 and 12 weeks after, starting anticonvulsant therapy for tonic/clonic seizures are shown in Table 2. In the case of phenytoin, there was a significant decrease in the area under the plasma concentration–time curve (AUC) for both EE_2 (42%) and LNG (40%). Such a change may well be sufficient to produce contraceptive failure in long-term oral contraceptive users. In contrast, sodium valproate had no detectable effect on the kinetics of EE_2 and LNG (Table 2). While phenobarbitone, phenytoin and carbamazepine are known to be enzyme-inducing agents in humans, sodium valproate has no enzyme-inducing action.

In a recent study by Klosterskov Jensen and colleagues[10], the effect of oxcarbazepine on the kinetics of EE_2 and LNG was investigated in 13 regular oral contraceptive users. The AUCs of both steroids were markedly decreased after 1 month of the antiepileptic (300 mg thrice per day) (see Figure 2). In addition to enzyme induction an additional factor in this interaction is the increase in sex hormone binding globulin (SHBG) concentration which limits the 'free' (and biologically active) progestogen. The decreased bioavailable steroid leads to breakthrough bleeding, as demonstrated by Sonnen[15] in four out of six women receiving oxcarbazepine with an oral contraceptive.

The molecular basis of the antiepileptic–oral contraceptive interaction is the ability of phenobarbitone, phenytoin, carbamazepine and oxcarbazepine to induce specific enzyme(s) responsible for steroid metabolism. The predominant route of oxidative metabolism of EE_2 is cytochrome P450-dependent 2-hydroxylation to form the catechol estrogen 2-hydroxyethinylestradiol. The major isozyme catalyzing this hydroxylation is CYP3A4[16], which is inducible. Ball and co-workers[17] studied EE_2 metabolism in a panel of human livers *in vitro*. The highest EE_2–2-hydroxylase activity was found in the liver of a subject who had received phenobarbitone and phenytoin for more than 25 years. Although synthetic progestogens undergo both reductive and oxidative pathways, it appears that hydroxylation becomes a more important metabolic pathway as a result of enzyme induction. Hence, both components of the pill are influenced by the enzyme-inducing antiepileptic drugs.

The antiepileptic drugs introduced into therapeutics in recent years (apart from oxcarbazepine) do not have significant enzyme-inducing

Table 2 Area under the plasma concentration time curve (AUC_{0-24h}) for ethinylestradiol (EE_2) and levonorgestrel (LNG) in patients taking either phenytoin, carbamazepine or sodium valproate

	Patient group		
	Phenytoin (*n* = 6)	*Carbamazepine* (*n* = 4)	*Sodium valproate* (*n* = 6)
Daily dose of antiepileptic (mg)	200–300	300–600	400
EE_2 AUC (pg ml^{-1} h)			
control	806 ± 122	1163 ± 466	880 ± 267
test	411 ± 132*	672 ± 211*	977 ± 319
LNG AUC (ng ml^{-1} h)			
control	33.6 ± 19.2	22.9 ± 9.4	29.1 ± 5.8
test	19.5 ± 9.3*	13.8 ± 5.8	29.2 ± 3.8

*, $p < 0.05$

potential. Lamotrigine is a weak inducer of the UDP-glucuronyltransferase, and by this mechanism increases its own plasma clearance after 3 weeks of administration[18], but it does not affect oral contraceptive plasma concentrations[19]. Vigabatrin does not undergo significant metabolism and has not been shown to induce hepatic metabolism[20].

STRATEGIES AND MANAGEMENT

Any patient who receives multiple drug therapy could be at risk of a drug interaction. However, an understanding of the antiepileptic–oral contraceptive interaction allows us to put forward a rational strategy for dealing with this problem.

(1)　When a woman with seizures seeks contraception, it is good clinical practice to determine that her seizures are due to recurrent epilepsy and confirm the necessity of maintaining antiepileptic medication[1]. For women with epilepsy, seizure control is of paramount importance.

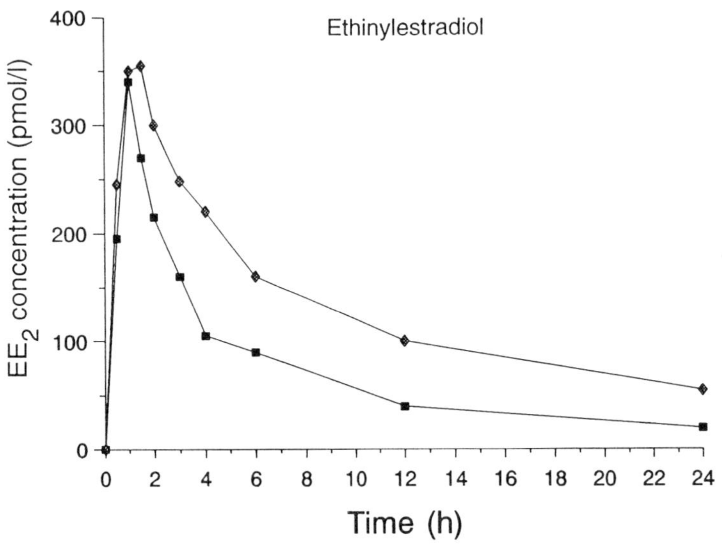

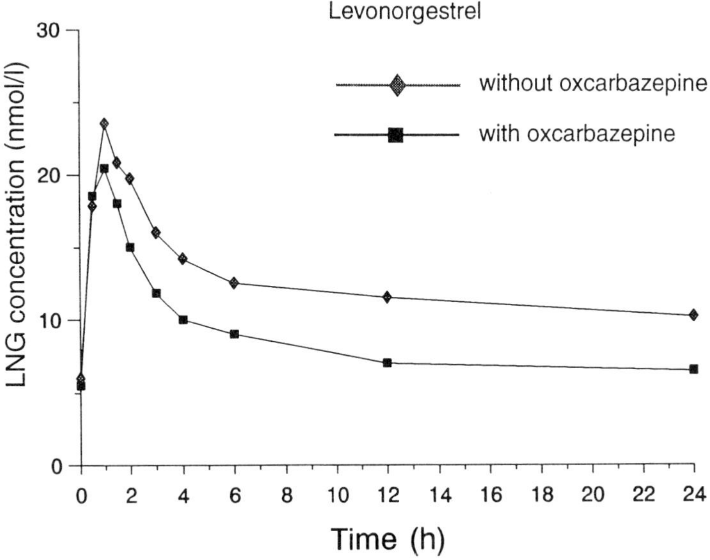

Figure 2 Effect of oxcarbazepine (300 mg thrice daily for 1 month) on plasma concentrations of ethinylestradiol (EE_2) and levonorgestrel (LNG). Results are mean data from ten women receiving a tricyclic oral contraceptive regimen (30, 40, 30 µg EE_2; 50, 75, 125 µg LNG). Adapted from reference 10 with permission

(2) If it is possible to use or substitute an antiepileptic drug which does not induce hepatic enzymes, this should be done. No dose adjustment of the oral contraceptive will then be necessary.

(3) If an enzyme-inducing antiepileptic drug is preferred for clinical reasons, the effect can be overcome by using a larger dose of the oral contraceptive than usual. Instead of starting with 30–35 µg EE_2, patients can be started on a 50 µg preparation (Ovran® is available in the UK). If breakthrough bleeding occurs into the second cycle of contraceptive use, then the dose of EE_2 can be increased to 80 µg (e.g. Ovran® plus Ovranette®) daily. In the majority of women, this dose will be adequate to achieve good cycle control and contraceptive efficacy.

CONCLUSION

There is a large quantity of literature on drug interactions with oral contraceptives[21–24]. However, comparatively few are of clinical significance. The interaction of some antiepileptic drugs and rifampicin (anti-tuberculous drug) with oral contraceptives is beyond dispute. The issue is not so clear with antibiotics where only a small percentage of women receiving co-medication are probably at risk[21]. Methods for predicting who these women are remain to be developed. Based on biochemical and clinical data, it is almost certain that erythromycin, co-trimoxazole and sulfonamides do not interact with the combined pill. However, as uncertainty remains with other antibiotics (particularly penicillins and tetracyclines), it will be prudent to recommend use of additional precautions when these drugs are used. Regulatory authorities demand oral contraceptive interaction studies for new drugs which will be taken by women of child-bearing age. Interaction problems, therefore, should be picked up in Phase II/III development. It is still important, however, that contraceptive service providers are vigilant when giving the pill to women already receiving other medications.

REFERENCES

1. Mattson, R.H. and Rebar, R.W. (1993). Contraceptive methods for women with neurological disorders. *Am. J. Obstet. Gynecol.*, **168**, 2027–32

2. Patsalos, P.N. and Duncan, J.S. (1993). Anti-epileptic drugs. A review of clinically significant drug interactions. *Drug Safety*, **9**, 156–84

3. Belaisch, J., Driguez, P. and Janaud, A. (1976). Influence de certains médicaments sur l'action des pilules contraceptifs. *Nouvelle Presse Med.*, **5**, 645–6

4. Coulam, C.B. and Annegers, J.F. (1979). Do anticonvulsants reduce the efficacy of oral contraceptives? *Epilepsia*, **20**, 519–26

5. Diamond, M.P., Greene, J.W., Thompson, J.M., Vanttooydonk, J.E. and Wentz, A. (1995). Interaction of anticonvulsants and oral contraceptives in epileptic adolescents. *Contraception*, **31**, 623–32

6. Gagnaire, J.C., Tchertchian, J., Revol, A. and Rochet, Y. (1975). Grossesses sous contraceptifs oraux chez les patients recevant des barbituriques. *Nouvelle Presse Med.*, **4**, 8

7. Hempel von, E., Bohm, W., Carol, W. and Klinger, W. (1973). Meditamentose enzyminduktion und hormonale kontrazeption. *Zentrab. f. Gynakol.*, **95**, 451–7

8. Janz, D. and Schmidt, D. (1974). Antiepileptic drugs and failure of oral contraceptives. *Lancet*, **1**, 113

9. Kenyon, T.E. (1972). Unplanned pregnancy in an epileptic. *Br. Med. J.*, **1**, 686–7

10. Klosterkov Jensen, P., Saano, V., Haring, P., Svenstrup, B. and Menge, G.P. (1992). Possible interaction between oxcarbazepine and an oral contraceptive. *Epilepsia*, **33**, 1149–52

11. Back, D.J., Grimmer, S.F.M., Orme, M.L.'E., Proudlove, C., Mann, R.D. and Breckenridge, A.M. (1988). Evaluation of Committee on Safety of Medicines yellow card reports on oral contraceptive–drug interactions. *Br. J. Clin. Pharmacol.*, **25**, 527–32

12. Lumley, C.E., Walker, S.R., Hall, G.C., Staunton, N. and Grob, P.R. (1986). The underreporting of adverse drug reactions seen in general practice. *Pharmaceut. Med.*, **1**, 205–12

13. Crawford, P., Chadwick, D., Cleland, P., Tjia, J., Cowie, A., Back, D.J. and Orme, M.L.'E. (1986). The lack of effect of sodium valproate on the pharmacokinetics of oral contraceptive steroids. *Contraception*, **33**, 23–9

14. Crawford, P., Chadwick, D.J., Martin, C., Tjia, J., Black, D.J. and Orme, M.L.'E. (1990). The interaction of phenytoin and carbamazepine with combined oral contraceptive steroids. *Br. J. Clin. Pharmacol.*, **30**, 892–6

15. Sonnen, A.E.H. (1990). Oxcarbazepine and oral contraceptives. *Acta Neurol. Scand.*, **82** (Suppl. 133), 37

16. Guengerich, F.P. (1988). Oxidation of 17α-ethinyloestradiol by human liver cytochrome P450. *Molec. Pharmacol.*, **33**, 500–8

17. Ball, S.E., Forrester, L.M., Wolf, C.R. and Back, D.J. (1990). Differences in the cytochrome P450 isozymes involved in the 2-hydroxylation of estradiol and 17α-ethinyloestradiol: relative activities of rat and human liver enzymes. *Biochem. J.*, **167**, 221–6

18. Anderson, G.D. and Graves, N.M. (1994). Drug interactions with antiepileptic agents. Prevention and management. *CNS Drugs*, **2**, 268–79

19. Orme, M., Back, D., Ward, S., Power, J. and Holditch, T. (1992). The lack of effect of lamotrigine on oral contraceptive steroid therapy. Abstract presented at *V[th] World Conference on Clinical Pharmacology and Therapeutics*, Yokohama, Japan, July, Abst. P408-16

20. Grant, S.M. and Heel, S.M. (1991). Vigabatrin: a review of its pharmacodynamic and pharmacokinetic properties and therapeutic potential in epilepsy and disorders of motor control. *Drugs*, **41**, 889–926

21. Back, D.J. and Orme, M.L.'E. (1994). Drug Interactions. In Goldzieher, J.W. (ed.) *Pharmacology of the Contraceptive Steroids*, pp. 407–25. (New York: Raven Press)

22. Shenfield, G.M. (1993). Oral contraceptives. Are drug interactions of clinical significance? *Drug Safety*, **9**, 21–37

23. Orme, M., Crawford, P. and Back, D. (1991). Contraception, epilepsy and pharmacokinetics. In Trimble, M.R. (ed.) *Women and Epilepsy*, pp. 145–58. (Chichester: J. Wiley and Sons)

24. Geurts, T.B.P., Goorissen, E.M. and Sitsen, J.M.A. (1993). *Summary of Drug Interactions with Oral Contraceptives*. (Carnforth, UK: Parthenon Publishing)

28

Can the pill be given to women with particular needs? Sickle cell disease, thalassemia and liver disease

S.P. Dourakis, I.X. Halikias, E. Vlachopapadopoulou and G. Tolis

LIVER DISEASE AND ORAL CONTRACEPTIVE USE

Introduction

Young women of childbearing age with liver diseases often ask if they can take oral contraceptives (OCs). Liver disease is often considered to be a contraindication to OC use but there is little information on this topic. Since long-term use of OCs may be associated with a small increased risk of certain types of liver disease (Table 1), their use is probably best avoided in patients with chronic hepatopathies, as there may be diagnostic problems if any complications develop. There seems to be a decreased incidence of adverse liver reactions in modern combined OCs with lower estrogenic and progestogenic contents[1].

Cholestasis with or without jaundice and oral contraceptives

Certain drugs containing the steroid (cyclopentanophenanthrene) nucleus are icterogenic. Both C-17-alkylated anabolic and androgenic

Table 1 Liver diseases in oral contraceptive users

Acute cholestasis
Benign hepatic tumors
    hepatic adenoma
    hemangiomas
    focal nodular hyperplasia
Hepatocellular carcinoma
Peliosis hepatis
Hepatic vein thrombosis
Portal vein thrombosis
Gallstones

steroids, and OC steroids, are capable of producing liver injury. Estrogens appear to have a dose-dependent effect on the hepatocyte surface membrane, including that lining the canaliculus. They reduce the excretory capacity for bilirubin, bile salts and bromosulfalein. Jaundice does not usually appear due to the large reserve capacity of the liver for the excretion of bilirubin, jaundice occurring only if the excretory capacity is reduced to less than 10% of normal[2–4].

Individual susceptibility means that mild adverse effects can result in clinically apparent jaundice in some OC users. A personal or familial history of jaundice in pregnancy will increase the chances of developing jaundice or pruritus if contraceptive steroids are used[5,6]. OC-associated cholestasis is rare in Great Britain. The clustering of cases of OC-associated jaundice in selected groups of women in Chile and Scandinavia (many of whom had cholestatic jaundice of pregnancy), strongly suggests a genetic susceptibility to this type of hepatic injury[7,8].

OC-induced jaundice appears to result from reduced bile excretion as a consequence of impaired uptake of bile acids from sinusoidal blood. There are a loss of membrane fluidity and decreases in Na^+–K^+-ATPase activity in the plasma membrane which are probably due to the estrogenic component of the OC[9]. The OC-induced jaundice is of the cholestatic canalicular type. No portal inflammation or parenchymal injury is found on liver biopsy. Contraceptive steroid jaundice usually has its onset within the first 1 to 6 months of treatment: its onset is insidious with pruritus, pale stools, dark urine and mild jaundice. Serum bilirubin is usually less than 5 mg/dl, with predominance of the conjugated form[10,11]. Rarely, the jaundice is deep and persists for months after the withdrawal of the drug[12]. The prognosis is excellent with complete recovery typically occurring within a few weeks. Serum alkaline phosphatase levels are only slightly elevated if at all, and aminotransferase levels are usually normal or slightly elevated[13,14]. There are case reports about OC-associated jaundice with high levels of aminotransferases mimicking viral hepatitis: this syndrome may recur in the third trimester of pregnancy. Death resulting from OC-induced jaundice has only been reported in patients who were debilitated or had underlying disease[15].

Oral contraceptives and liver adenomas

Oral contraceptive steroids have been implicated with the development of benign hepatic tumors, especially adenomas[16,17]. The causal connection between OCs and hepatocellular adenoma is quite convincing. Liver cell adenomas were relatively rare before the advent of the OC. During the past two decades their incidence has increased sharply. Since the first report in 1973[17] many similar cases have been published[18–20]. There is apparently a direct relationship between the duration of OC use and the incidence of liver adenoma. Liver adenomas usually develop in women above 30 years old (mean age 34) who have been taking OCs for more than 5 years, without a previous history of hepatopathy; some of them regress after discontinuation of the OC[21–24]. Their recurrence is possible upon reintroduction of the drug. Their behavior is usually benign, rarely transforming into hepatocellular carcinoma[25–27]. The finding of liver cell adenoma and hepatocellular carcinoma within the same lesion has been assumed by certain investigators to be strongly indicative of malignant transformation. However, on the basis of their cytomorphologic appearance, OC-associated liver adenomas are not frankly premalignant, as opposed to other liver abnormalities, such as liver cell dysplasia, which is an irreversible premalignant state, eventually progressing to frank hepatocellular carcinoma[28].

Hepatic adenomas are usually solitary, sometimes large in size. Hemorrhage occurs in as many as 30–50% of cases. About 10% of the tumors are pedunculated. They present as either an abdominal mass accompanied by localized pain, or more dramatically with shock due to their rupture and intraperitoneal hemorrhage. Large adenomas therefore should be resected[29].

Liver adenomas on biopsy appear as a collection of normal hepatocytes. The notion that too few, if any, Kupffer cells are present within the lesion and consequently no technetium is absorbed by it on liver scan has been shown to be mistaken. Often, in symptomatic patients, a characteristic hemorrhagic border around the lesion is observed, indicating local periadenoma hemorrhage as the cause of the abdominal pain. An association between liver cell adenomas and granulomas has also been described[30].

These tumors often regress when OCs are discontinued. However, cases in which hepatic adenomas did not regress after the discontinuation of the drug have been documented. In addition, a tumor that has apparently regressed may resume growth and rupture during pregnancy. Rarely, malignant transformation towards frank hepatocellular carcinoma may occur. Therefore, long-term follow-up of these patients is warranted to safeguard against this outcome, even if withdrawal of the OC has initially resulted in shrinking or even resolution of the adenoma.

Hepatocellular carcinoma and oral contraceptives

Since the 1970s several reports on the development of hepatocellular carcinoma (HCC) in young women using OCs have been published[21, 31–35], and a possible causal relationship suggested[31,36]. The risk of a woman developing HCC is very small[37]. Women receiving OCs for 8 years or more seem to have a small increased risk of HCC[38,39]. Others have postulated that the relative risk of HCC in women receiving OCs for 5 years or longer is 5.5; serologically determined viral hepatitis was not a confounding factor[40]. It should be noted that most of the evidence that combined OCs increase the risk of HCC comes from developed countries where the incidence of this disease is extremely low. As yet there is little information about the risk in countries where hepatitis B and/or C virus is endemic and HCC rates are high[41,42].

The OC-associated HCC usually develops on a non-cirrhotic liver, without infiltrating the surrounding tissues; distant metastases are rare. Compared to HCC in young adult women without a previous history of OC intake, this patient group has better survival, fewer symptoms and lower α-fetoprotein levels[43]. They tend to be more vascular and hemoperitoneum due to rupture occurs more commonly.

The causal relationship between HCC and the use of OCs has been challenged[44]. In a review of 128 cases of HCC in women reported to the Armed Forces Institute of Pathology no association between HCC and OCs could be demonstrated[44–46].

Hepatic vein thrombosis (Budd–Chiari syndrome)

The Budd–Chiari syndrome, caused by the obstruction of the hepatic veins, includes hepatomegaly, abdominal pain, ascites and zone 3 sinusoidal distension and blood pooling on biopsy. It has been suggested that hepatic vein occlusion might occur due to the thrombogenic effect of the estrogenic component of the OC preparations, especially in women predisposed to the development of thromboses[47–50]. Evidence in support of the association is insufficient to allow a definite conclusion. It has been reported, however, that the risk of hepatic vein thrombosis is more than doubled (relative risk = 2.37) by the use of OCs[51].

Portal vein thrombosis

Portal vein thrombosis can be an extremely rare complication of the OC's thrombogenic activity[52]. OCs are presumed to act synergically in women who are predisposed to arterial and/or venous thrombosis.

Liver hemangiomas

OC use apparently increases the size of pre-existing hemangiomas. Moreover, the recurrence of these tumors in patients who have hepatectomy followed by continuation of estrogen therapy is well established[53]. There is no evidence, however, to support the hypothesis that OC use results in the *de novo* formation of liver hemangiomas.

Focal nodular hyperplasia

Focal nodular hyperplasia (FNH) is a benign liver lesion comprising mainly hepatocytes and Kupffer cells; it has a central stellate scar with radiating septae surrounded by a capsule. There is no convincing evidence that the use of OCs has a role in the development of FNH: its incidence has not apparently increased since the advent of the OC and the lesion affects all ages and both sexes (although the female-to-male ration is 2 : 1). There is some concern, however, about the possibility of an increase in size of pre-existing FNH lesions following the use of OCs[54], since estrogens might have either a direct trophic effect or may induce vascular changes[55–58]. The prognosis of FNH is excellent; no case of malignant transformation has been described. It can usually be managed conservatively after discontinuation of the OCs.

Cholelithiasis

Oral contraceptives have lithogenic properties, evidenced by a rise in biliary cholesterol secretion and cholesterol saturation index[59]. There is a transient increase in the occurrence of gallstones following the administration of OCs, that does not accumulate beyond 10 years of use[60]. However, the association between the use of OCs and the risk for cholelithiasis has been challenged[61].

Hepatic peliosis

Oral contraceptive-associated liver sinusoidal ectasia (hepatic peliosis) is a rare abnormality of unknown pathogenesis. It may represent the telangiectatic precursor of a centrally scarred focal nodular hyperplasia[62].

Chronic liver disease

Amenorrhea is a well-recognized complication of all types of end-stage chronic liver disease. Nevertheless, several reports have documented successful pregnancies in women with chronic liver disease and adequate liver function. Chronic liver disease is widely considered as a contraindication for the administration of OCs, despite the lack of supporting evidence for the recommendation. In our view, since the long-term use of OCs may be associated with an increased, though small, risk of hepatic complications, their use is best avoided in patients with chronic liver disease, as diagnostic problems might arise in cases of liver complications.

If a woman with chronic liver disease insists on using a contraceptive pill, a trial of a low-estrogen or a progestogen-only preparation can be instituted. OCs should be avoided in jaundiced patients or in those with clear evidence of biochemical abnormality. Liver function tests (mainly bilirubin and aminotransferases) should be ordered regularly while the patient is on the pill, weekly for the 1st month, monthly for the next 3 months and every 3 months thereafter[63]. If there is a deterioration in any of these tests the drug must be stopped.

Oral contraceptive use after liver transplantation

A normal menstrual pattern is established soon after a successful liver transplant[64]. The need for contraceptive counselling immediately after the transplantation is therefore evident. Ideally, pregnancy should be deferred for at least 1 year following the operation. OCs can be prescribed; there are no data to show an increased incidence of cholestatic reactions in liver transplants. However, OCs might interfere with cyclosporin elimination and thus potentiate its hepatotoxicity; its levels should therefore be closely monitored.

OCs should not be prescribed in patients who had a liver transplant because of the Budd–Chiari syndrome, as they have an underlying thrombogenic propensity, even though they are usually on anticoagulants. Warfarin is teratogenic, and contraceptive counselling is therefore even more important in this context[65].

SICKLE CELL DISEASE AND ORAL CONTRACEPTIVE USE

Sickle hemoglobinopathies include the following entities: sickle cell anemia (SS disease) (homozygous or sickle cell disease, and heterozygous or sickle cell trait), sickle cell-hemoglobin C disease (SC disease) and sickle cell-β-thalassemia disease (S-β disease). Although the sexual development of this patient group is rather delayed, fertility is usually normal in females[66]. Pregnancy in patients with sickle cell disease carries an increased risk of maternal and fetal complications such as sickle cell crises, abortions, stillbirths and neonatal deaths, fetal growth retardation, pulmonary infarction and embolization, acute pyelonephritis and pneumonias and exaggeration of physiologic anemia of pregnancy. Consequently, pregnancy in patients with SS disease is considered to be high-risk pregnancy, with an estimated maternal mortality of 1–1.5%[66,67]. It is therefore evident that an effective means of contraception to safeguard against unplanned pregnancy is very necessary in this group of women.

Until recently, SS, SC and S-β disease had been considered to be absolute contraindications for the administration of OCs, despite the lack of convincing evidence to support this recommendation. The reason for this advice was the observation that this patient group has an increased risk for the development of thromboembolic episodes, a condition which is a well established absolute contraindication for the use of combined OCs. Recent advice, however, suggests that SS, SC and S-β disease should only be considered as relative contraindications, especially when balanced against the risks of pregnancy in these women[68]. There has not been a single prospective cohort or a case–control study on the risk of thromboembolic episodes in women with sickle hemoglobinopathies receiving OCs[69]. Patients with sickle cell trait have not been reported to have altered coagulation status and they are not at increased risk of thrombosis[70]. Thus, they should be regarded as being normal for the prescription of combined OCs.

Splenectomy, for whatever reason (including the treatment of sickle cell disease) is also considered to be a relative contraindication for the administration of OCs. In these women the platelet count should be closely monitored, and a count above $500 \times 10^9/l$ would absolutely contraindicate the use of estrogen-containing preparations[71].

The increased risk for thrombosis is attributed to the estrogenic part of combined OCs. Most of the available literature about the thromboembolic risk in women on OCs includes studies in which the first generation high-dose preparations, i.e. those containing more than 50 µg of ethinylestradiol, were used. A cohort study in 200 000 women enrolled from the Michigan Medicaid population demonstrated that the relative risk of deep venous thromboembolic disease in women taking OCs containing less than, equal to or more than 50 µg of estrogen, was 1 : 1.5 : 1.7 respectively[72].

In addition to these epidemiological data, several reports on the effect of OCs on the coagulation profile can be found in the literature, including increased procoagulant factor activities (such as the factor VII) and decreased activity of the intrinsic coagulation inhibitors (such as antithrombin III, protein S and protein C)[73,74]. These effects appear to depend on the dose of the estrogenic component of the OC, and it has been reported that modern low-dose OCs may actually increase the fibrinolytic activity and plasminogen activity, thus possibly reducing the risk of thromboembolism[75–77]. Similar alterations of the coagulation profile have been also reported in patients with sickle hemoglobinopathies[78–82]. However, these effects have been the subject of small studies with limited numbers of patients, and no prospective study has demonstrated that a change in a clotting protein is actually associated with an increased risk of thrombosis[83].

As an alternative to the combined OCs certain estrogen-free contraceptives have been evaluated in patients with sickle cell disease. In a retrospective study performed in the UK among patients with SS disease[84], 67 women (total 148 women years) were given combined OCs, 30 women (total 77 women years) were given progestogen-only pills (POPs), 28 women (total 140 women years) used intrauterine devices and 26 women (44 women years) had injections of medroxyprogesterone acetate (Depo-Provera®). Two women in the combined OC group developed deep venous thrombosis (DVT), whereas no DVT episodes were observed in the group who received the injectable progestogen. In another clinical trial of levonorgestrel implants (Norplant®) in women with sickle cell disease, no serious or unexpected adverse effects related to their use occurred during a mean observation period of 12.4 months (ranging from 1 to 29 months), and no pregnancies were reported[84]. Medroxyprogesterone acetate has been demonstrated to reduce the frequency of crises[84,86]. It thus seems possible that these alternatives may become the methods of contraceptive choice in women with sickle cell disease if properly organized prospective studies confirm their efficiency and superiority over the combined OCs.

THALASSEMIAS AND ORAL CONTRACEPTIVES

Women with thalassemia major usually have impairment of their hypothalamic–pituitary–ovarian axis, with primary or secondary amenorrhea and reduced fertility. The use of OCs in this patient group has not been studied and information regarding the risks and benefits is lacking.

REFERENCES

1. Lindgren, A. and Olsson, R. (1993). Liver damage from low-dose oral contraceptives. *J. Intern. Med.*, **234**, 287–92
2. Waters, B. and Riely, C.A. (1995). Drug and chemical induced hepatic injury. In Haubrick, W.S. and Schiffner, F. (eds.) *Bockus Gastroenterology 1985*. 5th edn, pp. 2158–89. (Philadelphia: W.B. Saunders)
3. Maddrey, W.C. (1985). Drug and chemical induced hepatic injury. In Berk, J.E., Haubrick, W.S., Kalser, M.H. *et al.* (eds.) *Bockus Gastroenterology 1985*. 4th edn, pp. 2922–56. (Philadelphia: W.B. Saunders)
4. Lewis, J.H. and Zimmerman, H.J. (1989). Drug-induced liver disease. *Med. Clin. North Am.*, **73**, 775–92
5. Adlercrutz, H. and Tenhunen, R. (1970). Some aspects of the interaction between natural and synthetic female sex hormones and the liver. *Am. J. Med.*, **49**, 630–2
6. Metreau, J.M., Dhumeaux, D. and Berthelot, P. (1972). Oral contraceptives and the liver. *Digestion*, **7**, 318
7. Kreek, M.J. (1987). Female sex steroids and cholestasis. *Semin. Liver Dis.*, **7**, 8–11
8. Orellana-Alcale, J.M. and Domingues, J.P. (1966). Jaundice and oral contraceptive drugs. *Lancet*, **2**, 1278
9. Reichen, J. and Simon, F. (1984). Mechanisms of cholestasis. *Int. Rev. Exp. Pathol.*, **26**, 232–40
10. Danan, G. (1988). Consensus meeting on causally assessment of drug-induced liver injury. *J. Hepatol.*, **7**, 132–6

11. Sherlock, S. (1986). The spectrum of hepatotoxicity due to drugs. *Lancet*, **2**, 440–4

12. Weden, M., Glaumann, H. and Einarsson, K. (1992). Protracted cholestasis probably induced by oral contraceptive. *J. Intern. Med.*, **231**, 561–5

13. Kaplowitz, N., Aw, T.Y., Simon, F.R. and Stolz, A. (1986). UCLA conference: drug-induced hepatotoxicity. *Ann. Intern. Med.*, **104**, 826–39

14. Pessayre, D. and Larrey, D. (1991). Drug-induced liver injury. In McIntyre, N., Benhamou, J., Bircher, J. *et al.* (eds.) *Oxford Textbook of Clinical Hepatology*, Vol. 1, pp. 876–902. (New York: Oxford University Press)

15. Lieberman, D.A., Keefe, E.B. and Stenzel, P. (1984). Severe and prolonged oral contraceptive jaundice. *J. Clin. Gastroenterol.*, **6**, 145–8

16. Ishak, K.G. (1981). Hepatic lesions caused by anabolic steroids. *Semin. Liver Dis.*, **1**, 116–20

17. Baum, J.K., Holtz, F. and Bookstein, J.J. (1973). Possible association between benign hepatomas and oral contraceptives. *Lancet*, **2**, 926–9

18. Klatskin, G. (1977). Hepatic tumors: possible relationship to use of oral contraceptives. *Gastroenterology*, **73**, 386–94

19. Vana, J. and Murphy, G.P. (1979). Primary malignant liver tumor: association with oral contraceptives. *NY State J. Med.*, **79**, 321–5

20. Shar, S.R. and Kew, M.C. (1982). Oral contraceptives and hepatocellular carcinoma. *Cancer*, **49**, 407–10

21. Gala, K.V. and Griffin, T.W. (1983). Hepatomas in young women on oral contraceptives: report of two cases and review of the literature. *J. Surg. Oncol.*, **22**, 11–14

22. Neuberger, J., Nummerly, H.B., Davis, M., Portmann, B., Laws, J.W. and Williams, R. (1980). Oral contraceptive-associated liver tumors: occurrence of malignancy had difficulties in diagnosis. *Lancet*, **1**, 273–6

23. Pryor, A.C., Cohen, R.J. and Goldman, R.L. (1977). Hepatocellular carcinoma in a woman on long-term oral contraceptives. *Cancer*, **40**, 884–8

24. Edmondson, H.A., Reynolds, T.B., Henderson, B. and Benton, B. (1977). Regression of liver cell adenomas associated with oral contraceptives. *Ann. Intern. Med.*, **86**, 180–2

25. Tesluk, H. and Lawrie, J. (1981). Hepatocellular adenoma: its transformation to carcinoma in a user of oral contraceptives. *Arch. Pathol. Lab. Med.*, **105**, 296–9

26. Gordon, S.C., Reddy, K.R., Livingstone, A.S., Jeffers, L.J. and Schiff, E.R. (1986). Resolution of a contraceptive steroid-induced hepatic adenoma with subsequent evolution into hepatocellular carcinoma. *Ann. Intern. Med.*, **105**, 296–9

27. Gyorffy, E.J., Bredfeldt, J.E. and Black, W.C. (1989). Transformation of hepatic cell adenoma to hepatocellular carcinoma due to oral contraceptive use. *Ann. Intern. Med.*, **110**, 489–90

28. Tao, L.C. (1991). Oral contraceptives-associated liver cell adenoma and hepatocellular carcinoma. Cytomorphology and mechanism of malignant transformation. *Cancer*, **68**, 341–7

29. Chequi, D., Rahmouni, A., Charlotte, F. *et al.* (1995). Management of focal nodular hyperplasia and hepatocellular carcinoma in young women: a series of 41 patients with clinical, radiological and pathological correlations. *Hepatology*, **22**, 1674–81

30. Le Bail, B., Jouhanole, H., Deugnier, Y., Salame, G., Pellegrin, J.L., Saric, *et al.* (1992). Liver adenomatosis with granulomas in two patients on long-term oral contraceptives. *Am. J. Surg. Pathol.*, **16**, 982–7

31. Henderson, B.E., Preston-Martin, S., Edmondson, H.A., Peters, P.L. and Pike, M.C. (1983). Hepatocellular carcinoma and oral contraceptives. *Br. J. Cancer*, **48**, 437–40

32. Glassburg, A.B. and Rosenbaum, E.H. (1976). Oral contraceptives and malignant hepatoma. *Lancet*, **1**, 479

33. La Vecchia, C., Negri, E. and Parazzini, F. (1989). Oral contraceptives and primary liver cancer. *Br. J. Cancer*, **59**, 460–1

34. Ferrara, B.E and Rutland, E.D. (1988). Liver tumor in long-term user of oral contraceptives. *Postgrad. Med.*, **84**, 107–9

35. Adami, H.O., Persson, I., Hoover, R., Schairer, C. and Bergkvist, L. (1989). Risk of cancer in women receiving hormone replacement therapy. *Int. J. Cancer*, **44**, 833–9

36. Forman, D., Vincent, T.J. and Doll, R. (1986). Cancer of the liver and use of oral contraceptives. *Br. Med. J.*, **292**, 1357–61

37. Forman, D., Doll, R. and Peto, R. (1983). Trends in mortality from carcinoma of the liver and the use of oral contraceptives. *Br. J. Cancer*, **48**, 349–54

38. Palmer, J.R., Rosenberg, L., Kaufman, D.W., Warshauer, M.E., Stolley, P. and Shapiro, S. (1989). Oral contraceptive use and liver cancer. *Am. J. Epidemiol.*, **130**, 878–82

39. Neuberger, J., Forman, D., Doll, R. and Williams, R. (1986). Oral contraceptives and hepatocellular carcinoma. *Br. Med. J.*, **292**, 1355–7

40. Yu, M.C., Tong, M.J., Govindarajan, S. and Henderson, B.E. (1991). Non-viral risk factors for hepatocellular carcinoma in a low-risk population, the non-Asians of Los Angeles County, California. *J. Natl. Cancer Inst.*, **83**, 1820–6

41. La Vecchia, C., Negri, E., Franceschi, S. and D'Avanzo, B. (1992). Reproductive factors and the risks of hepatocellular carcinoma in women. *Int. J. Cancer*, **52**, 351–4

42. Prentice, R.L. (1991). Epidemiologic data on exogenous hormones and hepatocellular carcinoma and selected other cancers. *Prevent. Med.*, **20**, 38–46

43. Hromas, R.A, Srigley, J. and Murray, J.L. (1985). Clinical and pathologic comparison of young women with hepatocellular carcinoma with and without exposure to oral contraceptives. *Am. J. Gastroenterol.*, **80**, 479–83

44. Goodman, Z.D. and Ishak, K.G. (1982). Hepatocellular carcinoma in women: probable lack of etiologic association with oral contraceptive steroids. *Hepatology*, **2**, 440–4

45. Abdi, E.A., Brien, W. and Venner, P.M. (1986). Autoimmune thrombocytopenia related to interferon therapy. *Scand. J. Haematol.*, **36**, 515–19

46. The WHO collaborative study of neoplasia and steroid contraceptives. (1991). Depot-medroxyprogesterone acetate and risk of liver cancer. *Int. J. Cancer*, **49**, 182–5

47. Lewis, J.H., Tice, H.L. and Zimmerman, H.J. (1983). Budd–Chiari syndrome associated with oral contraceptive steroids: review of treatment of 47 cases. *Dig. Dis. Sci.*, **28**, 673–5

48. Maddrey, W.C. (1987). Hepatic vein thrombosis (Budd–Chiari syndrome): possible association with the use of oral contraceptives. *Semin. Liver Dis.*, **7**, 32

49. Mitchel, M.C., Boitnott, J.K., Kaufman, S., Cameron, J.L. and Maddrey, W.C. (1982). Budd–Chiari syndrome: etiology, diagnosis and management. *Medicine*, **61**, 199–204

50. Sterup, K. and Mosbech, J. (1967). Budd–Chiari syndrome after taking oral contraceptives. *Br. Med. J.*, **4**, 660–2

51. Valla, D., Le, M.G., Paynard, T., Rueff, B. and Benhamou, J.P. (1986). Risk of hepatic vein thrombosis in relation to the recent use of oral contraceptives: a case control study. *Gastroenterology*, **90**, 807–11

52. Chu, G. and Farrell, G.C. (1993). Portal vein thrombosis associated with prolonged ingestion of oral contraceptive steroids. *J. Gastroenterol. Hepatol.*, **8**, 390–3

53. Conter, R.L. and Longmire, W. (1988). Recurrent hepatic haemangiomas. *Ann. Surg.*, **207**, 115–19

54. Wanless, I.R., Mawdsley, C. and Adams, R. (1985). On the pathogenesis of focal nodular hyperplasia of the liver. *Hepatology*, **5**, 1194–200

55. Nime, F., Pickren, J.W., Vana, J., Aronoff, B.L., Baker, H.W. and Murphy, G.P. (1979). The histology of liver tumors in oral contraceptive users during a national survey by the American College of Surgeons Commission on Cancer. *Cancer*, **44**, 1481–9

56. Scott, L.D., Katz, A.R., Duke, J.H., Cowan, D.F. and Maklad, N.F. (1984). Oral contraceptives, pregnancy and focal nodular hyperplasia of the liver. *J. Am. Med. Assoc.*, **251**, 1461–3

57. Zafrani, E.S. (1989). Update on vascular tumors of the liver. *J. Hepatol.*, **8**, 125–310

58. Mathieu, D., Zafrani, E.S., Anglande, M.C. and Dhumeaux, X. (1989). Association of focal nodular hyperplasia and hepatic haemangioma. *Gastroenterology*, **97**, 154–7

59. Van Berge Henegouwen, G.P. and Van der Werf, S.D.J. (1992). Serum bile acids and the bile acid tolerance test under oral contraceptives. *Hepatogastroenteriol.*, **39**, 177–80

60. Thus, C, Leffers, P. and Knipschild, P. (1993). Oral contraceptive use and the occurrence of gallstone disease: a case–control study. *Prevent. Med.*, **22**, 122–31

61. Basso, L., McCollum, P.T., Darling, M.R., Tocchi, A. and Tanner, W.A. (1992). A study of cholelithiasis during pregnancy and its relationship with age, parity, menarche, breast feeding, dysmenorrhea, oral contraception and a maternal history of cholelithiasis. *Surg. Gynecol. Obstet.*, **175**, 41–6

62. Oligny, L.L. and Lough, J. (1992). Hepatic sinusoidal ectasia. *Hum. Pathol.*, **23**, 953–6

63. Zimmerman, H.J. (1983). Hepatic disease and oral contraceptive therapy. *J. Am. Med. Assoc.*, **249**, 3241

64. Cundy, T.F., O'Grady, J.G. and Williams, R. (1990). Recovery of menstruation and pregnancy after liver transplantation. *Gut*, **31**, 337–8

65. Hall, J.G., Pauli, R.M. and Wilson, K.M. (1980). Maternal and fetal sequelae of anticoagulation during pregnancy. *Am. J. Med.*, **68**, 122–40

66. Alleyne, S.I., Rauseo, R.D. *et al.* (1981). Sexual development and fertility of Jamaican female patients with homozygous sickle cell disease. *Lancet*, **2**, 275

67. Cunningham, F.G., MacDonald, P.C. and Gant, N.F. (1994). *Williams Obstetrics*, 19th edn, p. 1179. (New York: Appleton & Lange)

68. Guillebaud, J. (1993). *Contraception: Your Questions Answered*, 2nd edn, p. 164. (Edinburgh: Churchill Livingstone)

69. Goldzieher, J.W. and Zamah, N.M. (1995). Oral contraceptive side effects: where's the beef? *Contraception*, **52**, 327–35

70. Platt, O.S. and Dover, G.J. (1993). Sickle cell disease. In Nathan, D.G. and Oski, F.A. (eds.). *Hematology of Infancy and Childhood*, 4th edn, pp. 732–82. (Philadelphia: W.B. Saunders)

71. Guillebaud, J. (1993). *Contraception: Your Questions Answered*, 2nd edn, p. 161. (Edinburgh: Churchill Livingstone)

72. Gerstmann, B.B., Piper, J.M., Tomita, D.K. *et al.* (1991). Oral contraceptive estrogen dose and the risk of deep venous thromboembolic disease. *Am. J. Epidemiol.*, **133**, 32

73. Abbate, R., Pinto, S., Rostagno, C. *et al.* (1990). Effects of long term gestodene-containing oral contraceptive administration on hemostasis. *Am. J. Obstet. Gynecol.*, **163**, 424–30

74. Tait, R.C., Walker, I.D., Islam, S.I.A.M. *et al.* (1993). Protein C activity in healthy volunteers – influence of age, sex, smoking and oral contraceptives. *Thromb. Haemost.*, **70**, 281–5

75. Jespersen, J. and Kluft, C. (1985). Increased euglobulin fibrinolytic potential in women on oral contraceptives low in oestrogen. Levels of extrinsic and intrinsic plasminogen activators, prekallikrein, factor XII and C1-inactivator. *Thromb. Haemost.*, **54**, 454–9

76. Jespersen, J. and Kluft, C. (1982). Decreased levels of histidine-rich glycoprotein (HRG) and increased levels of free plasminogen in women on oral contraceptives low in oestrogen. *Thromb. Haemost.*, **4**, 283–5

77. Massafra, C., Butini, P., Cavion, M.A. *et al.* (1993). Evaluation of risk of thrombosis during use of low-dose ethinylestradiol-desogestrel oral contraceptive. *Adv. Contracept.*, **9**, 195–203

78. Porter, J.B., Young, L., Mackie, I.J. *et al.* (1993). Sickle cell disorders and chronic intravascular haemolysis are associated with low plasma heparin cofactor II. *Br. J. Haematol.*, **83**, 459–65

79. Peters, M., Plaat, B.E., ten-Cate, H. *et al.* (1994). Enhanced thrombin generation in children with sickle cell disease. *Thromb. Haemost.*, **71**, 169–72

80. el-Hazmi, M.A., Warsy, A.S. and Bahakim, H. (1993). Blood proteins C and S in sickle cell disease. *Acta Haematol.*, **90**, 114–19

81. Foulon, I., Bachir, D., Galacteros, F. *et al.* (1993). Increased *in vivo* production of thromboxane in patients with sickle cell disease is accompanied by an impairment of platelet functions to the thromboxane A2 agonist U46619. *Arterioscler. Thromb.*, **13**, 421–6

82. Bokarewa, M.I., Falk, G., Sten-Linder, M. *et al.* (1995). Thrombotic risk factors and oral contraception. *J. Lab. Clin. Med.*, **126**, 294–8

83. Comp, P.C. and Zacur, H.A. (1993). Contraceptive choices in women with coagulation disorders. *Am. J. Obstet. Gynecol.*, **168**, 1990–3

84. Howard, J.R., Lillis, C. and Tucu, S.M. (1993). Contraceptives, counselling and pregnancy in women with sickle cell disease. *Br. Med. J.*, **306**, 1735–7

85. Ladipo, O.A., Falusi, A.G., Feldbum, P.J. *et al.* (1993). Norplant[®] use by women with sickle cell disease. *Int. J. Gynecol. Obstet.*, **41**, 85

86. Guillebaud, J. (1993). Sickle cell disease and contraception. *Br. Med. J.*, **307**, 506–7

29

Oral contraceptives and migraine

Ø. Lidegaard

INTRODUCTION

It is estimated that 65 million women around the world are currently using oral contraceptives (OCs). When considering the risks and benefits associated with OCs, much attention has been given to the vascular effects, including cerebral thrombosis and transient ischemic attacks.

Known risk factors for thromboembolic disorders are very different on the venous and arterial sides of the vascular system (Table 1). Migraine is one of the established risk factors for cerebral thrombosis and transient ischemic attacks. Since the use of oral contraceptives increases the risk of cerebral thrombotic events, and since many women suffer from migraine, it is important to assess the impact of OC-use among women with migraine.

STROKE AND TRANSIENT ISCHEMIC ATTACKS IN YOUNG WOMEN

Cerebral thrombosis and transient ischemic attacks before the age of 45 years account for approximately 4% of all cerebral thrombotic events occurring in women. Fortunately, the mortality rate is low in young women; the case fatality rate is 2–5%. Nevertheless, these diseases are important because they leave approximately one-third of the survivors with some form of disability.

299

Table 1 Risk factors for venous thromboembolism (VTE), myocardial infarction (AMI) and cerebral thromboembolic attcks (CTA) among young women. + indicates a risk factor, − indicates no risk factor

Risk factor	VTE	AMI	CTA
Age	+	+	+
Smoking	—	+	+
Hypertension	—	+	+
Diabetes	—	+	+
Family VTE	+	—	—
Family AMI	—	+	+
Family CTA	—	+	+
Body mass index >30	+	+	—
Migraine	—	—	+
Varicose veins	+	—	—
Leiden factor V	+	—	—

The incidence rate of cerebral thrombosis in the developed world rises nearly exponentially with age[1–3]. In Denmark, the annual rate increases from 2/100 000 among 15–19-year-old women to about 22/100 000 in women 40–44 years old (Figure 1)[1], a doubling of risk for every 5–6 years. The incidence of transient ischemic attack also increases exponentially with age, although the age-specific rates are about half those of cerebral thrombosis.

MIGRAINE IN YOUNG WOMEN

A history of regular migraine has been reported by 5% of women of reproductive age[4].

Migraine and OC use

A general association between migraine and the use of OCs has not been demonstrated[5].

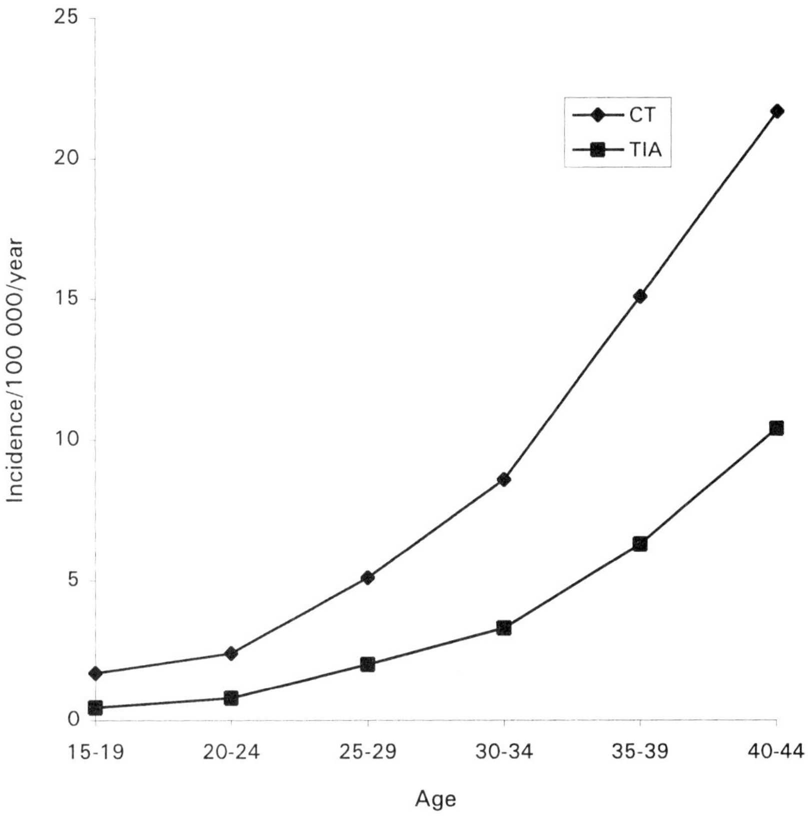

Figure 1 Cerebral thrombosis (CT) and transient ischemic attacks (TIA) among young women. Incidence rates according to age. Thrombotic stroke: only first-ever attacks. Denmark 1987–93, number of cases: 1071

MIGRAINE AND STROKE

Several studies have demonstrated a higher frequency of migraine among women with cerebral thromboembolism than among men with the same problem[6–9].

Several studies have found an association between migraine and stroke in young women[4,9–13]. Oleckno found that 11% of stroke patients (males and females, all cerebrovascular events including cerebral hemorrhages) had a history of migraine compared with none of the control group ($p < 0.001$)[9]. The Collaborative Group for the Study of Stroke in Young Women (CGSS) found that migraine was associated with a relative risk for thrombotic strokes of 2.0[10]. Bogousslavsky and colleagues demonstrated that 91% of women suffering from a thrombotic stroke during a migraine attack did not have any arterial or cardiac abnormalities compared with 9% of migraineurs with stroke remote from a migraine attack[11]. Tzourio and colleagues demonstrated in a case-control study of 72 women with ischemic stroke that migraine without aura gave a relative risk of 3.0 (1.5–5.8) while migraine with aura was associated with a relative risk of 6.2 (2.1–18.0)[12]. In a Danish case–control study, a history of migraine implied a relative risk of thrombotic strokes of 2.8 ($p < 0.01$)[4].

USE OF THE PILL AND THROMBOTIC STROKE

During the last two decades, several retrospective case-control studies and prospective cohort studies have reported a significantly increased risk of thrombotic strokes among current users of OCs. Some of the studies were conducted during a period when higher-dose OCs were widely used. The published relative risks have declined with time, indicating an effect of reductions in the hormonal content of the pill[1].

The overall relative risk of thrombotic strokes among users of OCs has been found to be between 1.8 and 4.4[13–15]. A Danish study demonstrated a dose–response relationship with the estrogen content: progestogen-only pills were not associated with any increased risk, 30–40 μg estrogen pills had a relative risk of 1.8 whereas OCs with 50 μg estrogen increased the risk 2.9 times (Figure 2)[14]. The same trend for estrogen content was found in a British study of all strokes (thrombotic and hemorrhagic)[13].

The influence of the progestogen dose and type has received less attention. Hannaford and colleagues found an increasing risk of stroke (thrombotic and hemorrhagic) with increasing doses of norethisterone: relative risks of 2.6, 3.6 and 6.7, respectively for pills containing 1, 2 or 4 mg norethisterone, all combined with 50 μg of ethinylestradiol[13]. Lidegaard found in the Danish series identical odds ratios for the progestogens, norethisterone, levonorgestrel or desogestrel when combined with 30–40 μg estrogen. None of the women had used OCs with gestodene which were introduced in Denmark in 1988.

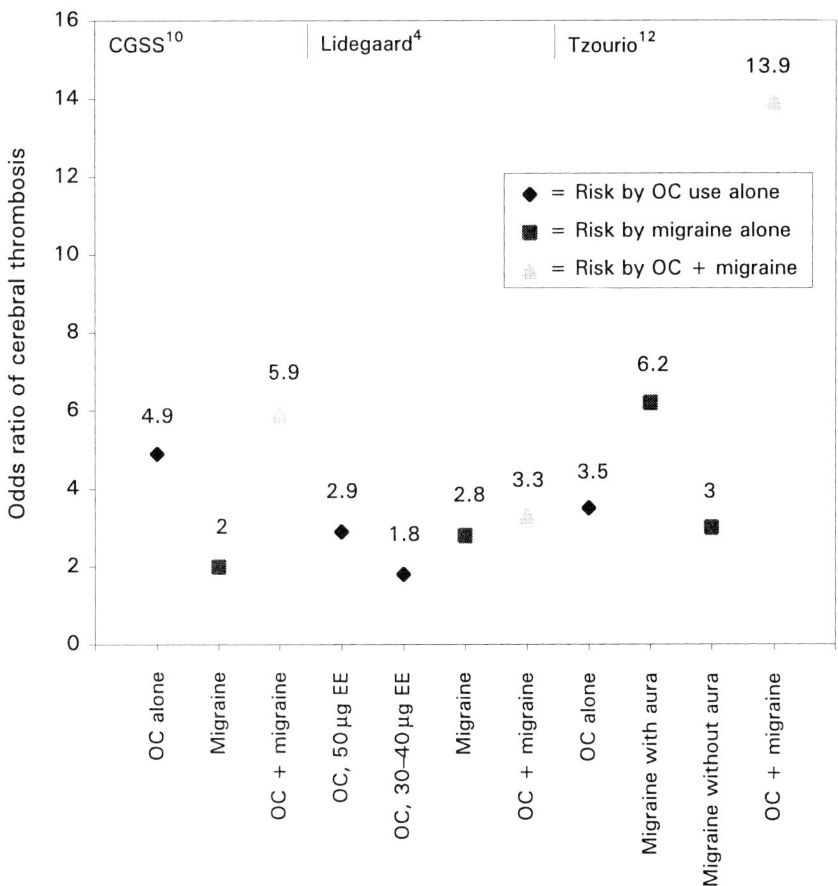

Figure 2 Cerebral thromboembolic risk according to use of oral contraceptives and presence of migraine

MIGRAINE, ORAL CONTRACEPTIVES AND THROMBOTIC STROKES

Are contraceptive pill users who have a history of migraine at greater risk of cerebral thromboembolism than users without such problems? As mentioned previously, a general association between migraine and the pill has not been established[5]. Any study of association between migraine, OCs and cerebral thrombosis is complicated by two important circumstances:

(1)   Women with migraine are often dissuaded from taking the pill. Study results, therefore should be stratified by pill use and history of migraine.

(2)   It may be difficult to distinguish between severe migraine and transient ischemic attacks. Case definition may therefore be a problem.

Only a few studies have been conducted on this matter, and the majority are uncontrolled. In 1978, Boisen reported on six female stroke patients (collected between 1968 and 1977) with associated migraine[16]. None of them were users of OCs. Bogousslavsky and Regli did not find more migrainous infarctions among stroke patients who were users of OCs than among other patients with stroke[17], and Bogousslavsky and colleagues found no excess of users of OCs among 22 migraine sufferers with ischemic stroke than among non-migraine sufferers with stroke[11]. Likewise, Rothrock and colleagues found only three users of OCs among 19 migraine-associated female stroke patients aged 15–44 years[18]. The CGSS study found that, while migraine was associated with a relative risk of thrombotic strokes of 2.0, the combination of migraine and OCs had a relative risk of 5.9 – a risk not higher than that for pill usage alone[10] (Figure 2). Tzourio and colleagues demonstrated that women with migraine and using OCs had a relative risk of ischemic strokes of 13.9 whereas use of the pill alone was associated with a four-fold increased risk, and migraine with aura a six-fold elevated risk[12]. Lidegaard demonstrated in the Danish case-control study that use of OCs was as common among migraine patients as among women without migraine, both among the controls and among the cases[14]. Women who at the same time were users of 30–40 μg estrogen OCs and suffering from migraine had a relative risk of thrombotic strokes of 3.3, indicating an additive rather than multiplicative effect for the combination of migraine and OC use (Figure 2).

RELATIVE AND ABSOLUTE RISK

It is important to remember that the incidence of thrombotic stroke increases with age. Since the relative risk (odds ratio) is constant over the age groups, the absolute increase in risk of cerebral thrombosis by use of OCs or by the presence of migraine is about 10 times higher for a woman aged 40 than for a woman aged 20 years. The absolute OC or migraine attributable risk is 2–4/100 000 annually at 20 years, and about 10 times as much among women 20 years older. This implies that, even though the risk of cerebral thrombosis is increased significantly by use of OCs or by the presence of migraine, the absolute risk for a young healthy woman is still very low.

CONCLUSION

Available data suggest that migraine increases the risk of thrombotic strokes by 2–6-fold, an effect which is independent of the OC status. No synergism appears to exist between OCs and migraine as regards thrombotic strokes. Migraine with aura may imply higher risk than migraine without aura.

A woman suffering from migraine who consults her doctor for contraceptive advice must be informed that she has an increased risk of cerebral thromboembolism because of her migraine history, a risk which will be further but not dramatically increased by the use of OCs at a young age. Women who have experienced improvement in their migraine (frequency and/or severity) while taking OCs probably could continue their use. Otherwise, women suffering from migraine with aura should not take combined oral contraceptives and those above 35 years who suffer regularly from migraine should also consider alternative contraception, especially if they smoke.

REFERENCES

1. Lidegaard, Ø. (1995). Decline in cerebral thromboembolism among young women after introduction of low-dose oral contraceptives: an incidence study for the period 1980–1993. *Contraception*, **52**, 85–92
2. Robins, M. and Baum, H. (1981). Stroke incidence. *Stroke*, **12** (Suppl. 1), 45–57
3. Bonita, R., Anderson, C.S., Broad, J.B., Jamrozik, K.D., Stewart-Wynne, E.G. and Anderson, N.E. (1994). Stroke incidence and case fatality in Australasia. *Stroke*, **25**, 552–7
4. Lidegaard, Ø. (1995). Oral contraceptives, pregnancy and the risk of cerebral thromboembolism: the influence of diabetes, hypertension,

migraine and previous thrombotic disease. *Br. J. Obstet. Gynaecol.*, **102**, 153–9

5. Benson, M.D. and Rebar, R.W. (1986). Relationship of migraine headache and stroke to oral contraceptive use. *J. Reprod. Med.*, **31**, 1082–8

6. Hindfelt, B. and Nilsson, O. (1977). Brain infarction in young adults. *Acta Neurol. Scand.*, **55**, 145–57

7. Klein, G. M. and Seland, T.P. (1984). Occlusive cerebro-vascular disease in young adults. *Can. J. Neurol. Sci.*, **11**, 302–4

8. Hilton-Jones, D. and Warlow, C.P. (1985). The causes of stroke in the young. *J. Neurol.*, **232**, 137–43

9. Oleckno, W.A. (1986). Selected factors and stroke in young adults, 15–40 years of age. *J. R. Soc. Hlth.*, **3**, 102–7

10. Collaborative Group for the Study of Stroke in Young Women. (1975). Oral contraceptives and stroke in young women. Associated risk factors. *J. Am. Med. Assoc.*, **231**, 718–22

11. Bogousslavsky, J., Regli, F., Van Melle, G., Payot, M. and Uske, A. (1988). Migraine stroke. *Neurology*, **38**, 223–7

12. Tzourio, C., Tehindrazanarivelo, A., Iglesias, S., Alpérovitchy, A., Chedru, P., Anglejan-Chatillon, J. and Bouser, M.-G. (1995). Case-control study of migraine and risk of ischemic stroke in young women. *Br. Med. J.*, **310**, 830–3

13. Hannaford, P.C., Croft, P.R. and Kay, C.R. (1994). Oral contraception and stroke. Evidence from the Royal College of General Practitioners' Oral Contraception Study. *Stroke*, **25**, 935–42

14. Lidegaard, Ø. (1993). Oral contraception and risk of cerebral thromboembolic attacks: results of a case-control study. *Br. Med. J.*, **306**, 956–63

15. Thorogood, M., Mann, J., Murphy, M. and Vessey, M. (1992). Fatal stroke and use of oral contraceptives: findings from a case-control study. *Am. J. Epidemiol.*, **136**, 35–45

16. Boisen, E. (1975). Strokes in migraine: report on seven strokes associated with severe migraine attacks. *Dan. Med. Bull.*, **22**, 100–6

17. Bogousslavsky, J. and Regli, F. (1987). Ischemic stroke in adults younger than 30 years of age. *Arch. Neurol.*, **44**, 479-82

18. Rothrock, J.F., Walicke, P. Swenson, M.R., Lyden, P.D. and Logan, W.R. (1988). Migrainous stroke. *Arch. Neurol.*, **45**, 63–7

30

Can the pill be given to women with cancers?

R. J. E. Kirkman

INTRODUCTION

As seen from Table 1 and Figure 1, the most common sites of cancer in women living in England and Wales of reproductive years are the breast, cervix, skin and ovary, in that order. All these sites respond to sex hormones and many would say that in order to avoid doing harm a good doctor would never prescribe hormonal contraception to women with these cancers. However, when giving contraceptive advice to patients with cancer, whether cured, in remission or currently undergoing treatment, the reliability and acceptability of the method, and compliance of the individuals, have to be taken into consideration. The risks of an unplanned pregnancy have to be balanced against the risks intrinsic to use of the combined pill in healthy women and in relation to the type of cancer and the treatment given for it.

Possible drug interactions and side-effects of cancer treatments will also influence the decision. Most cytotoxic drugs are teratogenic and therefore the effectiveness of contraceptive method has a high priority during the treatment stage. No increase in fetal abnormalities or abortion rate has been recorded in patients who remain fertile after cytotoxic chemotherapy[1].

Table 1 Commonest cancers in women 1983–87. Annual incidence per 100 000 by age group in England and Wales. Derived from WHO Research on Cancer[18] with permission

	25–29 years	*35–40 years*	*40–44 years*	*65–69 years*
Stomach	0.3	1.1	2.1	36.2
Colon	0.4	3.0	6.3	79.9
Rectum	0.3	1.8	3.8	44.0
Lung	0.5	3.2	6.8	144.2
Melanoma of skin	3.8	8.0	10.4	13.2
Other skin	2.5	9.5	16.6	115.1
Breast	6.2	47.6	92.1	210.6
Cervix	11.9	24.1	24.3	29.9
Ovary, etc.	2.0	5.8	12.8	49.6
Brain	1.6	3.3	3.7	13.5
Thyroid	1.5	2.3	2.1	3.8
Hodgkin's	2.8	1.7	1.6	2.2
Non-Hodgkin's lymphoma	1.6	3.2	4.8	22.3
Placenta	0.2	0.1	0.0	0.0

BREAST CANCER

There is evidence that breast cancer cells metastasize more easily when mastectomy is undertaken in the mid-follicular phase of the menstrual cycle[2]. The antiestrogen tamoxifen given postoperatively[3] reduced the overall annual risk of developing contralateral breast cancer by 39% with, as expected, most benefit in women with tumors which were estrogen receptor-positive. However, the overall reduction in annual risk of breast cancer recurrence by use of tamoxifen in estrogen receptor-negative women was still 16% ($p = 0.001$). The results suggest that it is advisable to refrain from prescribing combined oral contraceptives (COCs) to women who have had breast cancer.

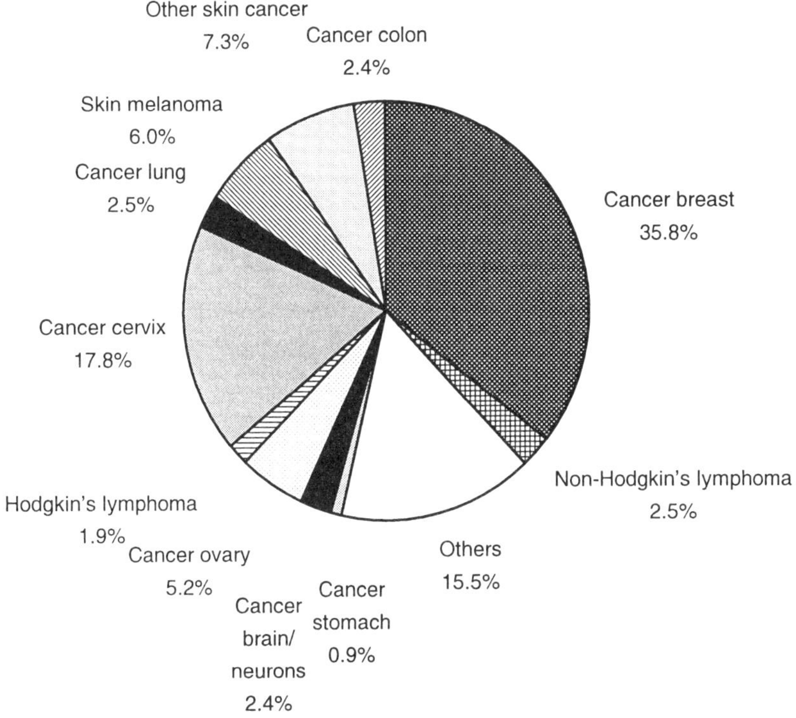

Figure 1 Site of origin of cancers in women aged 25– 44 years (England and Wales) 1983– 87. Source: Office of Population Censuses and Surveys (1989). OPCS Cancer statistics, registrations England and Wales. Series MB1 no. 22

CANCER OF THE CERVIX

The International Planned Parenthood Federation (IPPF) statement February 1995 on steroidal oral contraception advised that women with successfully treated premalignant disease of the cervix could use all contraceptive methods, including the pill. Women using COCs who are found to have positive smears should continue using the pill while undergoing investigation, since pregnancy at this stage poses much greater problems both in diagnosis and management. The number of fertile women requiring treatment for cancer of the cervix is small. There have, to my knowledge, been no studies concerning the risk of recurrence of cervical carcinoma and current use of COCs. However, cervical cancer cells are not thought to be hormonally dependent and therefore the pill is not contraindicated.

OVARIAN CANCER

Women with advanced cancers will have undergone one or a combination of three treatment regimens. Major surgery that may involve removal of the uterus and the ovaries obviously removes the need for contraception. Chemotherapy and radiotherapy may result in ovarian failure[4], although normal pregnancies following chemotherapy have been reported[5,6]. Unilateral oophorectomy may be carried out in a young woman with stage 1A grade 1 ovarian cancer where conservation of fertility is desired. Although combined oral contraceptives have a protective effect on the incidence of epithelial ovarian cancers, we have found no data on the effect of the pill on recurrence rates in women who have been treated conservatively. The estrogen and progestogen receptors in ovarian cancer tissue may be non-specific[7]. Since combined oral contraceptive pills and depomedroxyprogesterone acetate work mainly by ovulation suppression, it is probably safe to use them in this group of women.

MALIGNANT MELANOMA

Malignant melanoma is quite often diagnosed in women of childbearing age and may run an unpredictable course. Previously, pregnancy was regarded as an unfavorable prognostic factor in women with this disease and termination of pregnancy used to be recommended. This situation no longer applies[8] but, because the first 2–3 years after diagnosis is the period with the highest probability of relapse, it is recommended that pregnancy should be avoided during this period. The use of oral contraceptives does not appear to be contraindicated in patients with melanoma[9] but the side-effects of chemotherapy and radiotherapy, which often result in severe vomiting and nausea, may preclude their use in certain groups.

HYDATIDIFORM MOLE

Stone and co-workers[10] in 1976 reported that using COCs after evacuation of a hydatidiform mole increased the need for chemotherapy for trophoblastic tumor. Other studies, however, have refuted this finding. Curry[11], in 1989, reported a prospective study of 266 patients randomly allocated either to COCs or barrier methods after evacuation of hydatidiform mole. Post-molar trophoblastic disease was reported to have occurred in 23% of patients receiving oral contraceptives compared to 33% of those allocated to barrier methods. These are much higher rates than are recognized in the UK, where about 8% of post-molar patients have chemotherapy. Standard UK advice has been to avoid use of any hormonal methods until the β-human chorionic gonadotropin (β-hCG) levels have returned to normal[10]. More recent advice[12] is that oral contraceptives should be avoided until β-hCG levels have returned to normal for at least 6 months unless the patient is unlikely to comply with interim use of barrier or natural methods.

CHORIOCARCINOMA

Choriocarcinoma is a malignant tumor which can follow hydatidiform mole, an abortion or a normal pregnancy. Survival and cure rates are determined largely by tumor size and the interval between the antecedent pregnancy and the commencement of chemotherapy. Pregnancy after successful treatment of choriocarcinoma can and does occur[13]; therefore effective contraception is of paramount importance. It has been recommended that pregnancy should be avoided for 12 months after completing chemotherapy so that the risk of teratogenicity from the chemotherapy is minimized[14]. The combined oral contraceptive pill provides efficient contraception and suppresses pituitary luteinizing hormone (LH) which may cross-react with hCG in some assays. Advice concerning hormonal contraception is derived from the greater experience available in follow-up of those who have had hydatidiform mole.

HODGKIN'S DISEASE AND NON-HODGKIN'S LYMPHOMA

Irradiation is the main form of treatment for the majority of localized stages of Hodgkin's disease, that is stages 1, 2 and some 3A. Chemotherapy may be used in addition when apparently localized disease is associated with adverse prognostic factors. Temporary menstrual dysfunction is common and may lead to unplanned pregnancy if adequate contraception is not used, although pregnancy does not appear to accelerate Hodgkin's disease or to affect survival adversely[15]. Long-term remission may follow treatment of disseminated Hodgkin's disease with combination chemotherapy[16] and, because the majority of relapses will occur within 2 years, patients with active disease are usually advised to avoid pregnancy until the disease has been quiescent for this length of time. During this period, virtually all methods of contraception including the combined oral contraceptive pill may be used. The same considerations apply to non-Hodgkin's lymphoma.

THE LEUKEMIAS

Fertility after treatment for leukemia depends on the type of chemotherapy regimen used, since some are more likely to cause ovarian failure than others. Radiation also may produce ovarian failure unless the ovaries are shielded. Patients with thrombocytopenia as a result of either the malignancy or chemotherapy may have severe problems with menorrhagia and may gain specific benefit from the use of oral contraceptives or depo-medroxyprogesterone acetate.

LIVER CANCER

Combined oral contraceptives are contraindicated in patients with liver cancer and, although progestogen-only pills do not noticeably affect liver metabolism, authorities have suggested that a non-hormonal method should be the first choice[17].

OTHER ASPECTS

Most other cancers occur in women who are beyond their reproductive years, and there is a lack of information about the use of the COCs in women with these tumors. None of the cancers not specified in this article, however, are thought to be estrogen or progestogen dependent and so COC use is not contraindicated. For example, expert physicians advising the National Association of Family Planning Doctors (now incorporated into the Faculty of Family Planning) have in the past found no reason to refuse COCs to women with previous carcinoma of the thyroid or astrocytoma of the brain. Contraceptive choice will depend upon other health matters including possible interactions with chemotherapy. The only clear interaction of which we are aware is between progestogens and cyclosporin. This does not affect contraceptive efficacy but can result in a greater toxicity to the cyclosporin.

ACKNOWLEDGEMENT

I acknowledge with thanks the assistance of Dr B. Gbolade in the preparation of this paper.

REFERENCES

1. Van Theil, D.H., Russ, G.T. and Lipsett, M.B. (1970). Pregnancies after chemotherapy of trophoblastic neoplasms. *Science*, **169**, 1326–7
2. Badwe, R.A., Gregory, W.M., Chaudary, M.A., Richards, M.A., Bentley, A.E., Rubens, R.D. and Fentiman, I.S. (1991). Timing of surgery during menstrual cycle and survival of premenopausal women with operable breast cancer. *Lancet*, **1**, 1261–2
3. Early Breast Cancer Trialists' Collaborative Group (1992). Systemic treatment of early breast cancer by hormonal, cytotoxic or immune therapy. *Lancet*, **339**, 1–15, 71–85
4. Shalet, S. (1980). Effects of cancer chemotherapy on gonadal function of patients with cancer. *Cancer Treatment Rev.*, **7**, 141–52

5. Lee, R.B., Kelly, J., Elg, S.A. and Benson, W.L. (1989). Pregnancy following conservative surgery and adjunctive chemotherapy for stage III immature teratoma of the ovary. *Obstet. Gynecol.*, **73**, 853–5

6. Schneider, J., Erasun, F., Hervas, J.L., Acinas, O. and Gonzalez-Rodilla, I. (1988). Normal pregnancy and delivery two years after adjuvant chemotherapy for grade III immature ovarian teratoma. *Gynecol. Oncol.*, **29**, 245–9

7. Kaupila, A., Vierikko, P., Kivinen, S., Stenback, F. and Vihko, R. (1983). Clinical significance of estrogen and progestin receptors in ovarian cancer. *Obstet. Gynecol.*, **61**, 320–6

8. Slingluff, C.L. Jr and Reintgen, D. (1993). Malignant melanoma and the prognostic implications of pregnancy, oral contraceptives and exogenous hormones. *Semin. Surg. Oncol.*, **9**, 228–31

9. Osterlind, A., Tucker, M.A., Stone, B.J. and Jansen, O.M. (1988). The Danish case–control study of cutaneous malignant melanoma. III, hormonal and reproductive factors in women. *Int. J. Cancer*, **42**, 821–4

10. Stone, M., Dent, J., Kardana, A. and Bagshawe, K.D. (1976). Relationship of oral contraception to development of trophoblastic tumour after evacuation of a hydatidiform mole. *Br. J. Obstet. Gynaecol.*, **83**, 913–6

11. Curry, S.L., Schlaert, J.B., Kohorn, E.I., Boyce, J.B., Gore, H., Twiggs, L.B. and Blessing, J.A. (1989). Hormonal contraception and trophoblastic sequelae after hydatidiform mole (a gynecologic oncology group study). *Am. J. Obstet. Gynecol.*, **160**, 805–11

12. Newlands, E.S. (1994). Trophoblastic disease and hormones. *Br. J. Fam. Plann.*, **19**, 276–7

13. O'Neill, E., Pelegrina, I., Hammond, C.B., Vicens, R. and Almodovar, A.R. (1976). Normal pregnancy and delivery after cerebral metastasis of choriocarcinoma. *Cancer*, **38**, 984–6

14. Newlands, E.S. (1995). Clinical management of trophoblastic disease in the United Kingdom. *Current Obstet. Gynaecol.*, **5**, 19–24

15. Thomas, P.R.M. and Peckham, M.J. (1976). The investigation and management of Hodgkin's disease in the pregnant patient. *Cancer*, **38**, 1443–56

16. Rosenberg, S.A. and Kaplan, H.S. (1975). The management of stages I, II and III Hodgkin's disease with combined radiotherapy and chemotherapy. *Cancer*, **35**, 55–63

17. Guillebaud, J. (1993). *Contraception: Your Questions Answered*, pp. 204, 249. (New York: Churchill Livingstone)

18. Research on Cancer (WHO) (1992). In Parkin, D.M., Muir, C.S., Whelan, S.L., Gao, Y.-T., Ferlay, J. and Powell, J. (eds.) *Cancer Incidence in Five Continents*, Vol. VI, p. 773. (Lyon: IARC Scientific Publications)

31

A standardized patient information leaflet on oral contraception for Europe: just around the corner or never-ending circles?

T. Belfield

For years, medicines that were available on prescription were prescribed and dispensed with little or no information to patients. It was widely assumed that people would not be interested or have the intelligence or understanding, to benefit from receiving information about their treatments or drugs.

Today we know better – involving people in the management of their health, by enabling and empowering them through the provision of information and the parallel growth of patient and advocacy groups have resulted in people having access to information from a variety of sources. Some sources are accurate, providing up-to-date and impartial information, many are not – providing inaccurate, misleading and sometimes sensationalist misinformation.

Knowing about contraception and being able to make truly informed choices about methods are a fundamental issue for most of us at some point in our lives. But *how* contraception is considered, discussed and importantly delivered will determine just how well it is accepted and used[1].

Research into the care and consistency with which women use contraceptive methods highlights the importance of providing access to information which is understandable and relevant to the individual's own circumstances, and which addresses concerns and difficulties at an individual level. Women for the most part perceive contraceptive choices as a matter of finding the 'least worst' option, balancing effectiveness and ease of use with perceptions and expectations of side-effects and health risks. Increasing knowledge and confidence depends on identifying and countering misinformation and on promoting the benefits of contraceptive use through accurate, complete, consistent *and* memorable information about the method of choice.

Oral contraception is today by far the most commonly used reversible contraceptive method. The oral contraceptive pill is the most talked about, most worried about and most misunderstood drug, and is arguably one of the most researched products of our time. It is highly effective when taken correctly and consistently, giving a pregnancy rate of 0.12–0.34 pregnancies per 100 women years[2]. In practice however, failure rates for oral contraception range from 3% to 20% for diverse populations in developed and developing countries[3.] The gap between theoretical and actual efficacy of oral contraception relates mainly to non-compliance and discontinuation when still at risk of unintended pregnancy. Non-compliance occurs for many reasons, those relating to the individual: real side-effects, perceived side-effects, poor cycle control, and poor understanding of how to use the method correctly; and those relating to demographic, socioeconomic and behavioral factors: family views, peer pressure, media coverage, product package and labelling, product availability, societal attitudes, social class, and religion.

The Wyeth Ayerst Contraception Survey presented at the European Society on Contraception (ESC) June 1994 showed that, of the women surveyed:

(1) One in 5 women taking oral contraceptives forget to take their pill at least once every cycle;

(2) 34% of oral contraceptive users with an unplanned pregnancy forgot to take pills;

(3) 84% did not know that certain medications lessened the efficacy of the pill;

(4) 24% did not know about the positive health benefits;

(5)   27% discontinued their pill due to nuisance side-effects; and

(6)   69% of women did not consult a doctor before discontinuing oral contraceptive use.

The ESC Working Group on enhancing patient compliance and oral contraceptive efficacy[3] proposed that physicians interested in becoming advocates for oral contraception should be encouraged to take a leadership role in supporting its careful and consistent use, by:

(1)   Educating themselves and their peers about oral contraceptives;

(2)   Spending more time with clients providing counselling and information;

(3)   Selecting the best formulations for the individual; and

(4)   Improving the doctor/client relationship.

Providing information does much more than inform, it: generates awareness and understanding, corrects misinformation and misconception, helps demystify issues, updates people's knowledge, gives reassurance, minimizes or removes embarrassment, and backs up and reinforces advice given by health professionals.

Importantly, it enables and empowers people to seek help more effectively and to use their chosen method with confidence. The motive for providing information should *not* be to provide a safeguard against legal action for the provider or manufacturer.

Recognizing this important role and being aware that the current lack of harmonization provides for a high level of misunderstanding and confusion for both professionals and users, the aim for the future must be to produce harmonized information in Summary of Product Characteristics (SPCs), the new name for data sheets, and Patient Information Leaflets (PILs).

Discussion about the harmonization of information in Europe has been continuing since the first European Directive in 1965. Since that time considerable efforts have been made to harmonize the legislation and rules governing the marketing of pharmaceutical preparations. New procedures were put in place in 1995 to enable medicines to be authorized throughout the European Union (EU) through the European Medicines Evaluation Agency (EMEA).

The new system uses two licensing procedures: a centralized procedure via the EMEA which is now compulsory for new biotechnology products and a decentralized procedure which applies to most conventional products and is based on the previous system of mutual recognition of national authorizations. A product license obtained in one member state of the EU must be recognized in the others, unless they object to it within a fixed period. Disputed decisions go the Agency's Scientific Committee, the Committee for Proprietary Medicinal Products (CPMP). The end result of the these procedures is the production of consistent SPCs across the EU. The new licensing system will therefore ensure that PILs for individual medicines authorized through it will be effectively harmonized. Any difference should be minor and relate to the interpretation of language rather than substantive content[4].

Despite the existence of this system, we are a long way from achieving European harmonization of patient information and the PILs that are currently available are inconsistent, out of date, sometimes are too long, negative, non-user friendly, often aimed at health providers rather than users (Italy), lack full information (for fear of frightening patients) (Germany)[5], and in some areas lack evidence based data (UK hormone replacement therapy and progestogen-only pill data sheets).

Although a number of working groups have addressed these issues both at UK and European level, no concrete outcomes are apparent. The most effective work to date has emerged from collaborative approaches by Family Health International and the Food and Drug Administration in the USA. *We should learn from their experience.* Ley[6] wrote in 1982 'that the wisest method of improving compliance is to discover the features in the particular situation which are contributing to non-compliance and then do something appropriate about it'.

Developing more effective approaches to improving compliance demands more energy and more information than currently seem to exist. However, continued investigations into oral contraceptive non-compliance illustrates the need to provide more information, not less, contrary to the beliefs of those professionals who feel that consumers cannot deal with too much information[1]. At the very least, there is information that people have a *right* to know and *need* to know if they are to use their chosen method effectively and with confidence.

To explore the possibility of producing harmonized patient information in Europe, views were sought through a questionnaire of 30 respondents including leading family planning professionals in Europe and the USA, UK and European Regulatory Authorities and the oral contraceptive manufacturers. The questionnaire covered nine points on the subject of harmonized patient information and elicited a range of pragmatic views, a great deal of hope but a lack of consensus.

QUESTION 1 *Is it possible to produce a harmonized patient information leaflet for Europe?*

Key views

(1)   Considered possible in theory, but clear recognition of the real problems to date. 'Where there is a will there is a way.'

(2)   Considered definitely possible for core information to be standardized and for harmonization of all *new* product information for the future.

(3)   Recognition of the practical difficulties surrounding harmonized information, such as language, culture, labelling, design and content.

QUESTION 2 *Do you think that the different countries of Europe want standardized patient information leaflets?*

Key views

(1)   Recognition that Europe is moving towards harmonization with all new products.

(2)   Regulatory Authorities should be working more effectively and proactively towards having SPCs and PILs.

(3)   Recognition that to have harmonized PILs will require standardization in prescribing practice – not yet a reality.

(4)   Recognition of the very different views as to what PILs should contain.

QUESTION 3 *What advantages and disadvantages would there be in having a standardized patient information leaflet?*

Key views

Advantages

(1)   Consistency and clarity for providers, users and manufacturers;

(2)   Provide improvement in prescribing practice;

(3)   Recognition that inconsistencies in information can be exploited in product liability;

(4)   Provide medicinal information on oral contraceptives by gathering evidence-based data on all issues regarding risk and benefits and will allow for classification of controversial issues; and

(5)   It will provide for effective updating procedures.

Disadvantages

(1)   Conflict and lack of consensus in the decision-making process and questions regarding *who* will set the standards;

(2)   Harmonization will not allow for prevailing national differences and may cause cultural 'distance' from the user;

(3)   Final product may be too long, too bland, or too rigid;

(4)   Development will be at the speed of the slowest member.

QUESTION 4 *What steps in your opinion are needed to produce a standardized patient information leaflet?*

Key views

(1) Excellent and proactive liaison between Regulatory Authorities, leading organizations and professionals, manufacturers and clients/users – 'include all relevant partners';

(2) Set up a Task Force or Expert Committee using a major European organization, such as the ESC;

(3) Encourage and work with Regulatory Authorities to be more proactive;

(4) Speed up the work to standardized agreed SPCs which will lead to harmonization of PILs;

(5) Make evidence-based medicine a reality.

QUESTION 5 *What, if any, changes do you think will be required by any regulatory and licensing authority involved?*

Key views

(1) Need for better communication between national (i.e. country system) Regulatory Authorities and European Regulatory Authorities (i.e. centralized system);

(2) Need for better communication between organizations, professionals, manufacturers and Regulatory Authorities to understand fully the processes involved and the recognition of different national views and philosophies;

(3) Recognition that the EMEA are already working on harmonization of SPCs and PILs for new drug products (none on oral contraceptives yet);

(4)   Regulatory Authorities to become more proactive and work as advocates in the field of information improvement.

QUESTION 6 *How would any centralized European systems link in with individual country systems?*

Key views

(1)   Support and strengthen the centralized systems such as the EMEA which was set up to progress a new European drug registration system and aims to encourage co-operation, communication and transparency, among regulators, industry, health professionals and consumers; and

(2)   Educate country systems about the benefits of harmonized information in oral contraception.

QUESTION 7 *How would any changes in the license of a product be implemented into patient information leaflets?*

Key views

(1)   PILs must reflect the contents of the Product License – any changes to the SPCs will result in changes to the PILs;

(2)   Guidelines issued by the FPA or other equivalent European body would support and assist Regulatory Authorities to agree more easily to any recommended changes (based on evidence).

QUESTION 8 *What processes should be set up to ensure PILs can change quickly in the event of updated medical opinion and evidence?*

Key views

(1)   Use the same Task Force or Expert Committee set up to look into harmonization of PILs, to act as watchdog to monitor new evidence and facilitate *update and input* of changes in PILs;

(2)   Improve flexibility and remove bureaucracy;

(3)   Improve communication and liaison of all partners.

QUESTION 9 *If you believe it will be possible to produce a harmonized patient information leaflet for Europe what timescale do you think this will take to be a reality?*

Key views

(1)   To alter existing product information – SPCs and PILs – views ranged from not possible to many years – 'Have the year 2000 as a target';

(2)   Extremely dependent on how Europe is defined;

(3)   Recognition that if process is too bureaucratic, takes too long, provides too many reviews, and offers too many stages of consultation, the PIL would be too conservative and safe, and less effective for the user.

In conclusion, there is clearly strong support for the principle of harmonization of patient information for Europe, and also recognition of the difficulties of achieving this aim.

If we are to progress from never ending circles of hope and turn the corner, we will have to convert hope and pragmatism into action. We must recognize the need for much more effective and proactive collaboration, and accept responsibility for leadership.

We have a European Society of Contraception. The Society must be encouraged to establish an Expert Working Group which includes *all* the recognized partners in contraception. Only through this approach will the concept of harmonization of patients in Europe become a reality rather than a myth.

It should never be forgotten that 'patient information is not a target in itself, it is the means by which an individual is helped to achieve optimal use of the prescribed medicine'[7].

ACKNOWLEDGEMENTS

Thank you to those who who took the time to respond to the questionnaire and to Joan Walsh, FPA Health Policy/Research Officer.

REFERENCES

1. Belfield, T. (1992). Problems of compliance in contraception. *Br. J. Sex. Med.*, **19**, 76–8
2. Lachnit-Fixon, U. (1991). The role of oral contraception in population control. *Adv. Contracept.*, **7** (Suppl. 2), 9–17
3. ESC. International Working Group on Enhancing Patient Compliance and Oral Contraceptive Efficacy. (1992). *ESC Newsletter*, **2**, 1–4
4. Herxheimer, A. (1996). The EMEA – moving towards more transparent drug registration systems. *Br. Med. J.*, **312**, 394
5. Butler, S. (1995). Harmonisation of patient information: the European situation. *European Pharma Law Centre Update*, **45**
6. Ley, P. (1982). Satisfaction, compliance and communication. *Br. J. Clin. Psychol.*, **21**, 241–54
7. Munck, de H. (1991). Patient information in The Netherlands. In Mann, R. (ed.) *Patient Information in Medicine*, pp. 43–52. (Carnforth, UK: Parthenon Publishing)

Section 7

Effects of loss to follow-up on mortality data

The Royal College of General Practitioners' Oral Contraception Study has made a major contribution to our understanding of the health effects of combined oral contraceptives. The study began with the recruitment of 23 000 women who were using the pill and a similar number who have never used these preparations. Approximately 12 000 of the original count remain under observation. Such large losses to follow-up could introduce important biases, limiting the value of the study's results. The following paper examines whether mortality data from the study have been affected by loss to follow-up.

32

Mortality in relation to method of follow-up in the Royal College of General Practitioners' Oral Contraception Study

V. Beral, C. Hermon, C. Kay, P.C. Hannaford, S. Darby and G. Reeves

INTRODUCTION

The Royal College of General Practitioners' Oral Contraception Study is one of the largest studies of the effects of oral contraceptives on health in the world. During a 14-month period, starting in May 1968, 1400 general practitioners throughout the UK recruited 23 000 women who were taking oral contraceptives and a similar number of women who had never used them into a long-term study of the effects of oral contraceptive use on health[1]. All women were married or living as married, most (98%) were Caucasian and the average age at recruitment was 29 years. Since recruitment, participating general practitioners have been asked to provide information at 6-monthly intervals for each woman about her use of hormonal preparations, including oral contraceptives and about the occurrence of new episodes of illness, any surgery or pregnancy and, where appropriate, death. Over time many women have left their original general practice and some general practitioners have withdrawn from the study. Twenty years after recruitment, about one-third of the initial study population was still being followed regularly by their general practitioner. Such large losses could, in principle, affect conclusions about the effects of oral contraceptives on health, although theoretical arguments that such a bias is unlikely to have occurred have been advanced[2]. Attempts have therefore been made to find out whether the women who are no longer being regularly followed by participating general practitioners are alive or dead and, if so, their cause of death. In this paper, the mortality of women who have been regularly followed by their general practitioner is compared with the mortality of women who were not, to assess whether the rates in women who were followed by their general practitioner were similar to those of women who left the study, and whether analyses of the effects of oral contraceptives on mortality were biased by restricting analyses only to women who were under observation by their general practitioner.

METHODS

The method of recruitment and data collection has been described elsewhere[1]. At 6-monthly intervals since recruitment, general practitioners provided details about each woman still 'under observation' including prescriptions of oral contraceptives, new episodes of illnesses and, where appropriate, the date and cause of death. A woman is regarded as no longer 'under observation' by her general practitioner if the doctor withdraws from the study, if the woman leaves the practice or if she receives oral contraceptives from a family planning clinic. In the early stages of the study an attempt was made to maintain regular follow-up of women who moved by enlisting the help of her new general practitioner. It was found that fewer than 10% of women who moved could be kept in the study in this way and so this approach was abandoned. In the late 1970s, as many of the original study population as possible was 'flagged' on the National Health Service Central Registers (NHSCRs) in Southport and Edinburgh, so that deaths and cancer registrations could be reported automatically (no attempt was made to flag the relatively small number of women from Northern Ireland or the Isle of Man). The study team does not hold identifying details of the women and so general practitioners were asked to provide the necessary information directly to the Central Registers. This meant that patients of the general practitioners who had withdrawn from the study before the late 1970s could not be flagged. Nor could many women who had left their original doctors before then. Such women and women who could not be traced on the NHSCRs records have been classified as 'lost to follow-up'. For women who were flagged, flagging effectively began on 1 January 1977, and the NHSCRs report regularly about deaths among them after that date and supply copies of relevant death certificates. The date of death and underlying cause were ascertained from the death certificate and the cause of death coded to the 8th Revision of the International Classification of Diseases (ICD)[3].

For the women who were still under observation by their general practitioner, person years were calculated from the date of recruitment up to the date of death or 31 December 1988. For women lost to follow-up person years were recruited up to the date of the last 6-monthly report. For women who were lost to follow-up but who were subsequently flagged on the NHSCRs, person years were calculated up to the date of the last 6-monthly report by their general practitioner, and then from 1 January 1977, to the date of death or 31 December 1988. (For women who left their general practitioner before 1977, it is not appropriate to include the person years accumulated during the period between leaving their general practitioner and 1 January 1977, because these are available only for women who are known to have survived in the intervening period, and are not known for women who may have died during that period.)

The deaths and person years were subdivided into 5-year age groups (16–19, 20–24, up to 70–74) for single calendar years and according to whether the women were still under observation by their general practitioners and whether they had taken oral contraceptives. A woman who had never used oral contraceptives at recruitment, but whose general practitioner reported that she subsequently began using them, contributed person years to the 'never user' category up to the date when she began using oral contraceptives and thereafter contributed person years to the 'ever user' category. A woman who was still contributing to the 'never user' category at the time she left her general practitioner and who was flagged on the

Table 1 Follow-up status of women in the Royal College of General Practitioners' Oral Contraception Study on 31 December 1988, by method of follow-up

| | | *Oral contraceptive use* | |
| | | | |
Status	*All women*	*Ever*	*Never*
Dead	996 (2.1%)	599 (2.0%)	397 (2.3%)
under observation by general practitioner	673 (1.4%)	401 (1.4%)	272 (1.6%)
flagged on NHSCRs	323 (0.7%)	198 (0.7%)	125 (0.7%)
Alive	34 430 (73.3%)	21 618 (73.4%)	12 812 (73.1%)
under observation by general practitioner	15 799 (33.6%)	9745 (33.1%)	6054 (34.6%)
flagged on NHSCRs	18 631 (39.7%)	11 873 (40.3%)	6758 (38.6%)
Lost to follow-up	11 539 (24.6%)	7233 (24.6%)	4306 (24.6%)
Total	46 965 (100%)	29 450 (100%)	17 515 (100%)

NHSCRs remained in the 'never user' category until she left the study.

The expected numbers of deaths were calculated from age-specific mortality rates for women in England and Wales. Standardized mortality rates (SMRs) were calculated using a standard computer program[4]. Relative risks (RRs) and 95% confidence intervals were calculated using the Poisson regression module of EPICURE[5] to compare mortality in women who had used oral contraceptives with women who had not. For these analyses, as well as adjusting by age, adjustment was made for parity (0, 1–2, 3+; not known), social class at the time of recruitment into the study (I & II, III, IV & V, other), and cigarette smoking at the time of recruitment into the study (0, 1–14, 15+; not known).

RESULTS

Up to 31 December 1988, 996 (2%) women were reported to have died, 34 430 (73%) were known to be alive and 11 539 (25%) were lost to follow-up (Table 1). About half the women known to be alive were still under observation by their general practitioner and the other half were flagged on the NHSCRs. The proportions were similar in ever users and never users of oral contraceptives. Losses to follow-up were similar in women who had and had not used oral contraceptives (25% in both groups).

In Table 2 the characteristics of the women who were still under observation by their general practitioner at exit from the study, who were flagged on the NHSCRs, and who were lost to follow-up are compared. At entry to the study, women who subsequently remained under observation by their general practitioner tended to be older, less likely to be using oral contraceptives, of lower social class and of higher parity than women flagged on the NHSCRs or those lost to follow-up. The proportion who were smokers were similar in each group. There were, however, few differences in the characteristics at entry into the study between women flagged on the NHSCRs and women lost to follow-up, other than the timing and the way in which they ceased to be regularly followed by their general practitioners. The women flagged on the NHSCRs last saw their general practitioner on average 6.9 years after recruitment compared with 3.8 years for women lost to follow-up; and only 8% of those traced only on the NHSCRs compared to 31% of those lost to follow-up left the study because their general practitioner had withdrawn from it. The average duration of follow-up of women who remained under observation by their general practitioner was approximately 20 years, very similar to the total duration of follow-up for those only flagged on the NHSCRs. However, for those lost to follow-up the average duration of follow-up was very brief, i.e. less than 4 years. The reported average duration of oral contraceptive use differed considerably between the three groups, largely reflecting the differing length of time that women remained under observation by their general practitioner.

When all women were considered, mortality from all causes of death combined was 25% below the national average (SMR 75; see Table 3). All-cause mortality rates did not differ significantly in women who were under observation by their general practitioner and who were flagged on the NHSCRs (SMR 77 and 72, respectively; test for difference $p = 0.36$). Among the women flagged on the

Table 2 Characteristics of women at the time of recruitment and at the time of the last 6-monthly report by their general practitioner, by method of follow-up on 31 December 1988, or death if known to be earlier*

	Method of follow-up		
	Under observation by their general practitioner (n = 16 472)	*Flagged on NHSCRs* (n = 18 954)	*Lost to follow-up* (n = 11 539)
Characteristics at entry to study			
Average age (SE)	30.68 (0.05)	28.41 (0.05)	28.35 (0.06)
% oral contraceptive users (n)	45 (7395)	51 (9728)	54 (6183)
% smokers (n)	45 (7335)	45 (8466)	46 (5266)
Average no of cigarettes smoked (in smokers) (SE)	11.76 (0.08)	12.10 (0.08)	12.25 (0.10)
% social class I, II, III non-manual (n)	31 (5047)	40 (7557)	38 (4393)
Average number of children (SE)	2.02 (0.01)	1.71 (0.01)	1.73 (0.01)
Reason for no longer being under observation by their general practitioner			
% who left the practice (n)	n.a.	86 (16 252)	67 (7763)
% whose general practitioner withdrew from the study (n)	n.a.	8 (1607)	31 (3577)
% who obtained oral contraceptives from elsewhere (n)	n.a.	6 (1095)	2 (199)
Characteristics at time of last contact 6-monthly report by their general practitioner			
Average age (SE)	50.18 (0.05)	35.30 (0.07)	32.13 (0.07)
Calendar year of last contact with general practitioner			
% before 1976 (n)	1 (170)	58 (10 997)	82 (9469)
% during or after 1976 (n)	99 (16 302)	42 (7957)	18 (2070)

Continued

Table 2 *continued*

| | Method of follow-up | | |
	Under observation by their general practitioner (n = 16 472)	Flagged on NHSCRs (n = 18 954)	Lost to follow-up (n = 11 539)
Average duration of follow-up (in years)			
total duration (SE)	19.50 (0.02)	19.86 (0.01)	3.78 (0.03)
by general practitioner	19.50 (0.02)	6.89 (0.04)	3.78 (0.03)
on NHSCRs	n.a.	12.97 (0.04)	n.a.
% ever users of oral contraceptives (n)	62 (10 146)	64 (12 071)	63 (7233)
Average reported duration of oral contraceptive use (in months, users only) (SE)	76.34 (0.55)	49.93 (0.38)	39.10 (0.39)

* For each characteristic the small number of women coded as 'not known' for each variable are excluded. n.a., not applicable

NHSCRs mortality rates did not differ significantly in women who had left or whose general practitioner had withdrawn from the study (SMRs 71 and 84, respectively; test for difference p = 0.48). The SMRs for the major groupings of causes of death did not differ significantly in women who were under observation by their general practitioner and in women who were flagged on the NHSCRs (Table 4; p > 0.05 for all causes shown). In both groups, SMRs were significantly below the national average for most groupings of causes of death, except for violent and accidental causes.

In Table 5 SMRs in ever users and never users are shown, together with relative risks for ever users compared to never users (adjusted for age, smoking, social class and parity) by method of follow-up. In general the RRs are similar in women who were under observation by their general practitioner and those who were flagged on the NHSCRs; the only significant difference was for all circulatory diseases (RR = 1.95 for women under observation by their general practitioner; RR = 1.03 for women flagged on the NHSCRs; test for difference, p = 0.04). This difference is largely because there

Table 3 Standardized mortality ratios (SMRs) for all causes of death, by method of follow-up at exit from the study

Method of follow-up	Number of deaths	SMR (95% CI)
Under observation by their general practitioner	673	77 (71–83)
Flagged on the NHSCRs	323	72 (64–80)
woman moved from the practice area	297	71 (63–79)
GP withdrew from the study	26	84 (52–116)
Total	996	75 (70–80)

is a substantial difference in relative risk of deaths from circulatory disease before and after 1977 among women under observation by their general practitioner (see Table 6, RR = 3.74 and 1.55 respectively; test for difference $p = 0.03$). The high RR before 1977 is largely due to the fact that the excess mortality from circulatory disease is most evident in current and recent users[2], and the proportion of current and recent users has declined over time. Follow-up on the NHSCRs effectively began on 1 January 1977 and so there are no observations in that group before 1977. After 1977 there is no significant difference in circulatory disease mortality according to method of follow-up (RR = 1.55 and 1.03, respectively; test for difference, $p = 0.3$).

DISCUSSION

The Royal College of General Practitioners' Oral Contraception Study was set up in 1968 to record in detail the use of oral contraceptives and associated morbidity and mortality in women who were followed regularly by their general practitioners. Over the course of the study there have been inevitable losses from the original study population, mostly because women moved and thus changed their general practitioner, but also because some participating doctors themselves died or withdrew from the study. In addition some women obtained oral contraceptives from outside the practice.

Table 4 Standardized mortality ratios for main groupings of causes of death, by method of follow up

| | | | *Method of follow-up* | | | |
| | *All women* | | *Under observation by their general practitioner* | | *Flagged on NHSCRs* | |
Cause of death (ICD)	*Number of deaths*	*SMR (95% CI)*	*Number of deaths*	*SMR (95% CI)*	*Number of deaths*	*SMR (95% CI)*
All causes (000–999)	996	75 (70–80)	673	77 (71–83)	323	72 (64–80)
All cancers (140–209)	502	82 (74–89)	338	84 (75–93)	164	76 (64–88)
All circulatory diseases (390–458)	233	75 (65–84)	156	75 (63–87)	77	74 (57–90)
All respiratory diseases (460–519)	25	32 (20–45)	21	39 (23–56)	4	17 (0–33)
All digestive diseases (520–577)	38	81 (55–107)	19	62 (34–90)	19	116 (64–168)
All other diseases (1–139;210–389; 580–799)	79	57 (44–69)	59	62 (46–78)	20	44 (25–64)
Violent and accidental causes (800–999)	119	89 (73–105)	80	89 (69–108)	39	89 (61–117)

By the end of 1988, 34% of the women initially recruited were still under observation by a general practitioner, who continued to provide regular 6-monthly reports of their use of oral contraceptives and about new illnesses or deaths. In addition 2% of the study population had died and a further 40% could be traced on the NHSCRs, even though they were no longer under regular follow-up, by their general practitioner. The remaining 25% of the original study population were lost to follow-up, most of whom (82%) were last seen by their general practitioner before 1977 when flagging on the NHSCR effectively began. Apart from being lost earlier and hence being younger at the time of last contact with their general practitioner, women who were lost to follow-up tended to have similar characteristics to women flagged on the NHSCRs (Table 2).

Mortality rates were generally similar in the women under observation by their general practitioner and in women traced on the NHSCRs. Mortality from all causes combined was about 25% below the national average in both groups. Low mortality rates have been reported in other groups of women studied for the effects of oral contraceptives on health: for example in the Oxford/FPA study total mortality rates were 45% below the national average[6]. The reasons for the low mortality may be analogous to the 'healthy worker effect' often observed in occupational groups where the selection of people into a workforce on the basis of their health is known to be associated with total mortality rates that are below the national average[7]. The general practitioners volunteered to take part in this study and they selected the women to be recruited. These selection processes resulted in the recruitment of relatively healthy women.

The overall relationship of oral contraceptive use to mortality did not differ significantly in women under observation by their general practitioner and in women flagged on the NHSCRs. Thus there is no evidence that the women still under observation by their general practitioners are substantially biased with respect to the effects of oral contraceptives on mortality. These data support our previous arguments[2] that bias due to loss of subjects is unlikely to have occurred in respect of other measures of health. Continued observation of the cohort will therefore provide valuable information about the long-term effects of oral contraceptives.

Table 5 Standardized mortality ratios (number of deaths) in oral contraceptive ever users and never users and relative risk* of mortality in ever users compared with never users, by method of follow-up

				Method of follow-up					
	All women			*Under observation by general practitioner*			*Flagged on NHSCRs*		
	SMR (n)			*SMR (n)*			*SMR (n)*		
Cause of death (ICD)	*Ever users*	*Never users*	*RR (95% CI)*	*Ever users*	*Never users*	*RR (95% CI)*	*Ever users*	*Never users*	*RR (95% CI)*
All causes (000–999)	81 (581)	68 (382)	1.10 (0.96–1.25)	83 (401)	69 (272)	1.14 (0.97–1.34)	75 (180)	68 (110)	1.03 (0.80–1.31)
All cancers (140–209)	80 (271)	81 (212)	0.93 (0.77–1.11)	85 (186)	84 (152)	0.96 (0.77–1.20)	72 (85)	75 (60)	0.90 (0.64–1.26)
All circulatory diseases (390–458)	95 (158)	53 (72)	1.57 (1.18–2.09)	101 (112)	45 (44)	1.95 (1.36–2.80)	84 (46)	71 (28)	1.03 (0.63–1.68)
All respiratory diseases (460–519)	44 (18)	21 (7)	1.79 (0.74–4.35)	49 (14)	28 (7)	1.42 (0.56–3.58)	33 (4)	0 (0)	insufficient data
All digestive diseases (520–577)	97 (25)	56 (11)	1.67 (0.80–3.48)	65 (11)	58 (8)	1.31 (0.50–3.48)	159 (14)	51 (3)	2.63 (0.75–9.24)
All other diseases (1–139, 210–389, 580–799)	45 (34)	76 (43)	0.63 (0.40–0.99)	43 (23)	86 (36)	0.52 (0.31–0.90)	49 (11)	46 (7)	1.19 (0.46–3.09)
Violent and accidental causes (800–999)	101 (75)	72 (37)	1.36 (0.91–2.03)	105 (55)	66 (25)	1.56 (0.96–2.53)	92 (20)	88 (12)	0.99 (0.47–2.06)

* Relative risks are adjusted for age, parity, social class and cigarette smoking

Table 6 Standardized ratios (number of deaths) in oral contraceptive ever users and never users and relative risk* in ever users compared to never users, by calendar year of and method of follow-up

	Before 1977			1977 or later					
	Under observation by general practitioner			*Under observation by general practitioner*			*Flagged on NHSCRs*		
	SMR (n)			*SMR (n)*			*SMR (n)*		
Cause of death	*Ever user*	*Never user*	*RR (95% CI)*	*Ever user*	*Never user*	*RR (95% CI)*	*Ever user*	*Never user*	*RR (95% CI)*
All causes	77 (118)	61 (81)	1.29 (0.96–1.74)	86 (283)	73 (191)	1.09 (0.90–1.32)	75 (180)	68 (110)	1.03 (0.80–1.31)
Circulatory disease	130 (41)	35 (10)	3.74 (1.82–7.71)	89 (71)	50 (34)	1.55 (1.02–2.38)	84 (46)	71 (28)	1.03 (0.63–1.68)
All other causes	63 (77)	68 (71)	0.96 (0.69–1.34)	85 (212)	81 (157)	0.99 (0.80–1.23)	73 (134)	68 (82)	1.02 (0.77–1.35)

*Relative risks are adjusted for age, parity, social class and cigarette smoking
Flagging on the NHSCRs effectively began on 1 January 1977

ACKNOWLEDGEMENTS

We are grateful to the 1400 doctors who have contributed data to the Oral Contraception Study, which currently receives support from the Royal College of General Practitioners, Schering AG (Berlin), Schering Health Care Ltd (UK) and Wyeth-Ayerst International (USA). We thank Sarah Jones for assisting with the manuscript.

REFERENCES

1. Royal College of General Practitioners (1974). *Oral Contraceptives and Health*. (London: Pitman Medical)
2. Royal College of General Practitioners' Oral Contraception Study. (1981). Further analyses of mortality in oral contraceptive users. *Lancet*, 541–6
3. World Health Organization (1967). *International Classification of Diseases, Injuries and Causes of Death*, 8th Revision, 1965. (Geneva: WHO)
4. Coleman, M., Douglas, A., Hermon, C. and Peto, J. (1986). Cohort study analysis with a FORTRAN computer program. *Int. J. Epidemiol.*, **15**, 134–7
5. Preston. D.L., Lubin, J.H. and Pierce, D.A. (1993). *EPICURE User's Guide*. (Seattle: Hirosoft International Corporation)
6. Vessey, M.P., Villard-Mackintosh, L., McPherson, K. and Yeates, D. (1989). Mortality among oral contraceptive users: 20 year follow-up of women in a cohort study. *Br. Med. J.*, **299**, 1487–91
7. Beral, V., Carpenter, L., Booth, M., Inskip, H. and Brown, A. (1988). Paper 18: The 'healthy worker effect' and other determinants of mortality in workers in the nuclear industry. In *Health Effects of Low Dose Ionising Radiation*. (London: BNES)

Participants in the Workshop

The delegates who attended the International Workshop to determine evidence-guided prescribing of the pill are listed below. All persons were invited in their personal capacity rather than as representatives of the organizations for which they work. The names of those persons who acted as Chairpersons for the Sessions are indicated in bold type. The names of those persons who are employees of combined oral contraceptive manufacturers are indicated with an asterisk.

Dr J. Ahmad, Maidenhead, UK*

Dr Joan Austoker, Oxford, UK

Professor David Back, Liverpool, UK

Dr J. Bacon, High Wycombe, UK*

Dr G. Barker, Burgess Hill, UK*

Ms Toni Belfield, London, UK

Professor Valerie Beral, Oxford, UK

Dr Kitty Bloemenkamp, Leiden, The Netherlands

Dr David Bromham, Leeds, UK

Dr N. Bruyniks, Oss, The Netherlands*

Dr Eva Buiatti, Florence, Italy

Dr Carmen Coll Capdevila, Barcelona, Spain

Dr Philip Corfman, Rockville, USA

Professor George Creatsas, Athens, Greece

Dr David Crook, London, UK

Professor Howard Cuckle, Leeds, UK

Professor James Drife, Leeds, UK

Dr B. Düsterberg, Berlin, Germany*

Professor Max Elstein, Manchester, UK

Ms Susan Ferry, Manchester, UK

Dr Silvia Franceschi, Aviano, Italy

Dr Peter Frank, Manchester, UK

Ms Ann Furedi, London, UK

Dr D. Gibb, Cambridge, UK*

Dr Michael Gillmer, Oxford, UK

Mr Peter Greenhouse, Ipswich, UK

Dr Allan Hackshaw, London, UK

Dr Philip Hannaford, Manchester, UK

Dr Linda Heywood, Bury St. Edmunds, UK

Mr David Hicks, Sheffield, UK

Dr Kathleen Irwin, Atlanta, USA

Professor Jørgen Jespersen, Esbjerg, Denmark

Dr M. Kaffrisson, High Wycombe, UK*

Dr R. Kaper, Cambridge, UK*

Dr Clifford Kay, Manchester, UK

Dr Rosemary Kirkman, Manchester, UK

Dr S. Knijff, Oss, The Netherlands*

Dr U. Koch, Berlin, Germany*

Dr Ekke Kuenssberg, Edinburgh, UK

Dr Øjvind Lidegaard, Herlev, Denmark

Professor Per-Anders Mårdh, Uppsala, Sweden

Professor James McCormick, Dublin, Ireland

Dr Olav Meirik, Geneva, Switzerland

Dr A. Michaels, Philadelphia, USA*

Mr Stephen Morris, London, UK

Dr Nubia Muñoz, Lyon, France

Professor John Newton, Birmingham, UK

Dr T. Norpoth, Berlin, Germany*

Dr Björn Oddens, Brussels, Belgium

Dr Miguel Oliveira da Silva, Lisbon, Portugal

Dr G. Olsson, Oss, The Netherlands*

Dr Neil Poulter, London, UK

Dr Sarah Randall, Portsmouth, UK

Dr H. Reckers, Oss, The Netherlands*

Dr Gillian Reeves, Oxford, UK

Dr Sam Rowlands, Biggleswade, UK

Dr K. Schmidt-Gollwitzer, Berlin, Germany*

Dr Mary Short, Blackrock, Ireland

Professor Sven O. Skouby, Copenhagen, Denmark

Dr Bruce Stadel, Rockville, USA

Professor Meir Stampfer, Boston, USA

Dr Yvonne Stedman, Worcester, UK

Ms Lyn Thomas, London, UK

Dr Margaret Thorogood, London, UK

Dr George Tolis, Athens, Greece

Professor Martin Vessey, Oxford, UK

Dr Anne Webb, Liverpool, UK

Dr M. Weber, Philadelphia, USA*

Dr Bengt-Eric Wiholm, Uppsala, Sweden

Dr Christopher Wilkinson, London, UK

Dr Ulrich Winkler, Essen, Germany

Dr Pål Wölner-Hanssen, Lund, Sweden

Index